Perspectives in Paediatric Oncology Nursing

PERSPECTIVES IN PAEDIATRIC ONCOLOGY NURSING

Edited by

Faith Gibson PhD, MSc, RSCN, RGN, ONCCert, CertEd, RNT

Lecturer in Children's Nursing Research,
Centre for Nursing and Allied Health Professions Research,
Great Ormond Street Hospital for Children NHS Trust, London

Louise Soanes MSc, PG Dip(Ed), BSc, RSCN, RGN

Senior Sister for Children's Services,
Royal Marsden Hospital, Sutton, Surrey

Beth Sepion MSc, BEd(Hons), RSCN, RGN, SCM

Lecturer in Paediatric Oncology,
School of Nursing and Midwifery, University of Southampton

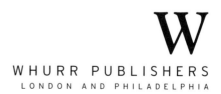

WHURR PUBLISHERS
LONDON AND PHILADELPHIA

© 2004 Whurr Publishers Ltd
First published 2004
by Whurr Publishers Ltd
19b Compton Terrace
London N1 2UN England and
325 Chestnut Street, Philadelphia PA 19106 USA

British Library Cataloguing in Publication Data

A catalogue record for this book
is available from the British Library.

ISBN 1 86156 293 4

Typeset by Adrian McLaughlin, a@microguides.net
Printed and bound in the UK by Athenæum Press Limited, Gateshead, Tyne & Wear

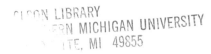

Contents

Foreword

Fiona Smith

This book brings together a unique body of knowledge about paediatric oncology nursing, charting developments, reflecting on the past and providing inspiration for the future. Paediatric oncology nursing has developed considerably over the last 20 years, with nurses leading and influencing both national and international policy and practice. Today nurses participate as equal members of the team providing care to children and young people with cancer, leading service provision, education programmes and research activities across the specialty.

The book is divided into 3 parts. Part 1 offers a perspective on education highlighting the crucial role of education to underpin clinical developments, role expansion and new ways of thinking and doing. The lack of specific education in many instances has acted as a key inhibitor preventing nurses from pushing the boundaries of their practice. Part 2 provides an insight into service provision, highlighting initiatives introduced to improve children's, young people's and families' experiences. In particular the needs of young people with cancer are acknowledged as often being overlooked by service providers. Part 3 considers current perspectives in paediatric oncology nursing practice, it includes chapters on various research studies, and emphasises the importance of facilitating practitioners to develop critical appraisal skills and expertise in undertaking research so as to provide the best possible care for children and young people.

The text clearly highlights the challenges for nursing leaders and practitioners within the field of paediatric oncology over the coming months and years. Undoubtedly there is a clear need for an agreed definition of future roles in paediatric oncology nursing, along with associated competencies. The plethora of roles and titles, without consistency in local application confuses not only other colleagues but children and their families as well. Meeting the needs of young people with cancer will continue to be a challenge for practitioners and managers alike. The future is likely to see new models of service provision and nurse leaders should be active in determining the shape of services to meet the specialist needs of their client group. The need to address mechanisms to enable practitioners to access education programmes to acquire specialist skills and knowledge to support clinical developments is also a key challenge, particularly in view of today's time pressures and workforce constraints. Of vital importance is the need clearly to demonstrate the impact that skilled nursing care has upon outcomes for the child or young person with cancer, as well as their family. The need for more in-depth clinically focused research cannot be over emphasised, particularly as future resources and services will undoubtedly be influenced by the available evidence to underpin decision-making. Practitioners must therefore recognise that developing research skills and knowledge is vital for the future, with research activities being seen by managers and others as a central component of clinical practice.

Lateral thinking and the development of a cohesive vision will be crucial to meet these challenges. This will entail even closer working between managers, practitioners and educators, as well as working in partnership with children, young people and their families to identify and promote best practice.

It was a pleasure to be invited to write this foreword and to have the opportunity to acknowledge the immense contribution the editors and authors have made over the years not only to paediatric oncology nursing, but to the entire field of children's nursing. It is only due to their undoubted commitment and enthusiasm that initiatives and developments have occurred.

Fiona Smith
Adviser in Children's Nursing
Royal College of Nursing

Personal reflections on the development of paediatric oncology nursing as a specialty

As a retired paediatric oncology nurse, I felt that the experiences and knowledge I have accrued and the changes I have witnessed as a nurse over the past four decades have provided me with sufficient material to offer a personal perspective on the development of paediatric oncology nursing, as an introduction to this textbook. Putting this narrative together has given me time to reflect on the challenges, resources and rewards encountered as the specialty has developed. As I have identified the significant changes in the treatment and care of childhood cancer, it was interesting to note the differences and similarities in nursing practice over the past four decades.

My first encounter with caring for a child with leukaemia was during a paediatric placement while in training as a general nurse in the late 1950s. In the 1950s to 1960s there were no major technological advances in the management of childhood cancer, apart from some attempts at drug therapy and limited use of radiotherapy for symptom control. At this time treatment generally consisted of steroid medication and blood transfusions. From a nursing perspective, I felt totally unprepared, with little knowledge about how to care for the child and family receiving cancer therapies. I would sit with a child and, when the family visited, I would also spend time with them. However, I was unable to answer their questions. Even if I had known the answer I could not have helped them, because the policy at that time was that only medical staff could offer information. Parents and family members of a very sick child were given special 'open visiting' status. Other families were restricted to visiting times. This was because childhood cancer was then viewed as a terminal illness. There was little or no acknowledgement of the need to prepare the child or the child's family for that death. As nurses we were left caring for children with cancer without adequate knowledge and specific training, and this resulted in a stressful and frightening experience. I was ill-prepared to cope with all aspects of the children's illness and at that time their inevitable death.

My experience was not, I am sure, too dissimilar to that of my medical colleagues. Although I felt inadequately prepared as a nurse in the face of caring for a dying child, I had a sense of feeling less hopeless. As a nurse I could at least provide physical and emotional support. The medical staff were unable to provide much in the way of treatment. Somehow, although frightening, it was this experience that stimulated me to train as a children's nurse and then to choose to work with children with cancer. Thankfully much has changed since the 1970s. The advent of new diagnostic tools and treatment techniques has considerably changed the nature and course of childhood cancer. The concerns of paediatric oncologists have shifted from terminal care, to cure and survival, and hence to an increased focus on the child and family's physical and psychological needs.

During the 1970s, I was working on a newly opened Paediatric Oncology Unit and new technology and trends in healthcare were rapidly changing. One trend that is now well established was the involvement of families in the care of the hospitalized child, with open visiting becoming the norm. Cure was now a possibility with up to 50% of children with leukaemia having a real chance of survival. Clinical trials were developing and well-conceived treatment protocols enabled treatment evaluations to be routinely undertaken. Much of this progress was as a result of a collaborative approach to studies and clinical trials coordinated locally by the United Kingdom Children's Cancer Study Group (UKCCSG) and at a European level by the International Society of Paediatric Oncology (SIOP).

This was also a time when supportive therapy was being developed for potential and actual side effects of treatment, such as pneumocystis carinii pneumonia (PCP). However, one of the most distressing problems that existed at this time was the nausea and vomiting children experienced post-chemotherapy treatment. Attempts were made with the available antiemetics to reduce this distressing side effect. Much of my nursing time was involved with comforting the child and family through this traumatic period. Frequent re-siting of intravenous cannulae added further distress and discomfort. I recall, on certain days, that children would attend as an outpatient for combination chemotherapy treatment and then be admitted to the inpatient area for monitoring and observation. This practice of giving a number of children similar treatment on the same day, roughly at the same time, meant that most of the nursing care for most of the inpatient children was to support and comfort both the child and the family through a distressing period of nausea and vomiting. Fortunately I worked with a supportive medical team who were willing to answer my numerous questions about changing this practice to one of a more staggered admission policy. By so doing, nursing resources were better used and, as a result, patient care was improved because closer monitoring and support for a small number of patients on different days could be accommodated.

My role and function continued to change and develop and, during the 1970s, I was involved not only in the physical care of the child but also in the mixing and administration of chemotherapy. This extension of my role also included undertaking the placement of intravenous cannulae. Training for these skills was developed 'in house' by committed nurse leaders. Some nurses argued that this development was nothing more than taking on doctors' tasks. Thankfully those who were more enlightened could see the benefit to patient care by extending our expertise. This was also a time when collaboration and teamwork began to develop and the role of the nurse was strengthened as credence was given to the nurse's contribution to the overall management: views on patient care were acknowledged and sought. Nurses at my institution and others were instrumental in the development of programmes to enable children to have painful procedures carried out under general anaesthesia. Before this development most centres were using a cocktail of sedative drugs; this combination was often ineffective for pain control and the effects left the child sleepy for the rest of the day.

This was also the time when patient and family education became a true reality and accepted as good practice. Nurses were now teaching parents about blood values and the effects of chemotherapy and other treatments on blood counts. Nurses were also beginning to look at their practice and early independent nurse research programmes were able to influence and change the way we practised. This also had an effect on the way we, and others outside the specialty, thought about childhood cancer.

One example was the work of Martinson (1976), a nurse working in North America who was instrumental in the development of home care for the dying child. Before this, children with a terminal illness would be admitted to hospital to die. In the UK, home care was slow to develop; recognition of the need was acknowledged but issues about funding and training for community staff had a detrimental effect by slowing down progress. It was also recognized that some curative treatment could be carried out in the home setting. This evolution began with the introduction of community liaison nurses who were employed to contact community staff over the telephone to advise on home care. It soon became evident that this approach to home care was less than satisfactory. Community nurses and other community staff stated that they were not sufficiently knowledgeable or did not have the clinical expertise to carry out this care without significant input from specialist nurses. Families and children with cancer were also finding that staff in the community lacked the specialist knowledge and expertise. As a result during the 1980s, paediatric oncology outreach teams based at specialist centres were developed. Again nurses were in the forefront of discussions and seeking funds for this much needed service. Funding for these posts was and remains a mixture of NHS and charitable organizations with Cancer Macmillan taking a significant role in supporting this development.

In the 1980s, more intensive therapies were developed and nursing acknowledged the need to underpin their practice with greater in-depth knowledge and training. The first steps were taken in the UK in 1984, when a cohort of paediatric nurses working in the specialty established the Royal College of Nursing's (RCN's) Paediatric Oncology Nursing Forum (PONF). The first paediatric oncology nursing conference, under the auspices of the RCN, was held in 1988. Simultaneously, nurses also held their first meeting at a SIOP conference where they met with medical colleagues to discuss issues of interest. Recognition of the need for specific nurse education in the care of children with cancer, at my institution, involved the development of a short 'in-house' paediatric oncology nursing course. This was followed by introduction of the English National Board (ENB) course and qualification (ENB 240) in a number of specialist centres (Gibson and Langton, 1998). Before these developments clinical nurse specialist posts were being introduced. These initiatives have been a powerful force in ensuring that nurses have a strong voice in the overall care and management of children and their families. Nurses were also becoming involved with clinical research and undertaking small-scale, single-site studies looking at specific issues, often related to symptom management.

Change continued apace with nursing care becoming more challenging as therapies became more complex. Thus, time spent managing patient care increased. At this time there were several advances that had a great impact on my nursing practice and the quality of life for patients; these were the introduction of tunnelled intravenous devices and the use of $5HT_3$ blockers ($5HT$ is 5-hydroxytryptamine or serotonin) for the control of nausea and vomiting. No longer were children suffering the frequent placement of intravenous cannulae and the prolonged exhausting bouts of nausea and vomiting. Nursing was still about direct patient care. However, nurses with expertise in the specialty were now involved in the administration of therapies, monitoring of side effects, and promotion of comfort and support for the child and family throughout their treatment trajectory. This included helping the child and family to understand the disease, understanding approaches to treatment, short- and long-term side effects, and care of the child at home. The use of central venous catheters, while improving the quality of life for the child on intensive regimens, increased the burden on home care and the need for further education. This education was of major importance for the child and family and the community-based staff because more children were receiving therapy as outpatients. Children were now discharged home with catheters in situ.

Another development was that of 'shared care'. This development has encountered many challenges, mostly related to the alleged lack of resources, expertise and knowledge of carers in the referring hospital, and the expectations of the now-empowered 'expert parent' and child. This situation continues to be a challenge and nurses are centrally involved in looking to resolve problems and improve collaborative relationships. This issue is addressed later in this textbook through exploration of the perceptions of parents.

In the 1990s, paediatric oncology nurses were employed in vital positions throughout the specialist centres. Educational programmes at diploma and degree level were developed to provide nurses with an academic qualification, further enabling them to take an essential role within the now established multidisciplinary team. New treatments continued to be developed and clinical trials became even more complex. The multi-faceted role of the nurse working with children undergoing clinical trials involved child and family education, direct care-giving and accurate data recording. Collaboration with the UKCCSG enabled nurses to be involved in decision-making such as in the New Agents Group (NAG) and in working parties looking at specific areas of interest, e.g. child and family consent to treatment, palliative and adolescent care. In 1995, I was personally invited to be the nurse member of a working party for the Department of Health, looking at the provision and treatment of care of the child with leukaemia. This invitation left me to reflect on how much the position and status of nurses has changed since my training days. Exciting other developments were the first multiprofessional conference in collaboration with the UKCCSG and PONF, which took place in 1997, and the fact that SIOP opened its membership to nurses in 1999.

New nursing roles were also being given consideration and the role of the advanced practitioner was established. During this decade specialist nurses continued to develop sophisticated and credible programmes of nursing research. Single-site studies designed to answer short-term questions have been undertaken, because care and procedures have aspects that are unique to each care setting. However, a concern within one paediatric oncology setting is more than likely to be of concern to others, and the sharing of outcomes has influenced and supported changes in practice more than single-site studies. Examples of single-site studies are to be found in this book.

Of particular interest during this decade was the result of a study reviewing the work of the paediatric oncology outreach nursing service.

The results of this study influenced and supported the continual development of the service at all specialist centres. A number of paediatric oncology nurses have also studied at PhD level and their research work has contributed to this specialist nursing body of knowledge. As we enter a new century, paediatric oncology nurse researchers/practitioners continue to provide and explore scientifically based care. Contributions to this book provide ample evidence of how the art and the science of paediatric nursing has been taken forward and the willingness of nurses to share their concerns and experiences through publication.

It has been interesting to reflect on my perceptions on the development of paediatric oncology nursing. As a student nurse I was totally unprepared when confronted with the care of a child with leukaemia. I then moved through decades of change in both the treatment and care of the child with cancer, approaches to healthcare, and the ever-changing role and status of the nurse. What has significantly changed is that nurses educated at diploma and degree level, with a firm knowledge-based clinical role, hold a central position in the multiprofessional team. What has not changed over the course of time is the presence of the nurse at the bedside providing comfort to the child and family. This development must in part be attributed to the timeless enthusiasm, dedication and the determination of nurses in the specialty striving to deliver improved knowledge-based care for children with cancer and their families. I hope that this book helps the nurses of the future, junior and senior, to continue with this work. I have no doubts that the specialty will continue to change; reflections over the next 50 years should look equally interesting.

Jenny Thompson

References and suggested reading

Bignold S, Ball S, Cribb A (1994) Nursing Families with Children with Cancer: the work of the Paediatric Oncology Outreach Nurse Specialists, A Research Summary, Department of Health. London: HMSO.

Forte K (2001) Paediatric oncology nursing: providing care through decades of change. Journal of Paediatric Oncology Nursing 18: 154-163.

Gibson F, Langton H (1998) Paediatric oncology nurse education; past present, current and future pathways for specialist preparation. European Journal of Oncology Nursing 2: 178-181.

Gibson F, Evans M (eds) (1999) Paediatric Oncology Acute Nursing Care. London: Whurr Publishers.

Hunt JA (1995) The paediatric oncology nurse specialist: the influence of employment location and funders on models of practice. Journal of Advanced Nursing 22: 126-133.

Martinson I (1976) Why don't we let them die at home? Research Nurse 39: 58-65.

Contributors

Alison Arnfield, MSc, RSCN, RGN, DMS, ONCCert, FETC Children's Nursing and Health care Consultant, London

Julie Bayliss, MSc, BSc, RGN, RSCN, Senior Nurse/Advanced Nurse Practitioner, Department of Haematology/Oncology, Great Ormond Street Hospital for Children NHS Trust, London

Karen Bravery, BSc, RSCN, RN, Senior Sister, Elephant Day Care Unit, Great Ormond Street Hospital for Children NHS Trust, London

Pippa Chesterfield, MSc, BSc, RGN, RSCN, ONCCert, RCNT, Macmillan Paediatric Nurse, Southampton General Hospital, Southampton

Tom Devine, MSc, BSc, RGN, RSCN, Oncology Research Fellow, Department of Paediatric Oncology, Royal Marsden Hospital NHS Trust, Sutton, Surrey

Jacqueline Edwards, MSc, BSc, RGN, RSCN, Dip Cancer Nursing, Research Fellow in Children's Cancer Nursing, Great Ormond Street Hospital for Children NHS Trust, London

Faith Gibson, PhD, MSc, RSCN, RGN, ONCCert, CertEd, RNT, Lecturer in Children's Nursing Research, Centre for Nursing and Allied Health Professions Research, Great Ormond Street Hospital for Children NHS Trust, London

Julianne Hall, BSocSc, Post Graduate Certificate in Rehabilitation, Senior Nurse Lecturer, School of Nursing Auckland University of Technology, Auckland, New Zealand

Julia Hannan, BSc, RGN, RSCN, Adv Dip Child Development, Clinical Nurse Specialist, Great Ormond Street Hospital for Children NHS Trust, London

Sharon Hayden, BSc, RGN, RSCN, Dip in Communication Studies, Assistant Director of Nursing, Nursing Administration, Our Lady's Hospital for Sick Children, Crumlin, Dublin, Ireland

Mariann Hedström, RN, Research Fellow, Department of Public Health and Caring Sciences, Section of Caring Sciences, Uppsala University, Uppsala, Sweden

Rachel Hollis, BA, RGN, RSCN, ONCCert, Senior Sister, Paediatric and Adolescent Oncology and Haematology Unit, St James's Hospital, Leeds Teaching Hospitals Trust, Leeds

Monica Hopkins, MSc, BNurs, NDN, RHV, RSCN, RGN, PG Dip Ed, PG Dip Adv Practice, Advanced Nurse Practitioner, Royal Liverpool Children's Hospital NHS Trust, Liverpool

Diane Huber, RGN, RSCN, ONCCert, Sister, St James's University Hospital, Leeds Teaching Hospitals Trust, Leeds

Louise Hooker, MSc, RGN, RSCN, Lead Cancer Nurse, Southampton University Hospitals Trust, Southampton

Jane Hunt, PhD, RGN, RSCN, DN, Cert FETC, Nursing and Health Services Research Consultant, Dunbridge, Hampshire

Helen Langton, MSc, BA, RGN, RSCN, RCNT, RNT, Associate Dean, School of Health and Social Sciences, Coventry University, Coventry

Guy Makin, PhD, BA, BM, BCh, MRCP, FRCPCH, Senior Lecturer in Paediatric Oncology, CRUK Molecular and Cellular Pharmacology Group, University of Manchester, Manchester

Sue Morgan, RGN, RSCN, ONCCert, Macmillan Clinical Nurse Specialist for Teenagers and Young Adults, St James's University Hospital, Leeds Teaching Hospitals Trust, Leeds

Charlotte Parsons, BSc, Health Studies, RGN, RSCN, ONCCert, Paediatric Oncology Outreach Nurse, Addenbrooke's Hospital NHS Trust, Cambridge

Linda Sanderson, MSc, BSc, RGN, RSCN, RNT, Sister, Yorkshire Regional Centre for Paediatric Oncology and Haematology, St James' Hospital, Leeds

Karen Selwood, MSc, BSc, RN, RSCN, RM, Advanced Nurse Practitioner, Oncology Unit, Royal Liverpool Children's Hospital NHS Trust, Liverpool

Beth Sepion, BEd, MSc, RSCN, RGN, SCM, Lecturer in Paediatric Oncology, University of Southampton, Southampton

Neil Shaw, RGN, RSCN, Dip HE, Senior Charge Nurse, St James's Hospital, Leeds Teaching Hospitals Trust, Leeds

Louise Soanes, MSc, PG Dip (Ed), BSc, RSCN, RGN, Senior Sister for Children's Services, Royal Marsden Hospital, Sutton, Surrey

Wilma Stuart, MSc, Former Nurse Lecturer, Auckland University of Technology, Auckland, New Zealand

Jenny Thompson, MSc, RGN, RSCN, Freelance Writer, Sussex

Louise von Essen, PhD, Associate Professor, Department of Public Health and Caring Sciences, Uppsala University, Sweden

Janet Williss, BSc, RSCN, SRN, DipN, Divisional Nurse Acute Medical Services, Great Ormond Street Hospital for Children NHS Trust, London

Howard Wilford, MSc, RGN, RSCN, Paediatric Oncology Nurse Specialist Child Health, Portsmouth Hospitals Trust, Portsmouth

Part 1

Perspectives on education

Helen Langton

As the care of children with cancer and their families becomes ever more complex and demanding, it is apparent that the specialty of paediatric oncology nursing is exploring and pushing the boundaries of practice. Nowhere is this more apparent than in the development of new roles and new ways of thinking and doing. This book offers a timely exploration of the history and development of new roles, based on current examples from practice. The book also shares ongoing research work to underpin these developments from an evidence-based perspective. Key issues are explored in relation to the complexities of professional practice, the influence of service delivery, and the role of education in supporting and developing practice in order to offer the reader an holistic overview of current perspectives in paediatric oncology nursing.

Chapter 1 presents a framework that can be used when developing new roles in paediatric oncology and sets the scene for the following two chapters which present the development of advanced roles in clinical practice. The chapter begins by demonstrating the value of networking and the vast resource that exists in terms of knowledge base and expertise within paediatric oncology nursing. This is in no small part the result of the Royal College of Nursing Paediatric Oncology Nursing Forum and the passion that exists among the members to develop practice for the benefit of children with cancer and their families. This chapter also demonstrates the value of using existing work in order to develop practice rather than unnecessarily reinventing the wheel. The value of this chapter is in the statements that are made around how to define advanced practice and the framework offered for role development. This chapter also offers a way through the often confusing implementation of such roles with a systematic and constructive approach. Service, management and education domains are all examined and pitfalls are identified; however, pointers for the future are also given and this chapter leaves the reader feeling that there may be light at the end of the tunnel.

Chapter 2 presents a useful exploration of the history and development of specialist nurses, both generally and in relation to paediatric oncology outreach nurse specialists within local communities and regional centres.

The literature is well evaluated and several key themes emerge. The overarching dilemma facing paediatric oncology nursing is the confusion of terminology around the concept and interpretation of the specialist nurse. This is seen at a variety of levels: Government, as expressed through policy; organizational, as expressed through service delivery; and at the point of delivery of care, as seen in the way in which the title 'specialist' is obtained and the perception of the user – the child and family. National guidelines give rise to multiple local interpretations, thus compounding the ability of the specialty to identify clearly the way forward. This impacts on career planning and career pathways, and it becomes difficult to advise and guide nurses new into the specialty without clear interpretations of role. However, what is clearly articulated within the chapter is the need to expand practice through development of these roles and this is explored more fully in Chapter 2.

The focus of Chapter 3 is the review of a specific role – that of the nurse practitioner as applied to a specific paediatric oncology unit. Again the clear theme arising from the literature is that of confusion over the concept and interpretation of the role. This chapter presents a literature review of this role, and then outlines the process and findings of participatory action research work that was undertaken within the unit. The role is identified as arising from a number of driving forces, in particular the reduction in doctors' hours (Greenhalgh & Co., 1994) and the need to develop career pathways for nurses (Department of Health or DoH, 1998). However, the action research demonstrated that focus on one role to the exclusion of staff development for all may be detrimental in the longer term. The chapter identifies the lack of clarity around the concept of advanced practice and is critical about the lack of education to enable development of the advanced practitioner. However, as the authors note, if there is lack of a clear concept of what an advanced practitioner is, then it is difficult to provide the right education to develop the skills required to be an advanced practitioner. This then impacts on the ability to offer clear career pathways for nurses within the specialty. The action research work did, however, demonstrate the need to develop all staff and also suggested that, in order to achieve this, a clear competency framework could be one way forward.

Chapter 4 commences with an overview of the history of competency development related to the literature regarding professionalism and the more recent debates around fitness for purpose and for practice. The authors present the difficulties surrounding the development and assessment of competency in nursing that is holistic and based on the concept of lifelong learning, using reflection in and on practice. However, the authors do not leave us frustrated with the debate but continue by presenting a tool that they have developed which identifies competencies and how to assess them in relation to qualified nurses undertaking a paediatric oncology course that incorporates practice and development of competency. This chapter also demonstrates the use of the nominal group technique as one way to generate competencies and to involve practitioners; it also demonstrates the value of an evaluation study to promote continuing refinement of such a tool.

Chapter 5 adds to the discussions exploring the need for new roles to be underpinned by education and competence; in this chapter the authors describe an educational programme for nurses working in paediatric palliative care. The programme described here demonstrates how collaboration between educators and practitioners aids the joint development of any initiative like this, and the suggestion that both parties need to be experienced in the field of paediatric oncology nursing in order for mutual regard and smooth working.

The theme of role development is maintained in Chapter 6, the final chapter of this part. Literature again demonstrates the lack of parity of interpretation of the concept of various roles, e.g. advanced nurse practitioner and clinical nurse specialist, and the education required to underpin these practice roles. The authors outline a case study undertaken locally that arose out of a perceived gap in continuity of care and communication across the multidisciplinary team. The reduction in doctors' working hours and the increasing complexity of care required by children with cancer and their families suggested that a detailed review of roles and education provision was required. The outcome of the review was the development of an advanced nurse practitioner role and the chapter is devoted mainly to a description of the implementation and subsequent development of the role. This chapter particularly emphasizes the clear need for relevant education to underpin the development into a role such as this which must include competencies in practice. It also emphasizes the value of the concept of teamwork if high-quality care is to be offered to users of the service. The authors comment on the lack of rigorous evaluation of the role, and indeed the development of new roles does offer an opportunity for evaluation, although it is well acknowledged that attempting to evaluate benefit to practice is difficult to achieve.

In conclusion, this part of the book offers paediatric oncology nurses the opportunity to develop insight into current thinking that is impacting on the specialty in relation to new roles and the issues that surround their development. At a national level, the profession has not agreed a clear definition of roles and this is resulting in confusion about the concept of various roles such as clinical nurse specialist, nurse/advanced nurse practitioner and nurse consultant. Furthermore, as a result of this confusion, these roles are interpreted at a service organizational level in a variety of ways, resulting in further confusion for colleagues and, more important-ly, for children with cancer and their families. Nursing roles are already experienced differently by these families as they move between shared care units, community care and the regional provider. The further intro-duction of new roles has the distinct probability of making this worse not better, and therefore the potential of fragmenting the patient experience, not providing greater continuity. If the concept of the user as central to care is to be maintained, this disparity needs to be addressed.

The value of this part of the book for paediatric oncology nurses is that, having explored the literature and exposed the confusion, it offers readers a framework within which to proceed when developing new roles. This framework is timely, and offers paediatric oncology nursing the opportu-nity to set its own house in order and to lead the way for nursing. The outline of various models already in existence also allows readers to bene-fit from the learning gained in these arenas and to translate this to their own area of practice in order not to reinvent the wheel or suffer the same pitfalls and difficulties. The advantage of paediatric oncology nursing, in being a relatively small specialty, is in the ability to network among prac-titioners. Readers need to capitalize on this in order to move practice forward at a greater pace and in a more coordinated way than may be pos-sible for others working within a larger arena. This particularly applies to the development of competencies. Nationally, cancer networks are pro-moting competency development and are keen not to reinvent wheels if best practice already exists. The close relationship between the Paediatric Oncology Nursing Forum and the Cancer Alliance may enable us to share with each other and thus address issues together where possible. This may also enable seamless delivery to occur nationally (DoH, 2000).

The final value is the way in which this part of the book demonstrates the use of a wide variety of research methods and methodologies as applied to the specialty. In this age of evidence-based practice it is encour-aging to see managers, practitioners and educators working together to identify and promote best practice through the generation of evidence. It is hoped that the reader will be motivated to explore the use of some of these tools in their own areas of practice and, as importantly, to share their findings.

References

Department of Health (1998) The New NHS – Working Together: Securing a quality workforce for the NHS. London: HMSO.

Department of Health (2000) The NHS Cancer Plan. London: HMSO.

Greenhalgh & Co. (1994) The Interface between Junior Doctors and Nurses. Macclesfield: Greenhalgh & Co.

Chapter 1

Defining a framework for advancing clinical practice

Faith Gibson and Louise Hooker

Paediatric oncology nurses today face challenges from both the profession itself and society to provide clinical expertise in a complex and rapidly changing specialty. Developments in the medical treatment of childhood cancer mean that the expected survival rates have never been better. Consequently, paediatric oncology nurses caring for children with cancer have had to keep pace with and respond to advances in treatment, as well as technological and service developments. The nature of the care provided in inpatient, outpatient and community settings has changed in recent years, and this change will continue, with an increasing number of children in all three settings requiring highly specialized care throughout their disease, e.g. the specialty of palliative care has grown significantly, with models of care for both children (Goldman, 1998) and adolescents in place (Edwards, 2001). In addition, long-term follow-up has become a major component of care as more children survive into adulthood (Stiller, 1994; Gibson and Soanes, 2001).

The changes that have taken place have altered the way in which healthcare is perceived and delivered. The roles involved in paediatric oncology nursing are now diverse, and offer scope for role development in direct clinical care, as well as education, management and research. In addition, there are a number of opportunities afforded by the variety of clinical specialisms within paediatric oncology, including clinical nurse specialist posts in bone marrow transplantation, care of adolescents, palliative care and intravenous therapy, to mention a few. Role development has taken place in response to changes in healthcare and local circumstances; the more recent additions of case managers and advanced nurse practitioners represent continuing innovations in the organization and delivery of care. These developments are to be welcomed if they ensure that outcomes are improved and that services continue to meet the needs of children and families. However, these changes are not without their problems, particularly where nursing roles have evolved in an unstructured or reactive way, or where full consideration has not been given to potential consequences.

Nurses have a significant contribution to make in ensuring a cohesive service, working as they do with other colleagues and across professional and organizational boundaries (NHS Executive, 2000). Such unstructured and reactive role evolution could benefit from a proactive and robust national framework that supports individual nurses in practice expansion, and provides safeguards for their patients. One such model is referred to as a 'safety net to support professional practice' (Royal College of Paediatrics and Child Health/Joint British Advisory Committee on Children's Nursing, 1996), and this has been adapted and applied to paediatric oncology nursing (Royal College of Nursing [RCN], 2000). This chapter details the approaches taken to define and develop the framework for role development in paediatric oncology nursing. It starts by setting the scene and placing role development within the context of policy and practice. The process of developing the framework is then outlined, followed by a discussion of the dimensions for role development that form the starting point in an exploration of the characteristics of paediatric oncology nurses. The framework presented is followed by an example of how it can be used in practice.

Setting the scene

The scope of paediatric oncology nursing practice

There are currently 21 United Kingdom Children's Cancer Study Group (UKCCSG) centres in the UK and one in Eire. This approach to the organization of care gives the family of the child with cancer access to the best medical treatment, supported by specialist nursing care (Gibson and Williams, 1997). There are a number of published documents that outline the standards required to offer a quality service to children with cancer (Expert Advisory Group on Cancer, 1995; Royal College of Pathologists, 1996; UKCCSG, 1997a, 1997b), all of which refer to the need for appropriately qualified and experienced nursing staff. In all, however, there is a distinct lack of detail about the nature and training of a paediatric oncology nurse. What is known, however, is that specialist areas of practice, such as paediatric oncology, need specialist nurses.

Specialization in nursing was noted by the International Council of Nurses (ICN, 1985) to have occurred because of:

- the need for more effective use of nurses
- the changing sociological, cultural and economic factors affecting health

- advances and changes in medical practice
- the specific health needs of a population
- developing national priorities in healthcare.

The process of this development was not, however, determined in a systematic way, and was often perceived to parallel developments in the disease-focused model of medical specialities (RCN, 1988). Problems and issues with increasing specialization were recognized by the ICN, with concerns revolving around the benefits of specialization and the forces driving them. The ICN was also anxious about the qualifications of nurses working in specialist areas, and their place within the structure of the profession and the healthcare system as a whole. One of the potential outcomes, if developments were to continue in a disorderly fashion, was thought to be fragmentation of nursing care and the splintering of the profession (Styles, 1989). Dalziel (1990) reinforced the concern about these potential outcomes and advocated that nurses define the specialities in nursing before the Government and other care workers seize that opportunity and impose frameworks more reflective of a medical than a nursing model.

In response to their growing concerns, and with the express aim of assisting the profession to develop a systematic means for designating specialities, the ICN (1991) detailed 10 essential features for orderly development of a specialization. The scope of paediatric oncology nursing expresses all the features detailed by the ICN and may therefore be defined as specialist practice:

1. *The specialty defines itself as nursing and subscribes to the overall purpose, functions and ethical standards of nursing.* Nursing practice is distinguished by a focus on holistic care, collaboration with families within a tradition of care and concern, and an ever-growing body of nursing knowledge.

2. *The specialty practice is sufficiently complex and advanced, and is beyond the scope of general nursing practice.* Although cancer and cancer nursing are represented in pre-registration curricula, the level of knowledge shared, together with the limited, and for some absent, clinical practice for children's nurses, equips nurses with only a very rudimentary knowledge and understanding of the area of practice. Further knowledge and skills of this complex area of care were initially acquired 'on the job' with nurses of children with cancer learning from role models and in-house training. It was soon recognized that this, although meeting local needs, was insufficient. Post-registration programmes were therefore developed to expand specialist knowledge and skills to complement core knowledge of child health and beliefs of how to care for children with cancer and their families.

3. *There is both a demand and a need for the specialty service.* Childhood cancer is a rare disease in the UK with an incidence rate for children under 15 years of only 110–130 per million per year. The referral to regional paediatric centres ensures that families receive care from healthcare professionals who are familiar with their specific needs. The holistic requirements posed by toxic and complicated treatment regimens demands a specialist service.

4. *The focus of the specialty is a defined population, which demonstrates recurrent problems and phenomena that lie within the discipline and practice of nursing.* Nursing focuses on the effects that cancer and its various treatments have on the individual family, observing side effects and managing symptoms. There is an understanding that nurses do undertake medical work that is appropriate but within the context of nursing. The therapeutic work of nursing is being developed throughout the specialty.

5. *The specialty practice is based on a core body of nursing knowledge, which is currently being expanded and refined through research. There are mechanisms for reviewing and disseminating research.* The charting of nursing knowledge within the specialty has been slow when compared with colleagues in the USA who established the *Journal of Association of Pediatric Oncology Nurses* (*JAPON*) in 1984. Nevertheless a core body of nursing knowledge is now being expanded through unidisciplinary, multidisciplinary, multicentre and collaborative research. There is increasing evidence that nurses publish and disseminate their work through both popular and academic nursing and medical journals.

6. *The specialty has established educational and practice standards, which are congruent with those of the profession and are set by recognized nursing body or bodies.* In the past, the English National Board regulated education programmes and the UKCC recorded specialist education. Both of these organizations have since been superseded by the Nursing and Midwifery Council (NMC). In contrast to colleagues in the USA, who set up standards of practice in 1979 and re-affirmed them in 2000 (Association of Pediatric Oncology Nurses, 2000), there are no nationally agreed published standards in the UK. Nevertheless, standards of care in the form of guidelines are being produced and endorsed in textbooks that detail the care of children with cancer. Clinical competencies are being developed locally (Gibson and Soanes, 2000) and the need for national competencies is being addressed (Long et al., 2001).

7. *The specialty adheres to the registration requirement for the general nurse.* Registration as a children's nurse is required as the first step to becoming a paediatric oncology nurse.

8. *Specialty expertise is obtained through a professionally approved advanced education programme, which leads to a recognized qualification. The educational programme preparing the specialist is*

administered by a nurse. The first specialist programme was a short programme developed in 1985. Longer English National Board for Nursing, Midwifery and Health Visiting (ENB) courses developed soon after to include a clinical component alongside theory (Casey, 1989). Since that time, nurse educators have introduced different and creative approaches to ongoing education. Access to core specialty knowledge for as many paediatric oncology nurses as possible has been provided through links with adult oncology courses, introduction of theory-only courses and production of short courses aimed at nurses in shared care centres (Gibson and Langton, 1998).

9. *The specialty has a credentialing process determined by the profession.* Registration as paediatric nurses and certification as paediatric oncology nurses are forms of credentialing.

10. *Practitioners are organized and represented within a specialty association or a branch of the National Nurses' Association.* Since 1984 the Paediatric Oncology Nurses' Forum (PONF), a forum of the RCN, has represented paediatric oncology nurses. The diverse areas of practice, such as direct clinical care, education, management and research, are represented in the Forum. It also provides a venue for communication where nurses can exchange new and alternative methods of nursing care provision, consider creative approaches to continuing education and identify a focus for research. All of these ultimately have an impact on improving the care for children and their families.

Changing the scope of nursing practice

Career opportunities have been enhanced through structured development of specialities in nursing. Since the appointment of the first infection control sister in 1974, the role of the clinical nurse specialist (CNS) in nursing specialities has grown (Tiffany, 1976; Humphris, 1994). These roles have developed from existing structures because of recognized patient need for more expert and specialized care, and by nurses who wanted to stay in a direct relationship with patients (Castledine, 1998). Specialization continues with advances in medical science and technology, resulting in a reappraisal of traditional roles within both nursing and medicine, and the boundaries between the clinical work of doctors and that of nurses being redrawn (Dowling et al., 1995). The team approach, in which doctors, nurses and other allied health professionals adapt and develop new skills, is being increasingly emphasized (English, 1997). For nurses, this has resulted in an increase in specialization, with some recent innovations clearly reflecting an expansion of the nurse's role, often at the interface between nursing and medicine (McKee and Lessof, 1992; Autar, 1996). Some of these areas of expansion have clearly had an impact on the workload of junior doctors; documents addressing the training of junior doctors, such as the 'New Deal' (NHS Management Executive, 1991) and that of Calman (1993), considered alongside the *Scope of Professional Practice* (UKCC, 1992), have provided tremendous opportunities and challenges to nurses in the UK (Pickersgill, 1993; Koefmann, 1995).

The demise of rigid practice boundaries heralded by the 'Scope' document (UKCC, 1992) led to nurses taking on an increasing number of tasks, e.g. venepuncture, cervical smears, taking blood samples and ECG recordings, defibrillation, catheterization of male patients, blood glucose monitoring, etc. (UKCC, 2000). This document ended the requirement for nurses to gain certificates for each extended role and placed the responsibility for competence within expanded practice boundaries for individuals. What was not addressed by the 'Scope' document was, however, how decisions are made about the scope of nursing practice, the education and training required, and how expansions into practice are monitored (Wainwright, 1994). The extent to which nurses achieve authority over the nature of their practice was also not addressed by the document. Nevertheless it played a significant role in encouraging the nursing profession to consider the development of roles that would encompass the complexities of role expansion, rather than simply absorbing medical tasks (Pickersgill, 1993). Although there is no explicit link between the document and the changes in nursing in relation to role development, they cannot be viewed separately (Finlay, 2000) because it provided a set of principles that have had a significant impact on how nurses' work is undertaken (Jowett et al., 1999). What remains, however, is some confusion about how far the expansion of nursing practice is associated with developing professional nursing practice (Bowler and Mallik, 1998; Cameron, 2000; Finlay, 2000; Woods, 2000).

Developing new roles

That nurses embrace the notion of role development is now implicit in a number of national strategy documents that have appeared over the last decade: *A Vision for the Future* (Department of Health [DoH], 1993), and *The Challenges for Nursing and Midwifery in the 21st Century* (The Heathrow Debate – DoH, 1994). More recently, the document *Making a Difference* (DoH, 1999a) has explicitly detailed a vision for how the current Government see nurses taking on more complex roles and having a greater responsibility for the delivery of patient care. A new modern career framework, linked to the Government's proposals to modernize the NHS pay system (DoH, 1999b), was proposed in *Making a Difference*, suggesting that delivery of a comprehensive service required the following: health support workers, registered practitioners, senior registered practitioners and consultant practitioners. Within this career structure, *The NHS Plan* (DoH, 2000) envisages further role expansion, which will give nurses the powers to prescribe, refer, admit and discharge patients. The profession is currently faced with the challenge of revealing this pattern of role development (Read, 1998; Shewan and Read, 1999; Bamford and Gibson, 2000; Read et al., 2001) and in particular the roles of nurse practitioner (Walsh, 2001), advanced nurse practitioner (Knowles and Kearney, 1998; Woods, 2000) and consultant nurse (NHS Executive, 2001).

This is a very exciting time for nursing in the UK, with many opportunities for nurses to shift the boundaries of their practice actively, to develop new roles and to expand existing roles in order to benefit their patient group. There is evidence that this is already taking place in cancer nursing (e.g. Moore et al., 1999; Oakley et al., 2000) and children's nursing (Dearmun and Gordon, 1999; Rushworth et al., 2000; Smart, 2001; Peter and Flynn, 2002). The pace of change will certainly increase in response to policy and demands of the service, but this will be received well only if nurses can avoid the crisis management that has plagued the profession in the past. Casey et al. (2001) highlight a number of significant concerns for children's nurses:

- Short cuts may be taken as new posts are established, with limited training for new roles compromising both quality and safety.
- There may be an issue about resources, with new tasks being adopted at the expense of the time available for nursing care of the child and family.
- There may be an increase in the problems caused by the varied and inventive terminology that is being used to describe the different roles.

Developing new roles in paediatric oncology nursing

As mentioned previously, we have seen the development of new roles within the specialty. On the whole, these roles have developed in response to local need and, although there has been open debate about new roles and the developments taking place here in the UK and in the USA at a number of conferences, there remains some confusion as to what advanced nurse practitioners 'actually' do. Practitioners in the UK have been liberated by the 'Scope' document and encouraged by the Government's new career pathway, but the structure, process and outcome of new roles remain a bit of a mystery to most nurses in clinical practice, e.g. practitioners in paediatric oncology nursing are left unsure about whether they should be considering such roles as:

- undertaking lumbar punctures and bone marrow aspirates

- prescribing blood products
- prescribing antiemetics
- admitting and discharging patients
- undertaking physical assessments
- running a nurse-led, long-term, follow-up clinic.

Questions are being asked about the benefits of such developments to patients, their families and the profession, and to service delivery in general. Although some questions remain unanswered, what is known is that paediatric oncology nurses are concerned that without a cohesive structure medical tasks may be handed down to nurses, resulting in fragmented care and the development of another type of medical role (such as doctors' assistants) which fails to maintain the holistic goals of nursing. In addition to these concerns, and in tandem with other areas of nursing, paediatric oncology nurses have witnessed an increase in the range of titles used to describe roles that remain unclear to most nurses in the specialty. As a result, confusion abounds, and paediatric oncology nurses in practice are unclear about the developments taking place in their specialty, managers remain uncertain about what roles are needed to develop their service, and, in education, requests for programmes to develop specialist practitioners continue and must reflect the muddle that previous professional bodies attempted to unravel (UKCC, 1998, 1999, 2002).

The steering committee of the PONF (RCN) were aware of this ongoing confusion and therefore arranged a series of meetings and commissioned a number of conference presentations to open up the debate across the specialty. In addition, as a group we had received a number of requests from our membership for guidance and clarification in relation to developing roles. Responding to the needs of our members, we began to clarify our thoughts, in debate as a group and with the help of other expert nurses, and added this to a synthesis of the growing literature. This recently culminated in our proposal to use a framework (the safety net) developed previously (Royal College of Paediatrics and Child Health/Joint British Advisory Committee on Children's Nursing, 1996; Coombs and Holgate, 1998), adapting it for use in our specialty (Gibson and Hooker, 1999). Development of the framework involved application, by a group of experienced paediatric oncology nurses, of the framework to the specialty and expanding the content to make it more applicable.

What follows is not an attempt to define nursing roles or competencies in any detail, but rather one to propose a common framework, which we can use to discuss, develop and study nursing roles. This process begins by looking at the constituent elements of the role of a paediatric oncology nurse.

Characteristics of paediatric oncology nursing practice

We considered what advanced practice meant to us and addressed nursing role development in paediatric oncology nursing within the notion of the following:

- labels and titles: description of the role
- dimensions of the role: values and focus
- area of specialty: specialist role
- level of expertise: expert and advanced practice
- medical and nursing models of care: expanded roles.

This list is used to present our deliberations so far.

Labels and titles: description of the role

In defining the role we recognize that a lot of the confusion stems from the increasing number of labels and titles being used to distinguish nursing roles. Reflecting on the role of the CNS, some would argue that in the UK there is no consensus about the title. For the role of a CNS there are a variety of levels of preparation and the criteria for these posts remain unclear, resulting in the title CNS describing a diverse group of individuals (Humphris, 1994). We are in danger of adding to that confusion with the introduction of titles such as nurse practitioner (NP) and advanced nurse practitioner (ANP). It is imperative to have an understanding of what these titles refer to. This should clarify the route of preparation, both clinical and educational, and the distinguishing features of those roles that relate to that title.

Titles for nursing roles have one main purpose: to communicate. As the most important people with whom nurses need to communicate are their patients, the titles we use must be meaningful to them. What do children and families want to know about the person with whom they are communicating? In the absence of concrete evidence, we are assuming that they want to know the following:

- you are a nurse
- whether you are a student, have some experience or are very experienced.

Given these assumptions we recommend that:

- All titles include the word nurse or words that the public understand as nurse, e.g. sister, charge nurse.

- The dimension of 'expertise' is reflected in simple titles, which are meaningful to patients and the public, e.g. staff nurse, sister and senior sister.
- All other aspects of the role, such as area of specialty, should be communicated by the nurse when she or he introduces her- or himself and explains the role in relation to the person with whom he or she is communicating.
- The title 'nurse practitioner' should be the only exception and should be used only where there is a significant element of decision-making about medical management in the role. This should be explained in clear and specific terms to patients and their families.

Dimensions of the role: values and focus

The framework (RCN, 2000) reaffirms the equal value of general and specialist knowledge and skills, and points to the fact that core abilities and qualities are shared by all nurses and by all children's nurses. We recognize that role development evolves over time, for both an individual and the profession. We also recognize that the core of nursing is not defined by the tasks that we perform. Nursing practice is distinguished by our focus on holistic care, collaboration with families within a tradition of care and concern, and an ever-growing body of nursing knowledge. As we expand our scope of practice, we incorporate new knowledge and skills, and thus advance our understanding of clinical nursing practice. We recognize that role development will be influenced by factors such as experience, level of expertise, personal and professional values, and place of work, specialty and aspects of role transition. Thus, role development will be dynamic, complex and context specific. Bearing these issues in mind we recommend that the role should:

- have a nursing focus (holistic care, family centred)
- be driven by the needs of children, young people and their families
- be appropriate to the client group, and the needs and values of society
- be relevant in your place of work or in your team
- include reviews to ensure continued usefulness and potential for further change
- only encompass tasks that nursing can influence
- have clear responsibility and accountability for decision-making, implementation and outcome of all aspects of the role, within agreed practice boundaries.

Area of specialty: specialist role

The paediatric oncology nurse applies both paediatric nursing expertise and specialist oncology (nursing and medical) expertise to the care of the child and the family. The specialty service has two dimensions: area of practice, i.e. patient group, e.g. adolescents, bone marrow transplant recipients; and location of the role, i.e. community, management and education. It may be necessary to distinguish major and minor parts of roles. We recommend that the role should:

- have a specific focus of specialist practice/client group
- have a role description that is explicit about clinical practice, as distinct from management, research and education responsibilities
- Describe a job that needs doing, as opposed to a specific person's attributes.

Level of expertise: expert and advanced practice

To help define the nature of practice, we wanted to distinguish here between general and specialty knowledge. To clarify this part of the framework, we have used Benner's levels (1984) of skill acquisition. At registration a nurse is deemed to be an advanced beginner in general paediatric nursing; however, the same nurse starting to work in nursing children with cancer would be considered a novice. This nurse would develop her or his expertise through preceptorship, clinical supervision, education and training, in order to progress on a continuum from novice to expert. It is this pathway, from novice to expert, that remains unclear in the specialty. While advancing specialist clinical practice, nurses concurrently advance their own knowledge and skills in paediatric nursing. This framework reaffirms the equal value of general and specialist knowledge and skills – those core abilities and qualities shared by all nurses and by all paediatric nurses.

We have clarified what we believe to be the defining characteristics of the *expert specialist*. We recognize that most nurses have the potential to become experts in their field, involved in advancing their own practice. In contrast, we feel that only a few paediatric oncology nurses will practise at an advanced level. Thus, the focus changes from the narrow concentration of the expert specialist to encompass additional features (Table 1.1). We recommend that:

- paediatric nursing practice be reaffirmed as the core nursing focus.

Medical and nursing models of care: expanded roles

Nursing focuses on the effects that cancer and its various treatments have on the individual family, observing side effects and managing

Table 1.1 Characteristics that discriminate between expert and advanced levels of practice

Expert

- Manages her or his own caseload
- Carries out medical/technical procedures within the narrow band of the specialty (within a nursing context)
- Uses expert decision-making, applying skills, and knowledge of the specialty and paediatric nursing
- Applies research, and evaluates and develops own practice
- Teaches/mentors less experienced staff in the clinical area
- Is recognized as an expert in the multiprofessional team providing care
- Recognizes skills of 'generalist expert' and refers to others as appropriate

Advanced

- Fulfils the above, and in addition:
- Brings breadth to the depth/thinks more globally, focusing on generalist and specialist, than the expert
- Will be masters (clinical) prepared with extensive clinical experience
- Identifies the need for and commissions research
- Sees and takes opportunities related to practice development for client group
- Is recognized in this role within the multidisciplinary team providing care across a broader field
- Is a leader within the specialty

symptoms. There is an understanding that nurses do undertake medical work that is appropriate but within the context of nursing. This would depend on the post and the individual; however, we would like to emphasize that all health care is teamwork and that each discipline has its primary focus. Whereas medicine focuses on investigations, diagnosis and treatment of diseases, nursing focuses on the effects of the disease and the various treatments on the individual and the family, observing for side effects and managing symptoms. In children's cancer care nurses do medical work every day that is appropriate; however, it is done within the context of nursing. We develop further the therapeutic work of nursing.

In relation to an expanded role, we have to decide what is appropriate and relevant for nurses to undertake, while ensuring that whatever role we expand into will make a difference to nursing, e.g. we might consider that an expert nurse should be able to prescribe antiemetics, because symptom management is clearly within the domain of nursing. In contrast, we might not consider that an expert nurse will be able to perform a lumbar puncture or bone marrow aspirate, asking ourselves whether nursing would make a difference in this situation. It clearly might under certain circumstances, such as when a child is having the procedure using distraction therapy, but would all experts undertake this role and is this advancing practice? We recommend that:

- the core values of nursing must be explicit in any role expansion
- improving patient care must be the purpose of any role expansion.

A different role that has emerged is the NP who has medical decision-making as the main element of the role (see Chapter 6). These nurses make autonomous decisions about medical management based on clinical examination, and use medical diagnostic skills. Such roles require further education in such areas as physical assessment of body systems, pharmacology, histopathology, etc., all undertaken within a child and family focus, which is the added value of NP-type roles (Smart, 2001).

The framework

After identifying some of the characteristics of the development of nursing roles in the specialty, the working party then considered it to be essential to apply these to the reality of clinical practice. The 'Safety Net' (Figure 1.1), initially developed by a team in Oxford and described in the document published by the Royal College of Paediatrics and Child Health/Joint British Advisory Committee on Children's Nursing (1996), proved a useful model as it encompassed rationale, context, accountability and evaluation. This model has been adapted for use as guidance for nurses and the teams in which they work when they are considering the possibilities for role development in their own service. The basic structure of the model remains the same; it is the additions that make the safety net very relevant to the specialty when considering role expansion.

Using the safety net

It is intended that this tool be used by nurses, in consultation with the appropriate members of the multiprofessional team, when planning developments in the scope of nursing practice. The proposed developments may involve minor or major changes; this framework was designed to be equally appropriate either when developing practice within an existing role or when considering a completely new role. Figure 1.1 is an overview of the framework's approach to the issues that should be addressed, and this tool provides a step-by-step guide through the framework,

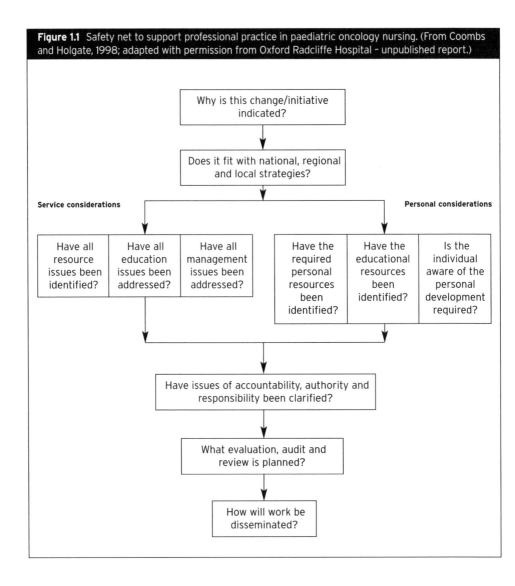

Figure 1.1 Safety net to support professional practice in paediatric oncology nursing. (From Coombs and Holgate, 1998; adapted with permission from Oxford Radcliffe Hospital – unpublished report.)

incorporating the two key components of planning for role development:

1. issues that relate to providing the clinical service
2. issues that relate to the individual.

The framework is provided as a template for discussion with colleagues, professional leaders and service managers, to plan future practice developments, and education/training and support needs, e.g. it could be used to develop an NP role in long-term follow-up.

A worked example of using the safety net

The general belief among paediatric oncologists is that all survivors of childhood cancer should be followed up for life (D'Angio, 1975). However, in the absence of evidence to support the view that follow-up has an impact on survival and quality of life, with an ever increasing number of long-term survivors, concern has been raised over the costs of providing this service (Brada, 1995). Not all survivors of childhood cancer require the same level of intervention from their primary, secondary or tertiary healthcare teams, nor do all these teams need to be involved with every survivor (Wallace et al., 2001). Gibson and Soanes (2001) considered alternatives in follow-up practice, to improve the current service in a more cost-effective and patient-centred way. They suggested three models of nursing – CNS, NP and consultant nurse – all of which could enable nurses to take a lead and oversee the long-term follow-up of children/young people with cancer, with evolution of the role being defined by the parameters of the specialist service and not constrained by role definitions. This would have implications for children/teenagers and their families, where the level of clinical surveillance would more closely match clinical need (Wallace et al., 2001), and care and information given at the clinic may be seen as more appropriate and useful (Eiser et al., 1996). Choice of role would depend on local need and must aim to preserve and improve the care, and therefore would need to be carefully introduced and evaluated (Brada, 1995). The safety net would provide a step-by-step approach for developing and evaluating an NP role in long-term follow-up that starts with:

- an examination of the current team and the needs of the patient group
- search of the literature to identify similar developments, to find out if there is any evidence to suggest that the proposed changes will have the desired effects
- consideration of Government and professional groups' strategies for nursing/healthcare.

After considering the above three points, the safety net would then direct the professional team to consider the service and resources required, and management and educational issues. There is a direct interrelationship of these three areas and therefore they must be considered together.

Service considerations

At this point a decision would need to be made about the model of NP role to be developed, because this would have implications for resources.

That decision may be quite difficult and would rely on the team having followed the initial step in the safety net, which asks about the current team and the needs of patients. In addition, it relies on the team having a clear understanding of the differences between various roles (e.g. CNS, NP, ANP and consultant nurse), and their purpose and function (NHS Executive, 2001; Reveley, 2001; Roberts-Davis and Read, 2001) and the level of care that needs to be delivered (Wallace et al., 2001). Each role would have a different effect on staffing provision, equipment required, time available to plan for the change in practice, support structures required and the 'knock-on' effects on other team members. Resource issues therefore require much consideration early on in the development process.

The role of the NP in the UK is fairly recent, and although the primary care NP is well defined, the role in acute care remains poorly defined. The team would need to consider established definitions of the role alongside the expectations of the role for their service. Of some help would be the guidance produced by the RCN's Nurse Practitioners' Association and RCN Council on the role and scope of nurse practitioners, identifying clearly the role within primary and secondary care settings (RCN Nurse Practitioners' Association, 1997, p. 2), defining a NP as someone who:

- makes professionally autonomous decisions, for which they have sole responsibility
- receives patients/clients with undifferentiated and undiagnosed problems; an assessment of their healthcare needs is made based on highly developed nursing knowledge and skills
- screens patients/clients for disease risk factors and early signs of illness
- develops with the patient/client a nursing care plan for health, with an emphasis on preventive measures
- provides counselling and health education
- has the authority to admit or discharge patients/clients from his or her own caseload and refer them to other healthcare providers as appropriate.

This definition indicates a level of autonomous nursing practice and accountability for that practice. A role that provides a full range of primary healthcare services with a holistic patient and family focus, using nursing and medical diagnosis to plan care, is very different to other practitioner roles (Reveley, 2001). Therefore, if this definition were accepted, with maybe some minor changes dictated by the nature of the clinical work, the team would need to give particular consideration to the following:

- a shift of medical input
- implications for other nursing roles

- types of interventions and where they would take place
- freedom to order investigations
- the need for new documentation
- initial and ongoing funding linked to a business plans
- changes in the activity on the service
- gaining support from nursing peers and medical colleagues
- gaining support from directorate and trust level management
- impact on the provision of holistic care
- implications for medical staff training and nursing staff development.

Management issues

Priorities for management would revolve around describing the NP role as distinct from other roles. Thoughts given to the level of previous experience required, mandatory and optional activities to be undertaken, and objectives for the role would lead to the development of a new job description. It would be important at this stage to consider how the NP role would fit into the existing team structure. Decisions would need to be made about pay scale and role title. It is at this point that information gained about similar developments elsewhere, and an awareness of Government and professional groups' strategies, would be crucial, e.g. nurse-led follow-up clinics have been in existence in the USA since 1983, coordinated by a paediatric nurse practitioner who specializes in cancer (Hobbie, 1986). Their experience and role evaluations have continued to refine a specific role that would be useful in any deliberations about an NP role. In addition, knowledge about role developments in the UK would be an important part of ensuring that the NP role corresponded to a national approach and strategy. A national approach has more benefits to patients and the profession by making clear the nursing contribution and placing the role within a well-defined career structure. In describing the NP role, a distinction would need to be made between other roles, particularly our medical colleagues. This is where a clear definition of the NP role and its functions would be crucial. Experience of developing an NP role in an adult surgical unit revealed that doctors were initially wary of the NP who was perceived as 'doing a doctor's job' and nurses were sceptical of the role (Reveley and Haigh, 2001). Role boundaries, responsibilities and clinical authority would therefore need to be addressed in relation to a NP role where there may be a confusion of accountability (Dowling et al., 1995, 1996). A priority for management would be to involve appropriate members of the multiprofessional team at all stages, ensuring that doctors and nurses are equal partners in planning and ultimately managing the new post (Dowling et al., 1996).

Education considerations

The education requirements for the post-holder pose a particular challenge, because there may or may not be a specific education programme already available (Woods, 1997; Crumbie, 2001). This has enormous implications on time where links may need to be made to the local education provider to work with the clinical team in developing an appropriate programme. Time would need to be allowed for the individual to undertake the programme, and this may include secondment to a programme at another institution. Planning at this stage would need to consider developing clinical competencies, agreeing on an assessment strategy (practical and theoretical), training required and/or education and clinical supervision. Many questions need to be asked at this point, in relation to the nature of the work to be undertaken and the preparation required. Initially, in 1993, the first NP course at the RCN was at diploma level. This moved to degree level in 1995. Since that time numerous courses have been developed in the UK, where an inconsistent approach has been revealed towards course content and academic levels (Read et al., 2001). It would be important, at this point in the safety net, to involve a member of the education team to help make sense of the education choices available, and to plan for initial and ongoing education and training that ensures that national standards and quality are assured.

Personal considerations

If there were a member of the team considering undertaking an NP role in long-term follow-up, once developed, there would be a number of specific questions that they would also need to ask such as:

- Who would act as their mentor?
- Is clinical supervision in place; if not how could this be arranged?
- Is there a process of staff appraisal, and how could this be used most effectively?
- Are expert practitioners available to offer help?
- Is there support of the multiprofessional team?
- Is there willingness, finance and time to invest in them as individuals?
- Is there appropriate education and training available?
- Why would they want to undertake the role?
- What are the risks and benefits of success and failure?
- How does this fit in with their longer-term plans?

These questions are crucial when matching the person to the post.

Accountability, authority and responsibility

These are fundamental to ensuring that the interests of service users are protected. Role expansion that would encompass the follow-up of children/teenagers includes more than increasing technical specialization. The scope of independence of judgement, decision-making and action would need to be clarified (Hunt, 1994). The safety net asks the professional team to consider important issues in the planning phase, e.g.:

- Who holds ultimate clinical responsibility?
- What is the trust/employer's position regarding risk management/ vicarious liability procedures, in relation to this planned development?
- Are there operational policies that clearly document the client group, professionals' responsibilities, activities and limitations to authority?
- How does the new role fit in with the trust/employers' clinical governance framework?

Evaluation, audit and review

Finally, evaluation, audit and review are considered to be crucial steps in the safety net: elements that have been lacking previously when new roles have been developed (Humphris and Masterson, 2000). This evaluation would need to include a range of perspectives, not just of the post-holder and those who have supported the development, because a change in the system will have a ripple effect. The introduction of a nurse playing a significant role in follow-up will impact on many people, and their views need to be sought, e.g. children/teenagers and families as consumers of care, other practitioners, managers, researchers and other team members. In addition, consideration will need to be given to when, how and what will be evaluated to give valid, unbiased and meaningful results that can guide future developments, e.g.:

- Do you need to collect information before the change as a baseline against which to measure its impact?
- When will you evaluate the impact of change?
- What quality standards are you going to audit against?
- How will the evaluation/audit results be used to influence the continued development of practice?
- What information will you need to collect to monitor the impact, such as waiting times and patient satisfaction?

All the areas discussed above would be of key importance when considering the development of an NP role in long-term follow-up. As evidenced in the example given, the safety net provides a useful framework to analyse, describe and evaluate role developments.

Conclusion

The aim for the RCN's PONF was to produce a framework that would enable nurses and organizations to act with confidence in devising and developing roles that are patient and service oriented. We believe that we have achieved this and that the framework described here provides practical guidance for developing practice in paediatric oncology nursing. The worked example suggests that the safety net can successfully direct those involved to consider all perspectives of role development. It is important that the safety net is used and evaluated, with developments clearly documented in order to be useful to practitioners and to develop the specialty locally, nationally and internationally. Overall, the framework provides a structure in which the specialty can be examined and described further. As Coombs and Holgate state (1998, p. 210): 'it is possible to learn in an orderly and constructive fashion, to have a sense of achievement from the past and not be overwhelmed by the possibilities of the future.'

Acknowledgements

Thanks to members of the PONF and the steering group who have contributed to the ongoing thinking and reflections on this framework for developing practice.

References

Association of Pediatric Oncology Nurses (2000) Scope and Standards of Pediatric Oncology Nursing Practice. Washington DC: American Nurses Publishing.

Autur R (1996) The scope of professional practice in specialist practice. British Journal of Nursing 5: 984-989.

Bamford O, Gibson F (2000) The clinical nurse specialist perceptions of practising CNSs about their role and development needs. Journal of Clinical Nursing 9: 282-292.

Benner P (1984) From Novice to Expert: Excellence and power in clinical nursing. Menlo Park, CA: Addison Wesley.

Bowler S, Mallik M (1998) Role extension or expansion: a qualitative investigation of the perceptions of senior medical and nursing staff in an adult intensive care unit. Intensive and Critical Care 14: 11-20.

Brada M (1995) Is there a need to follow-up cancer patients. European Journal of Cancer 31A:

655-657.

Calman K (1993) Hospital Doctors: Training for the future. London: HMSO.

Cameron A (2000) New role developments in context. In: Humphris D, Masterson A (eds), Developing New Clinical Roles: A guide for health professionals. Edinburgh: Churchill Livingstone, pp. 7-24.

Casey A (1989) Coping with cancer. Paediatric Nursing 1: 6.

Casey A, Gibson F, Hooker L (2001) Role development in children's nursing: dimensions, terminology and practice framework. Paediatric Nursing 13: 36-40.

Castledine G (1998) Clinical specialists in nursing in the UK: the early years. In: Castledine G, McGee P (eds) Advanced and Specialist Nursing Practice. Oxford: Blackwell Science, pp. 33-54.

Coombs M, Holgate M (1998) Developing a framework for practice: a clinical perspective. In: Rolfe G, Fulbrook P (eds), Advanced Nursing Practice. Oxford: Butterworth-Heinemann, pp. 199-211.

Crumbie A (2001) Educating the nurse practitioner. In: Reveley S, Walsh M, Crumbie A (eds), Nurse Practitioners: Developing the role in the hospital settings. Oxford: Butterworth-Heinemann, pp. 105-116.

Dalziel J (1990) Nursing specialities must be defined. Editorial. The Registered Nurse 2-3.

D'Angio G (1975) Pediatric cancer in perspective: cure is not enough. Cancer 35(suppl): 867-870.

Dearmun A, Gordon K (1999) The nurse practitioner in children's ambulatory care. Paediatric Nursing 11(1): 19-21.

Department of Health (1993) A Vision for the Future. The Nursing, Midwifery and Health Visiting contribution to health and health care. London: HMSO.

Department of Health (1994) The Challenges for Nursing and Midwifery in the 21st Century London: HMSO.

Department of Health (1999a) Agenda for Change: Modernising the NHS pay system. London: HMSO.

Department of Health (1999b) Making a Difference. London: HMSO.

Department of Health (2000) The NHS Plan. London: HMSO.

Dowling S, Barrett S, West R (1995) With nurse practitioners, who needs house officers? British Medical Journal 311: 309-313.

Dowling S, Martin R, Skidmore P, Doyal L, Cameron A, Lloyd S (1996) Nurses taking on junior doctors' work: a confusion of accountability. British Medical Journal 312: 1211-1214

Edwards J (2001) A model of palliative care for the adolescent with cancer. International Journal of Palliative Nursing 7: 485-488.

Eiser C, Levitt G, Leiper A, Havermans T, Donovan C (1996) Clinic audit for long-term survivors of childhood cancer. Archives of Diseases in Childhood 75: 405-409.

English T (1997) Personal paper: medicine in the 1900s needs a team approach. British Medical Journal 314: 661-663

Expert Advisory Group on Cancer (1995) A Policy Framework for Commissioning Cancer Services. London: HMSO.

Finlay T (2000) The scope of professional practice: a literature review to determine the document's impact on nurses roles. NTresearch 5: 115-126.

Gibson F, Hooker L (1999) Defining a framework for advancing clinical practice in paediatric oncology nursing. European Journal of Oncology Nursing 3: 232-239.

Gibson F, Langton H (1998) Paediatric Oncology Nurse Education; past present, current and future pathways for specialist preparation. European Journal of Oncology Nursing 2: 178-181.

Gibson F, Soanes L (2000) The development of clinical competencies for use on a paediatric oncology nursing course using a Nominal Group Technique. Journal of Clinical Nursing 9: 459-469.

Gibson F, Soanes L (2001) Long-term follow-up following childhood cancer: maximising the contribution of nursing. European Journal of Cancer 37: 1859-1868.

Gibson F, Williams J (1997) Network of care for children and teenagers with cancer: an overview for adult cancer nurses. Journal of Cancer Nursing 1: 200–207.

Goldman A (1998) Care of the Dying Child. Oxford: Oxford University Press.

Hobbie WL (1986) The role of the pediatric oncology nurse specialist in a follow-up clinic for long-term survivors of childhood cancer. Journal of the Association of Pediatric Oncology Nurses 3(4): 9–12.

Humphris D (1994) The Clinical Nurse Specialist: Issues in practice. London: Macmillan.

Humphris D, Masterson A (2000) Evaluating new role development. In: Humphris D, Masterson A (eds), Developing New Clinical Roles: A guide for health professionals. Edinburgh, Churchill Livingstone, pp. 185–201.

Hunt G (1994) New professional? New ethics? In: Hunt G, Wainwright P (eds), Expanding the Role of the Nurse. Oxford: Blackwell Science, pp. 22–38.

International Council of Nurses (1985) Report on the Regulation of Nursing: A report on the present, a position for the future. Switzerland: ICN.

International Council of Nurses (1991) Guidelines on Specialisation in Nursing. Switzerland: ICN.

Jowett S, Peters M, Reynolds H, Wilson Barnett J (1999) The impact of scope – practitioners' views on its relevance and potential for service development. NTresearch 4: 422–431.

Knowles G, Kearney N (1998) Advancing cancer nursing practice in the EU: an overview. European Journal of Oncology Nursing 2(3): 156–161.

Koefmann K (1995) Developing a new deal for nurses. Nursing Standard 9(44): 33–35

Long T, Hale C, Sanderson L et al. (2001) An evaluation of educational preparation for cancer and palliative care nursing for children and adolescents. Interim report to the ENB.

McKee M, Lessof L (1992) Nurse as doctor: whose task is it anyway. In: Robinson J, Gray A, Elkan RE (eds), Policy Issues in Nursing. Buckingham: Open University Press, pp. 60–67.

Moore S, Corner J, Fuller F (1999) Development of nurse-led follow-up in the management of patients with lung cancer. NTresearch 4: 432–445.

National Health Service Executive (2000) The Nursing Contribution to Cancer Care: A strategic programme of action in support of the national cancer programme. London: DoH.

National Health Service Executive (2001) Nurse Specialists, Nurse Consultants, Nurse Leads: The development and implementation of new roles to improve cancer and palliative care. London, DoH.

National Health Service Management Executive (1991) Junior Doctors: The new deal. London: NHSME.

Oakley C, Wright E, Ream E (2000) The experiences of patients and nurses with a nurse-led peripherally inserted central venous catheter line service. European Journal of Oncology Nursing 4: 207–218.

Peter S, Flynn A (2002) Advanced nurse practitioners in a hospital setting: the reality. Paediatric Nursing 14: 14–17.

Pickersgill F (1993) A 'New Deal' for nurses too? Nursing Standard 7(35): 21–22

Read S (1998) Exploring new roles for nurses in the acute sector. Professional Nurse 14(2): 90–94.

Read S, Lloyd Jones M, Collins K et al. J (2001) Exploring new roles in practice (ENRip): final report. Published on the world wide web, Sheffield University (www.sum.shef.ac.uk/research/enrip/enrip.pdf).

Reveley S (2001) Clinical nurse specialists, nurse practitioners and levels of practice: what does it all mean. In: Reveley S, Walsh M, Crumbie A (eds), Nurse Practitioners: Developing the role in the hospital settings. Oxford: Butterworth-Heinemann, pp. 28–37.

Reveley S, Haigh K (2001) Introducing the nurse practitioner role in a surgical unit: one nurse's journey. In: Reveley S, Walsh M, Crumbie A (eds), Nurse Practitioners: Developing the role in the hospital settings. Oxford: Butterworth-Heinemann, pp. 51–64.

Roberts-Davis M, Read S (2001) Clinical role clarification: using the Delphi method to establish similarities and differences between nurse practitioners and clinical nurse specialists. Journal of Clinical Nursing 10: 33–43.

Royal College of Nursing (1988) Specialities in Nursing: A report of the working party investigating the development of specialities within the nursing profession. London: RCN.

Royal College of Nursing (2000) A Framework for Developing Practice in Paediatric Oncology Nursing. London: RCN.

Royal College of Nursing, Nurse Practitioners' Association (1997) Nurse Practitioners: Your questions answered. London: RCN.

Royal College of Paediatrics and Child Health (1996) Developing Roles of Nurses in Clinical Child Health. London: RCPCH.

Royal College of Pathologists (1996) Provision of Care for Children with Leukaemia. London: HMSO.

Rushworth H, Bliss A, Burge D, Glasper EA (2000) Nurse-led pre-operative assessment: a study of appropriateness. Paediatric Nursing 12: 15-20.

Shewan JA, Read SM (1999) Changing roles in Nursing: a literature review of influences and innovations. Clinical Effectiveness in Nursing 3: 75-82.

Smart F (2001) The developing role of paediatric nurse practitioners in the hospital setting: plans and emerging issues. In: Reveley S, Walsh M, Crumbie A (eds), Nurse Practitioners: Developing the role in the hospital settings. Oxford: Butterworth-Heinemann, pp. 78-93.

Stiller CA (1994) Population based survival rates for childhood cancer in Britain. 1980-91 British Medical Journal 309: 1612-1616.

Styles MM (1989) On Specialization in Nursing: Toward a new empowerment. Missouri: American Nurses' Foundation, Inc.

Tiffany R (1976) Department of Nursing Studies, Royal Marsden Hospital Annual Report (Reference to the JBCNS course at the Royal Marsden Hospital and the concept of clinical nurse specialist). Nursing Mirror 141: 66-88.

United Kingdom Central Council for Nursing, Midwifery and Health Visiting (1992) The Scope of Professional Practice. London: UKCC.

United Kingdom Central Council for Nursing, Midwifery and Health Visiting (1998) Higher Level Practice, Dpecialist Practice Project Phase II. London: UKCC.

United Kingdom Central Council for Nursing, Midwifery and Health Visiting (1999) A higher Level of Practice: Report of the consultation on the UKCC's proposals for a revised regulatory framework for post-registration clinical practice. London: UKCC.

United Kingdom Central Council for Nursing, Midwifery and Health Visiting (2000) The Scope of Professional Practice – A study of its implementation. London: UKCC.

United Kingdom Central Council for Nursing, Midwifery and Health Visiting (2002) Report of the Higher Level of Practice Pilot and Project. London: UKCC.

United Kingdom Children's Cancer Study Group (1997a) The resources and requirements of a UKCCSG treatment centre. Unpublished report (www.ukccsg.org/members/index2htm).

United Kingdom Children's Cancer Study Group, Society of British Neurological Surgeons (1997b) Guidance for Services in Children and Young People with Brain and Spinal Tumours. London: Royal College of Paediatrics and Child Health.

Wainwright P (1994) Professionalism and the concept of role extension. In: Hunt G, Wainwright P (eds), Expanding the Role of the Nurse. Oxford: Blackwell Science, pp. 3-21.

Wallace WHB, Blacklay A, Eiser C et al. (2001) Developing strategies for long term follow-up of survivors of childhood cancer. British Medical Journal 323: 271-274.

Walsh M (2001) The nurse practitioner role in hospital: professional and organisational issues. In: Reveley S, Walsh M, Crumbie A (eds), Nurse Practitioners: Developing the role in the hospital settings. Oxford: Butterworth-Heinemann, pp. 12-27.

Woods LP (1997) Conceptualising advanced nursing practice: curriculum issues to consider in the educational preparation of advanced practice nurses in the UK. Journal of Advanced Nursing 25: 820-828.

Woods LP (2000) The Enigma of Advanced Nursing Practice. Wiltshire: Quay Books Divison, Mark Allen Publishing Ltd.

Chapter 2

Specialist nurse: identified professional role or personal agenda?

Jane Hunt

For the first half of the twentieth century the term 'specialist' denoted a nurse with extensive experience in a particular area of nursing and, in North America, nurses have been deemed 'specialist' since 1910 (Hamric, 1989). However, 'specialist' nurses such as 'Sister Dora', who became famous during the 1870s for her specialized nursing treatment of machinery accident victims in Walsall (Manton, 1971), have existed within the UK since the Nightingale era. Castledine (1994) argues that the creation of specialist nursing practice began during this period with both the establishment of the Florence Nightingale School of Nursing and the publication of Nightingale's second version of *Notes on Nursing*. These two initiatives, he suggests, identify and link nursing as a profession with that of a specialty in which two classes of nurse are described: the amateur and the professionally prepared hospital nurse.

In the history of nursing, however, it is more generally considered that the clinical nurse specialist (CNS) first emerged in North America, reaching the UK during the early 1970s. Storr (1988) suggested that 'specialists' in clinical nursing evolved when the term 'nurse clinician' was first adopted in 1943. Others have considered that the CNS title dates back to 1938 (Peplau, 1965). Elsewhere some confusion reigns as to the origins of the title (Hamric, 1989). It is agreed nevertheless that the title's beginnings arose, in North America, during the late 1930s or early 1940s. More commonly, the label CNS began to appear in the 1960s when, in North America, much of the early literature focused on the justification for master's level education for advanced clinical practice (Storr, 1988; Hamric and Spross, 1989; Fenton, 1992).

The rise in specialist nurses within the UK occurred in response to an increase in public demand for services, an expansion of knowledge and skills, in both medicine and nursing and particularly in technological interventions, and a desire on the part of nurses for a more varied career structure (Castledine, 1982, 1983, 1994). Early CNSs within the UK sometimes took on tasks previously undertaken by doctors, whereas others developed new skills to cope with new patient problems (Castledine, 1994). During the 1990s similar theories were assigned to the emergence of the advanced nurse practitioner (ANP) (United Kingdom Central Council for Nursing, Midwifery and Health Visiting [UKCC], 1994; Cassidy, 1996; Chan, 1996; Dowling et al., 1996; Cabellero, 1998). The emergence of the ANP in the UK compounded the continuing confusion about the CNS role and delineation between the two roles remains indistinct (e.g. Castledine, 1996; Castledine et al., 1996; Coyne, 1996; McGee et al., 1996; Mills, 1996; Wilson-Barnett et al., 2000).

In his earliest study of CNSs, Castledine (1982, 1983) identified 11 key aspects of the CNS role that no single CNS fully encompassed. These comprised: direct involvement in care, responsibility and accountability for nursing actions, to be highly educated, a researcher, an educator, a coordinator of care, an expert in both clinical assessment of patients and in her or his field, to be autonomous, to be a writer, and to form a liaison between the community and the hospital. This multiplicity of roles is reflected in a later survey conducted by the Daphne Heald Research Unit of the Royal College of Nursing (RCN) in which it was reported that 1016 CNSs nationally held 82 differing job titles (Wade and Moyer, 1989). Debating this confusion Steele and Fenton (1988, p. 45) wrote:

> Even though the role of the clinical nurse specialist (CNS) has been described in educational criteria, standards and the literature, some confusion still exists about the essential clinical practice skills needed for this advanced role. This situation may be due to the wide diversity of roles that CNSs assume in health care settings. In one institution a clinical nurse specialist may be involved primarily as an educator, in another as a consultant, and in another as an administrator or researcher or some combination of these roles.

A review of the literature undertaken during the mid-1990s in Britain, reflecting an earlier study (Storr, 1988), suggested six major components to CNS roles to which many healthcare professionals still subscribe, which comprise: clinical expert, resource consultant, educator, change agent, researcher and advocate (Miller, 1995). Many of these components have recently been ascribed to nurse consultants (NHS Executive, 1999) and this new role will inevitably further cloud boundaries between higher-level practitioners (Hesketh, 1999; Cox, 2000).

It has been recognized in the UK since the 1980s that nurse specialists: 'are prepared beyond the level of registration' (RCN, 1988, p. 6). However, in contrast to North America and despite support from the

UKCC (1999), distinctive criteria about educational attainments of CNSs remain unspecified. Moreover, educational accomplishments of all higher-level practitioners, including CNSs, have varied and, despite recommendations to the contrary (Wilson-Barnett et al., 2000), jobs have frequently been developed around the experiences of individuals (Smith, 1990). Although the UKCC recommended that nurses entering a specialty (as distinct from becoming a specialist, i.e. an 'expert') be appropriately trained (UKCC, 1996), there remain limited stipulations for attaining 'specialist' status.

Implicit within examinations of specialist nurses over the years is an assumption that a high degree of 'specialist' knowledge is acquired. Despite continuing confusion surrounding CNSs, ANPs and more recently nurse consultants, including both a lack of a clear definition of their roles and explicit educational criteria in the UK, 'specialist' knowledge pertaining to all higher-level practitioners has, for many years, been grounded in 'specialist', post-basic education. It is, however, also embedded within extensive clinical experience (Castledine, 1982, 1983; Benner, 1984; RCN, 1988; Hamric, 1992; Lipman and Deatrick, 1994; MacLeod, 1996; Wilson-Barnett et al., 2000).

This chapter draws on data from a study, undertaken during the 1990s, which examined the relationships between hospital- and community-based healthcare professionals and a group of specialist nurses collectively known as paediatric oncology outreach nurse specialists (POONSs). It suggests that, despite the continuing attempts of nursing to establish a professional agenda concerning the 'specialist' knowledge status of CNSs, healthcare professionals working with POONSs commonly disregarded professional agendas and conferred 'specialist' status on POONSs, according to their own personal agendas and experiences. The chapter therefore offers some new insights into defining 'specialist' practice. First, it provides multidisciplinary rather than nursing-specific definitions of 'specialist', through the perceived value of POONSs. Second, it proffers informal as opposed to formal definitions of 'specialist', which are not wholly enshrined in measurable criteria that have to be met, such as qualifications. Third, it tenders insight into the influence of work settings on the definitions of 'specialist' practice.

The nursing specialty of POONSs

POONSs emerged as a nursing specialty during the mid-1980s as a result of perceived gaps in services by both families caring for children with malignant disease and healthcare professionals in regional paediatric oncology units. They arose predominantly to support both families and carers through a child's terminal illness, at home. The successes of early posts led to a nationwide expansion of services, incorporating care through all stages of a child's illness and enhancing the philosophy of 'shared care' (Bacon, 1989; Orton, 1994; Bennett et al., 1994; Hooker and Williams, 1996; Gibson and Williams, 1997; Patel et al., 1997; Greener, 1998; Hunt, 1998a; Jones, 1998). POONSs act as the main contacts for families in their own homes during periods of treatment and post-treatment, enabling them to feel more secure (Bignold et al., 1994). In so doing they provide links for primary, secondary and tertiary care, offering local services information and support.

The degree to which POONSs fulfil the role of CNS, as identified within the literature, varies and is influenced by the different organizations associated with funding their work (Hunt, 1995, 1996, 1998a); during the period in which this study was undertaken, POONSs were either located within children's departments at district general hospital trusts or within specialist paediatric oncology units at tertiary referral centres. The funding arrangements and work location of POONSs, in turn, influenced service structure and POONSs worked either alone or in teams (Hunt, 1996, 1998a). The impact that differing work locations had on healthcare professionals' perceptions of 'specialist' are highlighted in this chapter.

The study

This chapter draws on qualitative interview data from the second stage of a large two-part study, which explored the impact of funding arrangements on the professional relationships between POONSs and other healthcare professionals (Hunt, 1996, 1998a). The first stage was designed to understand the structure, organization and working practices of POONSs better. Interviews were conducted with all POONSs in post in the UK and the Republic of Ireland during 1993, using a semi-structured interview schedule (n = 43). Findings from the first stage of the study have been reported elsewhere (Hunt, 1995, 1996, 1998a).

The second stage was designed to examine the perceptions and experiences of healthcare professionals working with POONSs. It comprised case studies at three locations in England (two regional, Southern Regional Hospital and Northern City Children's Hospital, and one district, Westlands District Hospital), consisting of focused interviews with a broad cross-section of community and hospital-based healthcare professionals. These included senior and junior medical and nursing staff, specialist social workers, general practitioners, health visitors (HVs) and district nurses (DNs). Sixty-five interviews took place between October 1994 and April 1995. The participants' details are summarized in Table 2.1.

Table 2.1 Interviews conducted at case study sites

Interviewees	Southern Regional Hospital	Westlands District Hospital	Northern City Children's Hospital
Hospital-based staff:			
Senior medical staff (consultants/associate fellows)	2 (I)	2 (I)	3 (I)
Junior doctors (SHO/registrar)	1 (G)	1 (I)	1 (I)
Ward sister/OPD sister	1 (G)	1 (I)	3 (I)
Junior staff nurses	1 (G)	1 (G)	1 (G)
Social workers	1 (I)	1 (I)	1 (G)
Community-based staff:			
GP (newly diagnosed patients)	5 (I)	4a (I)	4 (I)
GP (terminal care)	4 (I)	3a (I)	4 (I)
HV (depending on age of child)	4 (1G, 3I)	3 (2I, 1G)	1 (I)
DN (depending on disease status of child)	6 (2G, 4I)	3 (I)	6 (I)
Total no. of interviews	**25 (19I, 6G)**	**17ª (14I, 2G)**	**24 (22I, 2G)**

ª One GP included twice since interviewed in connection with both a newly diagnosed child and a terminally ill child.
I, individual interviews; G, group interviews (two to four interviewees). DN, district nurse; GP, general practitioner; HV, health visitor; OPD, outpatients department; SHO, senior house officer.

During the period in which the study was undertaken no ethical approval was required because interviewees of both stages of the research were consenting healthcare professionals. Ethical considerations mean, however, that hospitals and individual practitioners have been allocated pseudonyms to maintain their anonymity.

Analysis

Issues with analysing qualitative data are not concerned with generalizability or 'sample to population' representativeness, but with establishing theoretical links within each case and developing new theories (Brannen, 1992; Miles and Huberman, 1994). In this study, analysis of the interviews with healthcare professionals was conducted through the development of a conceptual framework that was generated using a data reduction, display and verification model (Miles and Huberman, 1994). Four major themes emerged from within the conceptual framework: teamwork, relationships between POONSs and other nurses, relationships between POONSs and doctors, and specialist knowledge. Only data pertaining to the theme of 'specialist knowledge' are drawn upon in this chapter. Other findings have been reported elsewhere (Hunt, 1996, 1998a, 1998b, 2000).

Conferring specialist status on POONSs

Disregarding nursing's professional agenda to ensure that specialist nurses are highly educated and experienced in their field, this study indicated that, in general, healthcare professionals conferred 'specialist' status to POONSs according to their own experiences and agendas. Perceptions of 'specialist' knowledge appeared to be contingent upon the level of experience that healthcare professionals had themselves gained in the specialty in question, the hospital location and the professional background of the POONSs with whom they worked. When 'specialist' status was conferred to POONSs, 'specialist' knowledge was seen to be derived from a combination of formal qualifications, hands-on technical skills, previous 'specialist' work experience, in-depth 'medical' knowledge and/or insight into families' dynamics. The relative contribution each of these made towards constructing a 'specialist' depended primarily upon the regional or district location of POONSs (Figure 2.1.) Different emphasis was placed on each conferred component of specialist knowledge, depending on the agendas of individual healthcare professionals working with POONSs. Here, examples of two personal agendas are described: (1) 'needs-driven agendas' and (2) 'peer-driven agendas'.

Needs-driven agendas

Some healthcare professionals who worked with POONSs had professional needs, either concerning caring for children with malignant disease, or helping them to pursue their own careers. This led to the identification of four personal 'needs-driven agendas' which contribute to healthcare professionals conferring 'specialist' knowledge and status on POONSs: (1) a knowledge gap, (2) resolving anxieties, (3) pursing 'specialist' nursing careers and (4) knowing families.

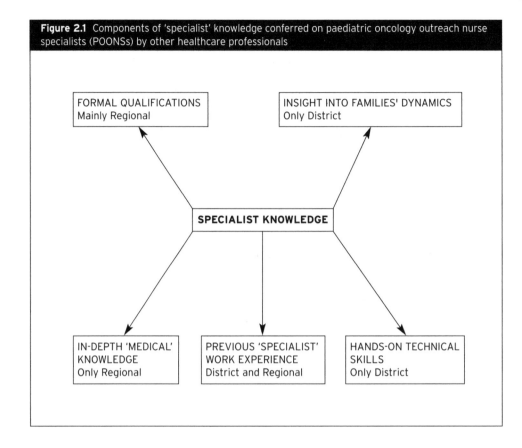

Figure 2.1 Components of 'specialist' knowledge conferred on paediatric oncology outreach nurse specialists (POONSs) by other healthcare professionals

A knowledge gap

Primary healthcare professionals' experience of working with children with malignancy, although different, are extremely limited (Halliday, 1990; Pinkerton, 1993; Hunt, 1996, 1998a, 1998b). These limited experiences are epitomized by one GP from this study who said:

> This particular patient was the first one . . . in general practice. I've not had anyone that's had a terminal illness. Yes, yes, I've not had anyone else.
>
> GP5, Northern City Children's area

The personal 'needs-driven agendas' of primary healthcare professionals relate to these limited experiences – primary healthcare professionals need to understand how to care for sick children and their families before comprehending the more 'specialist' problems associated with paediatric oncology. In this scenario emphasis is placed on two components of conferred 'specialist' knowledge: hands-on technical skills and 'specialist' work experience (see Figure 2.1). The definition of 'specialist' work experience depends not only on the past experiences of individual primary healthcare professionals, but also on where the POONSs with whom they worked were located. At one level, all POONSs achieved 'specialist' status because all had 'specialist' paediatric experience relative to primary healthcare professionals' needs. As one district nurse suggested: '[POONSs] are used to actually dealing with children' (DN9, Southern Regional area). Hence nursing sick children, irrespective of the disease 'needs somebody who's got experience of looking after children' (DN2, Northern City area).

At a second level, however, work experience takes on a 'specialist' perspective. A basic cognisance of paediatrics was seen as essential by all primary healthcare professionals. In contrast to those working with a POONS at a district general hospital trust, many primary healthcare professionals working with regional POONSs considered 'specialist' working practice to be derived specifically from paediatric oncology nursing experience. As one DN involved in the care of a newly diagnosed child commented: 'she's a specialist and I can't possibly keep up with the [cytotoxic] drugs, you know, the current ones' (DN15, Southern Regional area).

Resolving anxieties

A second 'needs-driven agenda' whereby 'specialist' knowledge was conferred on POONSs concerns resolving anxieties. District nurses, unused to nursing sick children, experience a great deal of anxiety when faced with caring for a child with malignant disease (Hunt, 1998a, 1998b). In this situation, anxieties may be resolved through the availability of 'specialists' with hands-on technical skills and previous work experience (see Figure 2.1), which they lacked.

For junior staff nurses (SNs) on a general paediatric ward, used to nursing sick children but less familiar with malignant disease, anxiety also arises when caring for children with cancer or leukaemia, and their families. The perceived 'specialist' status of POONSs, arising from SNs' anxieties, similarly draws on 'specialist' work experience and hands-on technical skills. It may also draw on formal training. 'Specialist' knowledge as identified by SNs is epitomized thus:

> I wouldn't be able to cope with the bereavement side of things – I just feel very inadequate and I'd need a lot of training in that direction I think, with parents, with knowing what to say and then saying it.
>
> SN8, Westlands District Hospital

Hence 'specialist' status was granted to POONSs through the 'needs-driven agendas' of both DNs and SNs at district hospitals, to resolve their anxieties. However, the stresses endured by these two groups of nurses, both inexperienced in paediatric oncology, arise from different baseline perspectives. Although DNs and SNs at district general hospitals conferred 'specialist' status on POONSs because of their 'specialist' work experience and hands-on nursing skills, their definitions differed. For DNs, these skills pertain to paediatric nursing, where the hands-on skills and work experience demanded by junior SNs at Westlands were specific to the needs of children with malignant disease.

Pursuing 'specialist' nursing careers

A third 'needs-driven agenda' in which 'specialist' status was accorded to POONSs concerns SNs pursuing careers – becoming a POONS is one option that was open to them. Contemplating future career pathways affected all junior SNs similarly, regardless of the environment in which they worked; work experience and further formal qualifications assist SNs up the ladder of seniority to attaining 'specialist' status. 'Specialist' status was conferred on POONSs according to the perceived deficits in the SNs' own knowledge, which they would have required before undertaking the work of a POONS (thereby becoming a 'specialist') themselves. It was this perceived need of SNs to rectify shortfalls in their own knowledge before attaining 'specialist' status that contributed to this 'needs-driven agenda'. However, 'specialist' knowledge was constructed differently according to the environments in which SNs worked, the formal training and experiences of the POONSs they worked with and, for those at regional centres, professional agendas concerning the professional and academic qualifications of CNSs. Furthermore, formal qualifications demanded by SNs to achieve the 'specialist' status of POONSs differed between regional centres and Westlands District Hospital.

Staff nurses at the district hospital overlooked professional agendas that attempt to dictate the formal post-registration training undertaken to attain 'specialist' status. Instead, reflecting the background of the POONS with whom they worked and their own working environment, they generally beheld 'specialists' as having extensive work experience and hands-on technical skills. In contrast, in addition to 'specialist' work experience, SNs at regional centres, mindful of the professional demands that nursing places on itself to achieve 'specialist' status, also emphasized the importance of formal post-basic qualifications.

Junior SNs at the district hospital considered that 'specialist knowledge' is gained through extensive work experience after the attainment of the Registered Sick Children's Nurse/Registered Nurse (part 15 UKCC registration, Child). It comprised 'specialist' hands-on nursing tasks (see Figure 2.1) such as handling central venous access devices and administering intravenous drugs. It may, for a limited number of SNs, have comprised formal post-basic training attained through a National Board Certificate in paediatric oncology nursing. One SN commented:

> You've got to have an overall paediatric knowledge . . . learning and knowing about oncology problems, of treatments . . .
>
> SN7, Westlands District Hospital

In contrast, SNs at regional centres envisaged that 'specialist' knowledge of POONSs comprised both formal post-basic community nurse training and 'specialist' experience in this field. Taking the premise that formal training and lengthy experience in both paediatrics and oncology were accomplished by all senior nurses working within the field of paediatric oncology, it was the community nursing experience and formal training in this area of work that was seen to separate POONSs from other senior nursing staff:

> You have to have a community qualification to be in the community; I mean that's a criterion to be a community nurse; you can't otherwise do it.
>
> SN11, Southern Regional Hospital

Knowing families

POONSs are seen to develop especially close relationships with families (Bignold et al., 1994, 1995a, 1995b; Hunt, 1998a). This arises through the abilities of POONSs to 'boundary hop' between hospital and the community. However, unique to the paediatric consultants at the district hospital, the in-depth knowledge of families' dynamics brought about through 'befriending' (Bignold et al., 1995b) families was seen as a skill of POONSs that should be drawn upon (see Figure 2.1). This gave rise to a fourth 'needs-driven' agenda in which consultants depend on this knowledge to assist them in making treatment-related decisions about patients. The reasons consultants at Westlands District Hospital depended on this knowledge were unclear, but it may lie in consultants' frequent provision of hands-on care to children, both in hospital and at home (Hunt, 1998a). In this situation, consultants were reliant on POONSs to teach them specialist technical 'nursing' skills such as accessing central venous access devices. To undertake such tasks required 'befriending' the child with malignant disease and his or her family in order to gain their trust. Consequently, in this 'needs-driven' agenda, consultants not only confer 'specialist' knowledge on POONSs through POONSs' relationships with families, but also draw on the latter's 'specialist' hands-on skills.

In summary, in this study 'needs-driven agendas' were derived from four perspectives: knowledge gaps of primary healthcare professionals, anxieties of some groups of nurses, career pathways of SNs and POONSs' knowledge of families. 'Needs-driven agendas' that drove healthcare professionals to confer 'specialist' status on POONSs were not only influenced by individuals' experiences and agendas. They differed predominantly according to the hospital location and the background of the POONSs with whom they worked.

Peer-driven agendas

A second type of personal agenda existed where 'specialist' knowledge was conferred by healthcare professionals who did not 'need' to draw on POONSs' knowledge. These personal agendas are referred to as 'peer-driven agendas', and two types are discussed here: (1) distinguishing between specialists, and (2) the professional status of POONSs. In the main, these existed for senior, hospital-based, healthcare professionals at regional centres, who, in the absence of POONSs, could (and previously did) provide a skeleton outreach service to children being cared for locally. In this scenario, 'specialist' was denoted by the attributes that distinguished one 'specialist' from another. However, 'peer-driven agendas' also existed for senior medical staff, regardless of their work location, whose concerns included the professional status of POONSs.

Distinguishing between 'specialists'

A major characteristic of 'peer-driven agendas' concerned distinguishing between 'specialists'. This arose from two perspectives: first it occurred when senior hospital-based healthcare professionals at regional centres distinguished the 'specialist' nature of POONSs' work from either their own or that of other senior hospital staff. Second, it transpired when healthcare professionals across both community and acute hospital settings distinguished the 'specialist' nature of POONSs' knowledge from that of community children's nurses.

Senior healthcare professionals at regional paediatric oncology centres achieve their own 'specialist' status such that both consultants and nursing sisters develop their own 'specialist' areas of practice, including bone marrow transplantation, long-term follow-up, adolescence and disease-specific areas such as brain tumours. In this situation 'specialist' knowledge was constructed among peers of POONSs as that which distinguished the nature of POONSs' work from their own, or that of other senior staff. In the main, 'specialist' knowledge was construed around the backgrounds of both the POONSs with whom they worked and, for some, the POONSs at other regional centres (through the professional bodies the Paediatric Oncology Nurses' Forum (PONF) of the RCN and the UK Children's Cancer Study Group, several senior staff at regional centres passed global insight into POONSs' backgrounds); it was reflected in post-basic qualifications and 'specialist' work experience (see Figure 2.1). One nursing sister indicated this by saying:

> The people I've worked with are people who've had a community background and paediatric training plus oncology . . . to me it appears to work well so therefore I feel that is what they need
>
> Sister 4, Southern Regional Hospital

In this 'peer-driven agenda' there was an axiom among nursing sisters and consultants that all senior nursing staff had attained previous work experience and formal training in paediatrics and oncology. The formal training and work experience that distinguished POONSs' 'specialist' knowledge from that of their nursing peers, as suggested above, concerned community nursing work:

> I think there is a dimension to care in the community, which we who work in hospital don't understand.
>
> Consultant 5, Northern City Hospital

Not only was great emphasis placed on formal training and 'specialist' work experience in community nursing, but this type of agenda uniquely recognized the importance of POONSs' in-depth, 'specialist', 'medical' knowledge. It is this in-depth 'medical' knowledge that distinguished the 'specialist' knowledge of POONSs from that of consultants. Here, consultants and nursing sisters alike overtly recognized that POONSs' 'specialist', 'medical' knowledge lay in symptom management during terminal care, which exceeded the knowledge of consultants. One commented:

> Nearly always they [POONSs] know more about pain control than the doctors do; they have a much better feel for it . . . beyond sort of straightforward antiemetics; you know, they're usually very good on second- and third-line antiemetics.
>
> Consultant 7, Southern Regional Hospital

A second feature of this 'peer-driven agenda' that separated POONSs from other 'specialists' distinguished between POONSs and community children's nurses. This arose when healthcare professionals across community and acute hospital sectors had experience working with both groups of outreach nurses. (Although Whiting [2000] noted that community children's services have developed substantially during 100 years of community children's nursing, nationally there had been a dearth of community children's nursing services [Whiting, 1995]. The Southern Regional Hospital was, however, located in a region that had been particularly well served by community children's nursing teams for a number of years.) Although it is formal training and experience in community nursing that stood POONSs apart from hospital-based healthcare professionals at regional centres, it was community nursing that linked POONSs with community children's nurses. However, there are components of conferred 'specialist' knowledge that distinguished POONSs from community children's nurses. The different experiences of primary healthcare professionals and acute hospital staff meant that professionals across the two healthcare sectors drew on different components of conferred 'specialist' knowledge to determine the specialist nature of POONSs.

Primary healthcare professionals predominantly distinguished the 'specialist' nature of POONSs' work from community children's nurses through hands-on technical skills. Although they acknowledged that both possessed 'specialist' technical skills relative to their own fields, the skills of POONSs were perceived to be more 'specialist' than those of community children's nurses. Hospital-based healthcare professionals, on the other hand, distinguished POONSs from community children's nurses because of their formal qualifications, previous 'specialist' work experience and in-depth 'medical' knowledge. One hospital doctor said:

> [POONSs] are likely to have had to have done more, longer, specialist training [than community children's nurses]
>
> SHO3, Southern Regional Hospital

whereas a consultant commented:

> I don't know how they [community children's nurses] get trained but I assume as part of their training they wouldn't have a lot of emphasis put on how you manage a child dying of cancer at home.
>
> Consultant 6, Southern Regional Hospital

The differences in formal training, specialist work experience and hands-on tasks were confirmed by a community children's nurse (CCN) interviewed during the course of this study who said:

> Nurses in that specialty usually have gone through courses for blood-letting and, you know, the practical things.
>
> CCN2, Southern Regional area

The professional status of POONSs

A second 'peer-driven agenda' concerns the professional status of POONSs. This feature of conferred 'specialist' knowledge was predominantly associated with senior hospital doctors who assumed a level of responsibility for the professional welfare of POONSs. The reasons why these perceived responsibilities arose are unclear. However, they were particularly developed in consultants who had procured charitable funds to establish POONSs' services (Hunt, 1998a). In this instance, consultants appeared to maintain a vested interest in the well-being of POONSs to ensure the success of the service. The concerns for the professional status of POONSs, which steer this 'peer-driven agenda', arose first from perceived 'specialist' knowledge required to establish successful relationships with local communities. Second, they existed for district-based consultants who are concerned that POONSs maintain professional credibility through sustaining 'specialist' knowledge.

Regional consultants, concerned for the professional status of POONSs, were troubled by relationships between POONSs and local communities. In this scenario, professional status was assumed by consultants to be gained through credibility with community nurses. This was achieved through POONSs accomplishing community nursing qualifications. Here, it was anticipated that POONSs required a community nursing qualification to make them: 'more acceptable to the local people' (Consultant 6, Southern Regional Hospital) and 'to the local paediatric teams' (Consultant 7, Southern Regional Hospital). Credibility as a 'specialist' was then established when it was perceived that the post-basic qualifications of POONSs both matched and exceeded those of community nurses. In this agenda great value was placed on post-basic formal qualifications (see Figure 2.1).

Concerns for the professional status of a district hospital-based POONS, by consultants, took a different form. Here, sustaining and updating knowledge was required in order to establish credibility among hospital-based healthcare professionals, thereby maintaining a 'specialist' status. In the main, this concerned keeping up to date with hands-on technical skills. When it was perceived that hands-on skills were kept up to date, professional credibility, and 'specialist' and consequently professional status were maintained. As one consultant commented:

> ... she's very good at going off and going into all the sessions and so forth.
>
> Consultant 2, Westlands District Hospital

Conclusion

Reflecting on the continuing confusion surrounding 'specialist' nurses, advanced practitioners and nurse consultants, this chapter has argued that healthcare professionals' perceptions of 'specialists' were subjective, being grounded in their personal experiences of, in this instance, childhood malignancy. They were also embedded in the hospital locations and individual backgrounds of the POONSs with whom they work. Disregarding nursing's professional agenda in which 'specialist' nurses are expected to attain a high degree of post-basic education, healthcare professionals generally conferred specialist status on anyone they perceived as more experienced or 'specialized' than themselves. These perceptions and experiences gave rise to two personal agendas that have been termed 'needs-driven agendas' and 'peer-driven agendas'. 'Needs-driven agendas' comprised: POONSs' abilities to fill a knowledge gap, resolving anxieties, pursuing 'specialist' nursing careers and knowing families. 'Peer-driven agendas' were drawn from the distinctions that regional senior hospital staff made between POONSs and other oncology 'specialists' and differentiations between POONSs and community children's nurses. Second, they were derived from senior hospital doctors' concerns about the professional status of POONSs.

Both 'needs-driven' and 'peer-driven' agendas drew on formal qualifications, hands-on technical skills, 'specialist' work experience, in-depth medical knowledge and/or insight into families' dynamics (see Figure 2.1). The relative contribution that each of these 'knowledge' components made to conferring specialist status on POONSs was primarily dependent on the regional or district work location of POONSs. In the main these concern distinctions between 'specialist' paediatric experience and education, and 'specialist' paediatric oncology and community nursing experience and education. These factors contribute to the adoption and adaptation of George Orwell's (1945, p. 114) slogan that: 'All nurse specialists are specialists, some nurse specialists are more specialist than others'.

Current policies present dichotomies for those working within the healthcare sector generally and in specialities such as paediatric oncology in particular. On the one hand, there is a national drive towards reducing the 'post code' lottery (Department of Health [DoH], 2000) and providing 'specialist' cancer services at designated 'specialist' centres (DoH, 2001). On the other hand, current health policy ensures that patients have access to health services within their local communities (DoH, 2000). In keeping with this dichotomy, this research has suggested that 'specialist' POONS status may be gained within both local 'general' and regional 'specialist' settings. Nurses seeking specialist status within paediatric oncology should be mindful of this and the ways in which other healthcare professionals confer 'specialist' status on nurses. Those wishing to acquire 'specialist' status without undergoing more 'specialist' training beyond first level registration may chose to work within a district general hospital trust. In contrast those aspiring to have 'specialist' status conferred on them within a specialist centre would be advised to gain both extensive experience and post-basic 'specialist' education in their selected 'specialist' field.

Acknowledgement

This chapter first appeared in the Journal of Advanced Nursing and is reproduced with permission of Blackwell.

References

Bacon CJ (1989) Shared care in paediatrics. Archives of Disease in Childhood 64: 148-149.

Benner P (1984) From Novice to Expert: Excellence and Power in Clinical Nursing Practice. Menley Park, CA: Addison-Wesley.

Bennett L, May C, Wolfson DJ (1994) Sharing care between hospital and the community: a critical review of developments in the UK. Health and Social Care 2: 105-112.

Bignold S, Ball S, Cribb A (1994) Nursing Families with Children with Cancer: The Work of the Paediatric Oncology Outreach Nurse Specialist. A report to the Cancer Relief Macmillan Fund. Basildon: HMSO.

Bignold S, Cribb A, Ball S (1995a) Creating a 'seamless web of care': the work of paediatric oncology nurse specialists. In: Richardson A, Wilson-Barnett J (eds), Nursing Research in Cancer Care. London: Scutari Press, pp. 67-82.

Bignold S, Cribb A, Ball S (1995b) Befriending the family: an exploration of the nurse-client relationship. Health and Social Care in the Community 3: 173-180.

Brannen J (1992) Mixing Methods: Qualitative and quantitative research. Aldershot: Avebury.

Cabellero C (1998) The role of the laparoscopic nurse practitioner. Nursing Standard 12: 43-44.

Cassidy J (1996) Job swap. Nursing Times 92(28): 20.

Castledine G (1982) The role and function of clinical nurse specialists in England and Wales. Unpublished MSc dissertation, University of Manchester.

Castledine G (1983) The nurse for job. Nursing Mirror 19: 43.

Castledine G (1994) Specialist and advanced nursing and the scope of practice. In: Hunt G, Wainwright P (eds), Expanding the Role of the Nurse. Oxford: Blackwell Science, pp. 101–113.

Castledine G (1996) Extremes of the nurse practitioner role. British Journal of Nursing 5: 581.

Castledine G, McGee P, Brown R (1996) A survey of specialist and advanced nursing practice. The Nursing Research Unit, University of Central England in Birmingham.

Chan JS (1996) An evaluation of the night nurse practitioner. Nursing Times 92: 38–39.

Coyne P (1996) Developing nurse consultancy in clinical practice. Nursing Times 92: 34–35.

Cox CL (2000) The nurse consultant: an advanced nurse practitioner? Nursing Times 96: 48.

Department of Health (2000) The NHS Plan. London: HMSO.

Department of Health (2001) The NHS Cancer Plan – www.doh.gov.uk/cancer/cancerplan.htm

Dowling S, Martin R, Skidmore P et al. (1996) Nurses taking on junior doctors' work: a confusion of accountability. British Medical Journal 312: 1211–1214.

Fenton MV (1992) Education for the advanced practice of clinical nurse specialists. Oncology Nurses Forum 19(1): 16–20.

Gibson F, Williams J (1997) Network of care for children and teenagers with cancer: an overview for adult cancer nurses. Journal of Cancer Nursing 1: 200–207.

Greener T (1998) Children's and families' perceptions of paediatric oncology shared care. Unpublished BSc dissertation, University of Surrey.

Halliday J (1990) Malignant disease in children: the view of the general practitioner and parent. In: Baum JD, Dominica F, Woodward RN (eds), Listen, My Child has a Lot of Living to Do. Oxford: Oxford University Press, pp. 19–27.

Hamric AB (1989) History and overview of the CNS role. In: Hamric AB, Spross JA (eds), The Clinical Nurse Specialist in Theory and Practice, 2nd edn. Philadelphia: WB Saunders, pp. 1–18.

Hamric AB (1992) Creating our future: challenges and opportunities for the clinical nurse specialist. Oncology Nursing Forum 19: 11–15.

Hamric AB, Spross JA (1989) The Clinical Nurse Specialist in Theory and Practice, 2nd edn. Philadelphia: WB Saunders.

Hesketh J (1999) None the wiser. Nursing Times 95: 56–57.

Hooker L, Williams J (1996) Parent-held shared care records: bridging the communication gap. British Journal of Nursing 5: 738–741.

Hunt JA (1995) The paediatric oncology nurse specialist: the influence of employment location and funders on models of practice. Journal of Advanced Nursing 22: 126–133.

Hunt JA (1996) Paediatric Oncology Outreach Nurse Specialists: the impact of funding arrangements on their professional relationships. A Report to PONF and the Paediatric Oncology Outreach Nurses Special Interest Group, RCN and the UKCCSG. London: Royal College of Nursing.

Hunt JA (1998a) Mixed funding within the British healthcare system: an examination of the effects on professional relationships between paediatric oncology outreach nurse specialists and other health care professionals. Unpublished PhD thesis, University of Surrey.

Hunt (1998b) Empowering health care professionals: a relationship between primary health care teams and paediatric oncology outreach nurse specialists. European Journal of Oncology Nursing 2: 27–33.

Hunt JA (2000) Relationships between outreach nurses and primary healthcare professionals. In: Muir J, Sidey A (eds), Textbook of Community Children's Nursing. London: Baillière Tindall, pp 103–110.

Jones CEM (1998) Shared care for children with acute lymphoblastic leukaemia. Unpublished BSc dissertation, Roehampton Institute, University of Surrey.

Lipman TH, Deatrick JA (1994) Enhancing specialist preparation for the next century. Journal of Nursing Education 33: 53–58.

McGee P, Castledine G, Brown R (1996) A survey of specialist and advanced nursing practice in England. British Journal of Nursing 5: 682-686.

MacLeod MLP (1996) Practising Nursing - Becoming expert. Edinburgh: Churchill Livingstone.

Manton J (1971) Sister Dora: The life of Dorothy Pattison. London: Methuen.

Miller S (1995) The clinical nurse specialist: a way forward? Journal of Advanced Nursing 22: 494-501.

Mills C (1996) The consultant nurse: a model for advanced practice. Nursing Times 92: 36-37.

Miles HB, Huberman AM (1994) Qualitative Data Analysis, 2nd edn. London: Sage.

National Health Service Executive (1999) Nurse, Midwife and Health Visitor Consultants. HSC, 1999/217. London: NHSE.

Orton P (1994) Shared care. The Lancet 344: 1413-1415.

Orwell G (1945) Animal Farm. London: Penguin.

Patel N, Sepion B, Williams J (1997) Development of a shared care programme for children with cancer. Journal of Cancer Nursing 1: 147-150.

Peplau HE (1965) Specialisation in professional nursing. Nursing Science 3: 268-287.

Pinkerton CR (1993) Multidisciplinary care in the management of childhood cancer. British Journal of Hospital Medicine. 50: 54-59.

Royal College of Nursing (1988) Specialities in Nursing: A Report of the Working Party Investigating the Development of Specialties Within the Nursing Profession. London: RCN.

Smith M (1990) Making the most of CNSs. Senior Nurse 10: 6-8.

Steele S, Fenton M (1988) Expert practice of clinical nurse specialists. Clinical Nurse Specialist 2(1): 45-51.

Storr G (1988) The clinical nurse specialist: from the outside looking in. Journal of Advanced Nursing 13: 265-272.

United Kingdom Central Council for Nursing, Midwifery and Health Visiting (UKCC) (1994) The Future of Professional Practice - The Council's Standards for Education and Practice Following Registration. London: UKCC.

UKCC (1996) Guidelines for Professional Practice. London: UKCC.

UKCC (1999) A Higher Level of Practice. London: UKCC.

Wade B, Moyer A (1989) An evaluation of clinical nurse specialists: implications for education and the organisation of care. Senior Nurse 9: 11-15.

Whiting M (1995) Directory of Paediatric Community Nursing Services, 12th edn. London: RCN.

Whiting M (2000) 1888-1988: 100 years of community children's nursing. In: Muir J, Sidey A (eds), Textbook of Community Children's Nursing. London: Baillière Tindall, pp. 15-30.

Wilson-Barnett J, Barriball KL, Reynolds H, Jowett S, Ryrie (2000) Recognising advancing nursing practice: evidence from two observational studies. International Journal of Nursing Studies 37: 389-400.

Chapter 3

The development of nursing roles in a day-care setting

Louise Soanes, Karen Bravery, Julie Bayliss, Faith Gibson and Emmie Parsons

For some time nurses have sought to refine and develop their roles within the clinical setting, in response to the changing needs of society and pressures outside and within the profession (Frost, 1998). Hence, a plethora of titles has emerged, both nationally and internationally. Roles such as clinical nurse specialist (CNS), nurse practitioner (NP), physician's assistant, advanced nurse practitioner (ANP) and nurse clinician are cited as examples. In the UK, some of these roles are more established and prolific than others.

One role, the paediatric nurse practitioner (PNP), was of particular interest to nurses working within a London hospital. The general feeling was that there could be a future role for the PNP in both inpatient and outpatient settings, with an emphasis on the day-care unit. In establishing the project the working party recognized two issues: first, that in the interests of patient care the developments of nursing roles should not be undertaken in an ad hoc manner; second that the evolution of roles would be dependent on the setting, the staff working in that setting, the specific needs of the organization, unit and trust, as well as the needs of the families who used the clinical area.

This chapter aims to present the findings of an action research project established to explore these issues. The first part of the chapter explores the literature surrounding the NP role, and then outlines the aims and objectives of the research project. The subsequent section briefly discusses the research methods used, and last the findings and recommendations for future practice are analysed in detail.

Literature review

International

The NP role was first conceived in the 1960s and was fuelled largely in response to the shortage of physicians in primary care (Hamric et al., 1996). From the outset, the NP role encompassed an expansion into the discipline of medicine, with the NP performing health histories and physical examinations, ordering and interpreting diagnostic tests, and initiating routine treatments (Hamric, 1998). NPs provided comprehensive, collaborative primary and specialty care for individuals, families and communities in a variety of settings, with an emphasis on community-based care for medically under-served populations (Romaine-Davis, 1997). The role provided an opportunity to focus on more autonomous and responsible functions, allowing the nurse to operationalize their expanded role within the scope of nursing practice (Ford, 1979). PNPs are employed in a number of clinical settings in the USA (Barnes and Sharu, 1998; Pitts and Seimer, 1998), including paediatric oncology (Christensen and Akcasu, 1999), e.g. the PNP role is well established at Texas Children's Hospital (USA), where 12 PNPs work in the paediatric oncology day-care unit.

Educational programmes for NPs were initially outside the mainstream of nursing education (Hamric et al., 1996). The first PNP programme was established at the University of Colorado School of Nursing. Other programmes quickly followed, and focused on care of the adult, family and older client. They offered certificate preparation and were predominantly taught by physicians (Hamric, 1998). The introduction of federal grants for NP education led, however, to the formulation of graduate programmes within schools of nursing (Cronenwett, 1995). Romaine-Davies (1997) identifies that the introduction of Masters' preparation parallelled the development of the NP as an advanced practice nurse. Over the years the number of Masters' programmes has steadily increased in line with the growth of NP roles within both primary and acute care settings (Hamric et al., 1996).

National

The role of NP in the UK initially followed the same pattern of development as in the USA. NPs were first introduced in the primary healthcare setting, under the auspices of Stilwell (1983). Furthermore, similarities are evident with regard to the clinical component of the NP role (Manley, 1996), with an expansion into parallel areas of technical and medically oriented practice. Sparrow (1997) identifies, however, that the NP role in the USA is more advanced than that witnessed in the UK. This is unsurprising, because the emergence of NPs, ANPs and others has been reported only within the last 15 years. The emergence of these roles, in the UK, has been driven by a number of external factors (Shewan and Read, 1999), which within the wider environment exert significant control on the initiation of change to nursing roles. One approach for the systematic examination of external influences is the PEST analysis (Bowman and Asch, 1987). Using the four headings political, economic, social and technological, a PEST analysis was used to address the external influences on the development of NP posts in the UK, and to place these activities within the context of current healthcare provision (Table 3.1).

In the UK, no universal definition of the role of the NP has yet been accepted (Castledine, 1995; Hicks and Hennessey, 1999). Likewise, consensus about role boundaries, education and skill levels has not been reached (Hicks and Hennessey, 1999). It is believed that this has resulted in variation in both the nature and the level of care offered by the NP (Read et al., 1998, cited by Hicks and Hennessey, 1999). A study by Hicks and Hennessey (1999) identified, however, that there are difficulties in providing a generic description of the NP role when NPs operate in different healthcare domains. Since their birth within the community setting in the 1980s, the UK has witnessed a steady growth of NPs in both primary (Salvage, 1991; Coopers & Lybrand, 1996; Kaufmann, 1996) and acute care (Read and George, 1994; Hodgkiss-Lagan, 1996; Mayled, 1998) with some blurring of their roles. When addressed independently, the definition of NP roles in primary care is much clearer than that of the acute sector. The most recent general definition of the role and scope of NP within primary and secondary settings was produced by the Royal College of Nursing (RCN) Nurse Practitioners Association and RCN council (1997). The NP was identified as a nurse who is responsible for professionally autonomous decisions, uses skills not usually exercised by nurses in making a differential diagnosis to screen patients for disease risk factors, develops preventive care management, provides health education and counselling, and makes referrals and discharges patients.

Within the same document, educational criteria for the NP role were also cited, recommending specific educational preparation of at least a degree level (RCN, 1997). Barton et al. (1999) refer to the increasing number of NP programmes of education, which were initially introduced at diploma level and are now first degree and Masters' level qualifications. New programmes are constantly being developed, but on the whole they have been criticized for failing to meet the needs of those working in acute settings (Jones and Smith, 1998). Barton et al. (1999) identify, however, that, although programmes of NP education initially concentrated on

Table 3.1 PEST analysis: external influences on nursing role development

External influence	Description
Political (governmental)	
New Deal (NHS Management Executive, 1991) Calman Report (Calman, 1993)	Reduction in junior doctors hours In response to reforms in medical specialist education, regional task-forces were formed to tackle implications related to the reduction in working hours of doctors. Funds were provided from the NHS Executive to pump prime innovative roles, many of which incorporated NP in their title (Read and Graves, 1994)
Greenhalgh Report (1994)	Emphasized the need for nurses and doctors to share responsibilities, for the benefit of quality of patient care
Making a Difference (DoH, 1998b)	Strengthened the nursing, midwifery and health visiting contribution to health and healthcare. Introduced the latest concept of a career framework for nurses and the idea of the consultant nurse
Professional	
New Horizons in Clinical Nursing (RCN, 1975)	Put the case for an advanced clinical role and proposed the development of a clinical nurse consultant (Albarran and Fulbrook, 1998)
Code of Professional Conduct (UKCC, 1992)	Addressed the issues of accountability and responsibility in nursing
Clinical grading (Nursing and Midwifery Staff's Negotiating Council, 1988)	Intended to reward nurses for clinical advancement
Exploring New Roles in Practice (ENRiP)	A database containing details of 603 roles carried out by nurses that were seen as innovative in 40 NHS Trusts in England (Levenson and Vaughan, 1999)
Higher Level of Practice (UKCC, 1999)	Outlined the development of a revised regulatory framework for post-registration clinical practice
Economic	
Rationalization of healthcare spending	Resulting in 'a review of traditional practices, with an examination of the effectiveness and efficiency of different means of delivering care' (Sparrow, 1997, p. 64)
Social	
Changes in healthcare needs	Changes in causes of mortality and morbidity. Infectious and acute diseases replaced by chronic, age- and stress-related illnesses. Focus on health education. ANPs can play a leading role in providing health education for patients and families
Demographic changes	Increase in the elderly population/decrease in birth rate
The healthcare consumer	Increased consumer expectation and demands for high-quality health-care
Technological	
Advances in medical science and technology and division of medicine into specialties	Reappraisal of traditional nursing and medical roles, redrawing the boundaries between the clinical work of doctors and nurses (Dowling et al., 1995)

primary care, the learning needs of acute sector NPs are now being acknowledged.

Evaluation of NP roles has only recently started to appear in the UK. Much of the literature available has reported on the immediate effects of posts developed to reduce junior doctors' hours of work (Read and Graves, 1994; Kendall et al., 1997; Cash and Hannis, 1998; Doyal et al., 1998). A limited number of studies have been undertaken, however, to confirm satisfaction with the NP role, viewed from the perspective of both the consumer (Stilwell et al., 1987, cited by Hicks and Hennessey, 1999; Touche Ross & Co., 1994) and the NP (Bailey and Cassidy, 1996).

The NP role has been the target of considerable criticism. The main source of concern has been the risk of the NP focusing on the development of medical tasks as opposed to developing nursing practice and patient care (Castledine, 1995; Cahill, 1996; Manley, 1996), literature that echoed initial arguments against the role when it was first developed in the USA (Rogers, 1972). Cahill (1996) describes the NP movement as the production of second-class doctors as opposed to first-class nurses, and warns of the danger of losing the art of nursing. This argument is, however, contradicted by a study undertaken by Bailey and Cassidy (1996, p. 43), whereby NPs found that, rather than losing the art of nursing, they were beginning to 'integrate their artistry with more scientific aspects of nursing care'. Barton et al. (1999) also recognize that the notion of nurses shifting the boundaries or scope of practice is not new, because nurses have always responded to changes in healthcare delivery. It should be remembered that both temperature taking and blood pressure reading used to be the exclusive preserve of medicine.

The development of such roles as NP could, therefore, be viewed as a very exciting time for nursing. Opportunities are available to nurses to shift the boundaries of their practice in order to benefit their client group. The NP movement has targeted several nursing domains, including paediatrics (Kobryn and Pearce, 1991; Dearman and Gordan, 1999). New roles have also emerged in paediatric oncology, with two nurses titled ANP in evidence in Liverpool; this work is discussed in Chapter 6.

In the UK, the title 'advanced nurse practitioner' is not exclusive to paediatric oncology (Redshaw and Harris, 1995; Dillon and George, 1997). This title has, however, introduced confusion about what this role refers to and how it differs from an NP. In contrast to the USA, the term ANP is not used as an overarching title referring to all nurses in advanced practice roles. The confusion is not surprising, however, because in the UK there is an ongoing debate about what constitutes advanced practice. Clarification of the meaning of an ANP would therefore be difficult at this time.

Local

The development of nursing roles within the trust is comparable with the situation nationally. The role of the CNS has been evident for several years at Great Ormond Street Hospital for Children (GOSH), covering a number of specialty areas: intravenous therapy, acute and chronic pain, neuro-oncology and infection control, to mention but a few. In addition to these well-established roles, there has also been a recent introduction of a variety of new nursing roles, such as patient care coordinator, nurse sedationist and practice educator (Beringer, 1999).

Looking at the existing and potential models of advanced clinical nursing roles in two trusts, Glen (1996) used a variety of research methods including semi-structured interviews, case studies and reviews of both job descriptions and current literature. Three roles were clearly identified as being used within these trusts. These were CNS, clinical specialist and nurse practitioner. The NP role included the role of medical assistant and the treatment of minor injuries. Glen (1996) identified a high degree of overlap between these roles with no policy or legislation providing clarification. This resulted in the titles being used differently by clinical directorates. In addition some of these posts were consultant, rather than nurse, led. Posts were being developed in response to a local need, with absence of strategic planning. Recommendations in the report focused on education, training and development, reflecting the development of clinical roles nationally, as well as within the trusts. Glen (1996) noted that the development of clinical nursing roles required careful planning of personnel, education and training; these factors are also seen as key issues in the work of Bamford and Gibson (1997).

Beringer (1999) explored the implementation of case management at GOSH. This study used a variety of approaches to data collection. It recommended that the creation of new case manager posts throughout the trust would be inappropriate. The local arrangements that have developed in some areas are working well to provide coordinated care. Beringer (1999) suggests that what is needed is for case management to become an integral part of current roles, such as CNS, senior nurses, lead consultants and the ward sister. Within the day-care unit there had been much discussion about the development of nursing roles. The post of patient care coordinator was introduced in 1998 to coordinate admission and discharge on one of the wards, and since the completion of this work this post has evolved into that of an NP. However, at the time this project was undertaken the establishment of NPs on the day-care unit was seen as a fundamental way forward in nursing role development.

The research design

Participatory action research

Action research is increasingly seen as a way of doing research and solving a problem at the same time (Lauri, 1982; Hunt, 1987; Coates and Chambers, 1990; Webb, 1990; Owen, 1993; Titchen and Binnie, 1993a; Rolfe and Philips, 1995; Jones, 1996; Gibson et al., 1997; Nichols et al., 1997). As a method it has much to offer because it can be used to analyse problems, carry out and evaluate plans, and learn more about research in the process (Hart and Bond, 1995a, 1995b; Webb, 1996). Action research focuses on the developmental aspects of research, with results fed back into the change process while research is ongoing (Webb, 1996).

The central characteristics of all forms of action research are collaboration between researcher and practitioner, solution of practical problems, change in practice and development of theory (Holter and Schwartz-Barcott, 1993). The potential for action research to be both collaborative and empowering (Street, 1995) increased its appeal to the working party. Selecting participatory action research (PAR) as opposed to other approaches was deliberate because PAR emphasizes that research is done with and for team members. Hart and Bond (1995a, 1995b) describe it as a bottom-up approach to implementing change in nursing. Greenwood (1994) warns, however, of the psychosocial costs of emancipatory change within a multidisciplinary setting, where nurses may be dealing with team members perceived to be more or less powerful than themselves. Attention should also be paid to the ethical implications of PAR. As action research is reliant on collaboration for the successful implementation of change, individuals may feel obliged to participate (Meyer, 1992; Lathlean, 1996).

The role of the researchers is also an important consideration in PAR. The working party adopted the 'insider' model of action research. Here, the role of researcher is undertaken by a practitioner working within the research setting, as opposed to using an 'outsider' model with a researcher external to the clinical setting (Titchen and Binnie, 1993a). Nursing studies indicate that the insider model has been more successful at meeting desired change (Titchen and Binnie, 1993b). A senior staff nurse from day care (DC) was therefore released to undertake the research nurse role, supervised by the two nurse academics from the working party. The potential shortcomings of this role were, however, acknowledged. These included the risk of reduced objectivity and bias as a result of using a researcher who could not be regarded as neutral (Titchen and Binnie, 1993a; Williams, 1995) and participant reluctance to disclose thoughts and opinions to another stake-holder (Lathlean, 1989, cited by Titchen and Binnie, 1993a). Attention therefore needed to be paid to the process as well as to the outcome of innovation (Meyer and Batehup, 1997).

Case study

A case study is defined as: 'a strategy for doing research which involves an empirical investigation of a particular contemporary phenomenon within its real life context using multiple sources of evidence' (Robson, 1993, p. 2).

Case studies have been described as 'the bedrock of scientific investigation' (Bromley, 1986, cited by Coolican, 1994, p. 85). The rich data produced can contribute uniquely to the knowledge of individuals, organizations, and social and political phenomena. Robson (1993) believes that case studies are most suited to understanding the context of an unexplored area that is in need of intervention or change. The relevance of this approach to the enquiry was considered very important.

The use of multiple methods of data collection was considered to expand the understanding of the phenomena under study greatly. Both qualitative and quantitative approaches can be used in case studies, interviews and observation, and the analysis of records is a commonly employed method (Robson, 1993). The value of 'triangulating' methods of data collection is also advocated in action research (Webb, 1990; Meyer, 1992; Waterman, 1995; Bellman, 1996). Data produced are generally intensive in nature and as a result the number of cases studied is often small (Robson, 1993). Questions may therefore arise as to how representative case study findings are (Robson, 1993). This was not, however, viewed by the working party as problematic. The enquiry did not attempt to achieve external validity and represent the development of nursing roles in all paediatric oncology day-care units. It was clearly specific to nurses in DC. The working party also understood that, although the generalization of study findings in the statistical sense is not appropriate, generalizing the findings to theory should be possible (Burns and Grove, 1997). The aims and objectives for this work are shown in Table 3.2.

Procedure

The sample for this study was taken from the key stakeholders in DC; they and their involvement are shown in Table 3.3. As the research involved the parents and staff at GOSH, approval from the Institute of

Table 3.2 Aims and objectives of the action research project to develop nursing roles on Elephant Day Care

To develop nursing roles that were well thought out, systematic and had been devised in consultation with members of the multiprofessional team

To provide an opportunity to talk to families about the service that they already received and to gain their views on potential changes to the role of the nurse

To identify education and training issues for the proposed developments

To increase the understanding of where nurses were and where they wanted to go

To raise the awareness and interest in nursing role development by disseminating the approach and findings of this work to the international, national and local audience

To provide a framework for the planning, implementation and evaluation for future role development throughout the trust

To facilitate consideration of nursing roles in light of statutory, professional body and government initiatives

---

Child Health and the GOSH Ethics Committee was sought and obtained. The rights of all participants not to take part in the project were acknowledged, with parents assured that this would not influence future treatment and care. National and local guidelines for research were adhered to throughout this project.

The following methods of data collection were used:

1. Semi-structured interviews were used as the primary method of data collection. This technique appeared well suited to exploring in depth the perceptions and feelings of participants, with regard to the development of nursing roles in DC. All participants were asked the same five open questions. Questions were asked in the same sequence for all participants, with probes and prompts used by the researcher as necessary. Interviews were undertaken with the nurses in DC, members of the multiprofessional team with an involvement in DC, and a sample of parents of children seen in DC.

2. A focus group was undertaken with the nurses in DC. There were several reasons for electing to involve DC nurses as a group. First, this aimed to encourage group ownership of the project and feelings of autonomy and control. Second, focus groups appeared to be well suited to the nursing team dynamics in DC. The nurses already interacted well during meetings, brainstorming and sharing ideas, feelings and opinions.

3. The SWOT analysis tool was used with the nurses working in DC, with the aim of further addressing the development of nursing roles. Three separate group discussions were undertaken, systematically assessing the strengths, weaknesses, opportunities and threats of the following options:

Table 3.3 Study sample

Sample	Rationale
Parents	
Parents attending DC with their children during a randomly selected clinic week were invited to take part in a semi-structured interview; 19 parents consented to the interview: 13 mothers and 6 fathers and both parents of 4 children	The views of users of a service are paramount in any case study involving an organization The decision to use this sample also reflects GOSH initiatives to seek the opinions and views of parents and families
Nurses working in Elephant Day Care	
The seven nurses working in DC were participants in a focus group and SWOT analyses Two nurses were also observed for a shift	As the group of individuals most likely to be affected by the proposed changes in DC, it was vital that their opinions were sought, throughout this process This allowed for a more complete understanding of current nursing roles in DC
Qualified nurses identified as users of DC	
Fourteen nurses identified as users of DC participated in a semi-structured interview. This sample predominantly consisted of CNSs, although the HDU senior nurse, practice educator and private patient liaison nurse were also included in this sample group	This choice aimed to obtain views from a group of users whose own role was likely to be impacted upon by future developments of nursing roles in DC
Doctors	
Nine HDU consultants, the DC registrar, and two registrars undergoing clinical rotation within the unit participated in a semi-structured interview The DC registrar was observed for a day	The issue of changing professional boundaries was also relevant to this group and hence their views and opinions were vital to any future success of role development in DC Observational study allowed for a clearer interpretation of medical responsibilities in DC
ANPs, NPs and nurse clinicians currently working in the UK and the USA	
Visiting and discussing nurses in expanded paediatric clinical role in London, Liverpool and Oxford The Olivia Hodson Fellowship granted an award for the visit of Marilyn Hockenberry-Eaton, Associate Professor and Director of Advanced Nurse Practitioners, Texas Children's Hospital	The effectiveness of nursing role development was assessed through the expert views, opinions and ideas of current practitioners Marilyn Hockenberry-Eaton's visit allowed her to observe and comment on current nursing roles in DC and to share her practical experience and expertise of developing ANP roles in a similar setting

What if the role of the nurse in DC stays the same?
What if all of the nurses in DC developed their roles?
What if nurse practitioners were introduced in DC?

4. Observation was performed on two nurses and one registrar in DC. The aim of this was to achieve a fuller understanding of the current nursing and medical roles in DC. Unstructured observation was chosen because it was in keeping with the qualitative nature of the study.

5. Documentary analysis was undertaken of the following written and recorded material: DC staff activity analysis (Senior Nurse Workforce Planning, 1996). This measured the proportion of time spent by nurses on nursing and non-nursing activities, thereby questioning time management issues and skill mix within the nursing team. The job descriptions of nursing staff in DC provided an overview of how the organization describes the role of the nurse DC and acted as a benchmark against which other data could be compared.

6. The literature on the advancement of nursing roles in the UK and the USA was re-visited to ensure that the reported development of nursing roles on both sides of the Atlantic had been identified and could be compared with the current roles of nurses working in DC.

Data analysis

The use of a case study design collecting multiple sources of evidence, although all contributing to the 'whole picture', did make data analysis and the organization of findings complex. Data were analysed using the steps identified by Strauss and Corbin (1998) and Dey (1993) as a guide. This involved the following:

- open coding
- creating categories
- assigning categories
- axial coding.

To structure the process a decision was made by the working party initially to identify themes and patterns from the semi-structured interview data. These themes and categories were then used to structure the examination of other data collected.

Results

In this section relevant findings identified throughout the data collection period are presented.

The current role of the nurse on DC

The role of the nurse in DC was recognized by all as being multifaceted, complex and, on occasions, undoable and therefore difficult to describe.

Practical/technical care was the most frequently mentioned role by interviewees. This included tasks such as taking blood (peripheral and central), siting a port needle, administering intravenous drugs and performing procedures (central line care and glomerular filtration rates). The list was often expansive; non-nursing staff generated a list of 15 items. In contrast nurses working in DC were unable to describe clearly their role in terms of practical/technical care, mentioning only coordination, organization, advocacy and liaison.

From all the interviews the nurse's role as support was divided into three main areas: talking and listening to families, and counselling and sitting in on 'bad news consultations'. Doctors in particular highlighted the pastoral role of nurses, and they and parents mentioned support in terms of assisting the doctor. The role of named nurse was seen by parents as being supportive, providing continuity and an advocate for families:

> To have a named nurse is quite nice . . . . There is someone to relate to rather than having a different nurse. Easier to open up, discuss problems. . . . Helps you build up a relationship.
>
> Parent no. 11

It was, however, identified that the named nurse role could be more consistent. When in place it worked well, but it was ineffective in some cases:

> Not every patient had a named nurse; when there is, it's a good system . . . due to the number of nurses it seems to have broken down.
>
> Doctor no. 8

All interviewees mentioned education; this included providing information to parents about treatment protocols and the side effects of drugs. Parents emphasized the amount of advice given to them by nurses in DC, both face to face and over the telephone. Although this advisory role was recognized by the non-nursing staff in DC, it was given less priority. Doctors did, however, note that the nurses in DC were often called on to interpret information that they had given to parents.

The liaison role was only briefly mentioned by the nurses working in DC; nurses with involvement in DC, doctors and parents all emphasized the importance of this role, although in different ways. The nurses with involvement in DC highlighted the liaison within the unit, throughout the rest of the hospital and shared care hospitals. Doctors and parents focused mainly on liaison with shared care hospitals. The parents also considered the nurses in DC as being effective in coordinating the many services needed to ensure that their and their child's experience of DC was as smooth as possible. However, at times this was perceived by other groups not to be as efficient as it could be, with poor communication between staff members resulting in nursing staff duplicating the work of others.

Echoing this, confusion arose in the interviews, particularly with parents, between the role of the healthcare assistant and the nurse in DC. In several interviews parents described nurses weighing and measuring children, distributing lunches and supervising children while parents were away from DC. Although on occasion nurses may undertake these tasks, they are more often the roles of healthcare assistants. As both groups wear the same uniform, the confusion is understandable and may have influenced parents' responses to other questions.

The interview findings reflected the job descriptions of the nursing staff within DC. Role expectations were, however, clearly dependent on the grade of the nurse and his or her level of knowledge and experience, e.g. although the job description of more junior nurses specifies competence in the administration of intravenous therapy and phlebotomy, within a negotiated timeframe the senior staff nurse is required to demonstrate clinical expertise in performing these skills. The findings of the DC activity analysis (Senior Nurse Workforce Planning, 1996) both supported interviewee's descriptions of the nurse's role on DC and correlated with the activities seen during the observation periods.

Finally, in this section, DC nurses were asked in SWOT analysis the question: 'What if the nurses' role in DC stayed the same?' Their overall responses seemed to indicate that their role was underused and undeveloped, and that their role could be developed further.

The statement for change

The notion of change and the changing role for nurses make up a loud voice in current nursing literature and government reports (see Table 3.1). On being asked the question 'Is there anything concerning the nurses' role in DC that you would change?' there was an overwhelming feeling from interviewees that nursing in DC was already over-stretched and understaffed. Nevertheless, interviewees were able to identify a number of factors that could be put in place to improve the service.

One of these was the development of the named nurse role. All interviewees shared their views on how they felt that this role could change and be developed to benefit families. One, considered by nurses with involvement in DC and medical staff, was to introduce a specific focus for DC nurses. The specialty focus was described as enabling DC staff to develop specific knowledge and skills for a patient group, so improving the link between these groups and offering more support to families. Medical staff described a similar development with DC nurses being linked to a particular consultant or clinic room. This was described as a process of encouraging teamwork, ensuring clarity of treatment plans, improving consistency of information given and avoiding duplication of work.

Introducing this focus was also considered in terms of DC nurses taking more responsibility for the overall care of a patient group, i.e. a case management role, thus allowing for an expansion of their current role, improving liaison with shared care hospitals and facilitating individual development. Medical staff, nurses involved in DC and parents addressed the notion of families being seen by a nurse before being seen by a consultant, or on some occasions being seen only by the nurse. However, medical staff and parents felt that this would be appropriate only when patients were not 'too complicated' and to be treated on a standard protocol. One of the doctors interviewed mentioned that this change in role could ultimately improve DC nurses' job satisfaction, impacting on retention and recruitment. The focus of many of the comments, about changes in the role of nurses in DC, centred on improvement of the overall experience of DC for children and their families. Specifically mentioned were reducing waiting times and improving continuity of care. There was also a general feeling that any change should encompass all DC nurses.

The potential for change

As one of the main aims of this study was the feasibility of introducing similar roles to those described above to DC, one of the questions asked of the sample related to the proposed expansion of the nurses' role in DC, a role that could include tasks once considered as medical; unsurprisingly this suggestion raised many questions.

One of the questions asked was: 'If these roles were to be introduced where would the role of the DC nurse begin and end?' Doctors listed mainly technical tasks that nurses could undertake in expanding their role, whereas nurses involved in DC highlighted the importance of avoiding simply taking over medical tasks to the detriment of developing nursing skills. A number of the interviewees stressed that psychosocial care of families was a fundamental role of the DC nurse and that this should not be sacrificed by the undertaking of more technical skills. The priority of technical skills over other aspects of the role of DC nurses was apparent in many of the interviews. Parents focused, however, on the caring aspects of the role, identifying these as important to their overall experience. Where the nurse could still bring the caring element of nursing to a technical role, this was considered to be acceptable. One of the medical staff felt that a designated nurse with a high level of expertise should be formally trained in DC to give advanced advice to shared care services. This role with shared care hospitals was also the focus for some parents, the focus being to identify a means to share knowledge and skills, as well as increase communication in both directions. Some parents considered that their role could also be expanded, including greater involvement with central lines/ports, taking bloods and decision-making. It was felt that, in redefining the role of DC nurse, all other roles in the team would need to be redefined, and only then would it be possible to identify the best person for the job.

Whatever changes occur it was agreed that these would need to be underpinned by appropriate education and training, with the addition of clinical support and supervision from the medical team. Doctors commented that there was no limit to role expansion as long as training was provided. In addition it was felt that education was needed to ensure that role expansion did not become just a series of tasks, but that holistic and family-centred care must remain the focus of nursing.

Even with education and training some areas of role expansion were considered by medical staff and parents to be beyond the scope of a nursing role. Specifically mentioned were the risks of mistakes, and the question of who has overall responsibility, who would assess clinical competence and who would have the time. Parents distinguished between some medical tasks that they thought nurses could undertake, and tasks that they considered too complex, e.g. one parent distinguished between ordering scans and interpreting scans. The first a nurse could do, but the latter, a diagnostic role, only a consultant could perform:

> Anything diagnostic I'd rather a doctor do. Anything practical and procedural I do not mind a nurse doing.
>
> Parent no. 2

Surrounding this issue seemed to be the notion of the difference between medical and nursing knowledge. This was considered by many parents already to be vague, with DC nurses undertaking roles that they had not experienced nurses in their shared care hospitals doing:

> No comparison with the nurses here and the ones at [my shared care hospital]. There are nurses and there are nurses . . . you could almost not call you nurses.
>
> Parent no. 12

Parents were, however, very clear about the role of doctors and nurses, and what they wanted from each. They also distinguished between which nurses should be further expanding the boundaries of their practice:

> You need experienced nurses . . . knowledge comes with experience.
>
> Parent no. 9

In considering the expansion of nurses' role in DC, nurses were asked, in SWOT 2 and 3 respectively, 'What if all of the nurses in day care developed their roles?' and 'What if we had nurse practitioners in DC?'. Although there was initial confusion about the definition of an NP, referring to the role as an 'unknown quantity', responses to these questions were that, although development of all the nurses working in DC seemed democratic and would enhance nursing care and service provision, in reality such a development would be difficult in the light of human and financial constraints. The group also recognized that not everyone wanted to expand her or his role and enforcing such a change on everyone was not an option. The second proposal was met with much debate but the group felt that, if clearly defined, an NP working in DC would bring the benefits mentioned above to bridging the gap between nursing and medicine, and lead to the definition of other nursing roles on DC. The disadvantages of such a post were seen to be mainly pragmatic although surmountable.

The group also felt that if only one NP post was introduced it would be difficult to change practice in any real shape or from. A better choice would be to introduce two NPs, thus providing greater support for each other and the nursing team, and having a greater impact on practice. Two (or more) nurses working in an advanced role was also strongly recommended by the post holders visited, for many of the reasons given by the group.

Discussion

From the project's outset, the role of the NP was of particular interest to the members of the research working party. The general feeling was that there could be a future for a paediatric NP in DC. It was recognized, however, that in the interests of patient care the development of nursing roles should not be undertaken in an 'ad hoc' fashion. The evolution of roles should be dependent on the setting and the staff within that setting, as well as the specific needs of the organization, unit and trust, and in response to Government and statutory body initiatives (UKCC, 1992, 1994; Department of Health, 1993, 1994).

From the data presented in this chapter and the extensive literature review undertaken during the project, it would appear that there is a lack of clarity in defining advanced roles and advanced practice both locally and nationally (Arnfield, 1996; Bamford and Gibson, 1997; Hicks and Hennessey, 1999). As this work finished the Trust announced a major reorganization of nursing and service provision, so it was thought unwise to introduce new roles until this reorganization was complete and the unit was re-established in its new place in the Trust.

At the time of the study six senior staff nurses (SSNs) working within the unit had developed an interest and expertise in specific areas of haematology, oncology, immunology and bone marrow transplantation. The working party felt that these roles offer a key area for development in line with the findings discussed earlier. The SSNs could choose an area of interest to focus on; education and multiprofessional facilitation would support their specialization in this area. This role is referred to as specialist named nurse (SNN). Working closely with the consultants and CNSs in their chosen area, the SNN would be seen as the lead nurse for that client group, acting as the main contact for families when telephoning for advice. The SNN would also coordinate appropriate clinics for that client group. On days when there are no clinics for that specialty, the SNN would work as an associate nurse for other client groups. SNNs are seen as the future group of nurses who could develop the skills and practice of a PNP. For this to be achieved it is necessary for an education package (whether BSc or MSc level) to be identified and clearly supported. Education as an integration of this development is viewed as a major aspect not only for the success of these proposals, but also for the recruitment and retention of senior staff working in DC.

For staff nurses it is proposed that they will initially work as an associate named nurse (ANN) in each of the four specialist areas as part of a rotational package. At a stage of their career in DC (using the preceptorship period and their professional development plan) when they feel confident, a decision would be made to remain in one of the specialist areas. Once again an education package and facilitation by the nurse practice educator is needed to enable the professional and personal growth necessary at this time. These proposals, in general terms, are outlined in Figure 3.1.

Critique of method

The multi-method approach used in this work offered distinct advantages. It not only met the aims and objectives of the study, but also addressed both the current and the future role of the nurse in DC from a number of different perspectives. This, combined with the broad sample

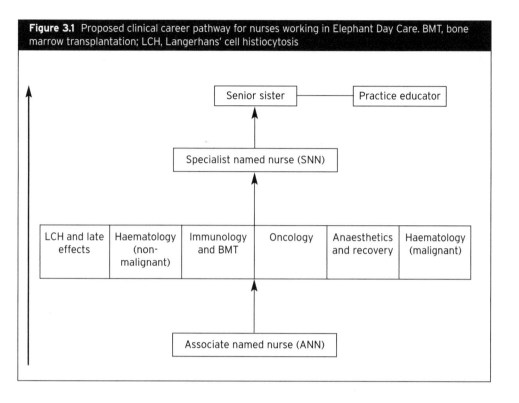

Figure 3.1 Proposed clinical career pathway for nurses working in Elephant Day Care. BMT, bone marrow transplantation; LCH, Langerhans' cell histiocytosis

selection, supported the opinion that nursing role development should not be undertaken in an ad hoc manner. The complementary nature of the multi-method approach (Robson, 1993) was also evident with, for example, the quantitative evidence in the activity analysis (Senior Nurse Workforce Planning, 1996) clearly enhancing the validity of the semi-structured interview data.

The main difficulties encountered in using this method of approach were the enormity and diversity of the data gathered. This heavily impacted on time scales, not only for data collection but also for the complex analysis involved. The adoption of the multi-method approach resulted partly from the enthusiasm of the working party and inexperience in using the case study approach. In hindsight data collection methods should have been balanced against time scales and resources.

The success of methods for data collection also varied. The observational analysis was less beneficial than expected. First, the individual nursing observations were unintentionally biased towards senior nurses and thus did not reveal a clear picture of the current roles in DC. Second, the period of time spent observing the registrar working in DC unfortunately provided few data of value to the study. Such data were not, however, discarded because the ongoing, cyclical nature of action research may warrant its use at a later stage.

Recommendations

The following recommendations have been made by the working party from this project:

- to develop a clinical career pathway for nurses working in day care
- to develop the current senior staff nurse role in day care
- to review the education and support needed for this development, and identify resources required
- to undertake role analysis, clarify job descriptions and develop clinical competencies for nurses working in day care
- to introduce a nurse practice educator post into day care at a later date
- to establish a telephone helpline for parents
- to evaluate any changes and plan for the future
- to encourage ongoing collaboration between education and practice to identify and support role development
- to consider future role development using the safety net outlined in PONF (2000).

Conclusion

This chapter presented the findings of an enquiry into the development of nursing roles within DC. Although the working party began with the notion of considering the development of a new PNP-type role, it soon became clear that there was a need to consider ongoing role development for all nurses in DC, and not simply the introduction of a new role. However, the research design enabled the enquiry to reveal views on current and new roles by encompassing not only nurses in DC, but also other nurses from within the unit, members of the multiprofessional team and parents who currently attend DC.

The results from the range of data collected would seem to be unanimous in stating that DC is not yet ready for a PNP-type role. The SWOT analysis alone reflects the quest for role development that improves patient care, but that development is surrounded by hesitation for a clear description of the roles that might be required to meet the needs of families in the future. The semi-structured interviews were illuminating and will guide the Senior Sister and the rest of the nursing team in developing a comprehensive action plan to facilitate ongoing role development, with the ultimate aim of improving the service.

The uncertainty and apprehension in challenging the present professional role reflect the debates in the literature, and ultimately represent the ongoing confusion that there is in the profession as a whole. Challenging established boundaries of practice is complex; nevertheless the recommendations presented in this report must provide a starting point from which innovation and creativity will result. Documented within this report is evidence from the whole sample that they would respond positively to change. The challenge will be to manage this change effectively through a shared vision, reflecting on current roles within the whole team, and establishing a realistic timeframe for personal and professional development to occur in tandem with any agreed change.

The use of participatory action research endorses the cyclical notion of change. Following on from the analysis of data from this study the next steps would be to re-plan, take action and collect data on action. As developments occur and the new career pathway begins to take shape in DC, the process of action research can once again be used to evaluate and continue to facilitate nurses to be proactive and take a lead in planning their future.

References

Albarran G, Fulbrook P (1998) Advanced nursing practice: an historical perspective. In: Rolfe G, Fulbrook P (eds), Advanced Nursing Practice. Oxford: Butterworth-Heinemann, pp. 11-32.

Arnfield A (1996) Clinical Nurse Specialists at Great Ormond Street Children's Hospital NHS Trust, unpublished report.

Bailey J, Cassidy A (1996) Using nursing theory to introduce change in practice. Nursing Standard 10: 40-43.

Bamford O, Gibson F (1997) Advanced Nurse Practitioner: The role and development of the Clinical Nurse Specialist. London: South Bank University.

Barnes K, Sharu K (1998) Advanced practice in the US: Part One: the paediatric nurse practitioner. Paediatric Nursing 10: 30-32

Barton T, Thome R, Hoptroff M (1999) The nurse practitioner: redefining occupational boundaries? International Journal of Nursing Studies 36: 57-63.

Bellman L (1996) Changing nursing practice through reflection on the Roper, Logan and Tierney model: the enhancement approach to action research. Journal of Advanced Nursing 24: 129-138.

Beringer A (1999) GOS 2000 and beyond: case management project, unpublished report.

Bowman C, Asch D (1987) Strategic Management. Basingstoke: Macmillan Education.

Burns M, Grove S (1997) The Practice of Nursing Research: Conduct, critique and utilisation, 3rd edn. Philadelphia: WB Saunders.

Cahill H (1996) Role definition: nurse practitioners or clinicians' assistants. British Journal of Nursing 4: 1382–1386.

Calman K (1993) Hospital Doctors: Training for the future. London: HMSO.

Cash K, Hannis D (1998) The evaluation of nurse practitioners funded under junior doctors' hours initiative: the Durham model. Leeds: Leeds Metropolitan University.

Castledine G (1995) Will the nurse practitioner be a mini doctor or a maxi nurse? British Journal of Nursing 4: 938–952.

Christensen J, Akcasu N (1999) The role of the pediatric nurse practitioner in the comprehensive management of pediatric oncology patients in the inpatient setting. Journal of Pediatric Oncology 16: 58–65.

Coates VE, Chambers M (1990) Developing a system of student nurse profiling through action research. Nurse Education Today 10: 83–91.

Coolican H (1994) Research Methods and Statistics in Psychology. London: Hodder & Stoughton.

Coopers & Lybrand (1996) Nurse Practitioner Evaluation Project: Final report – executive summary. London: Coopers & Lybrand.

Cronewett LR (1995) Moulding the future of advanced practice nursing. Nursing Outlook 43: 112–118.

Dearman A, Gordan K (1999) The nurse practitioner in children's ambulatory care. Paediatric Nursing 11: 18–21.

Department of Health (1993) A Vision for the Future. The nursing, midwifery and health visiting contribution to health and healthcare. London: DoH.

Department of Health (1994) The Challenges for Nursing and Midwifery in the 21st Century. London: DoH.

Department of Health (1998a) Review of Prescribing, Supply and Administration of Medicines: A report on the supply and administration under group protocols. London: HMSO.

Department of Health (1998b) Making a Difference: Strengthening the nursing, midwifery and health visiting contribution to health and healthcare. London: HMSO.

Denscombe M (1998) The Good Research Guide for Small-scale Social Research Projects. Buckingham: Open University Press.

Dey I (1993) Qualitative Data Analysis: A user friendly guide for social scientists. London: Routledge

Dillon A, George S (1997) Advanced neonatal nurse practitioners in the UK: where are they and what do they do? Journal of Advanced Nursing 25: 257–264.

Dowling S, Barrett S, West R (1995) With nurse practitioners, who needs house officers? British Medical Journal 311: 309–313.

Doyal L, Dowling S, Cameron A (1998) Challenging Practice: An Evaluation of Four Innovatory Posts in the South West. Bristol: University of Bristol the Policy Press.

Ford LC (1979) A nurse for all settings: the nurse practitioner. Nursing Outlook 27: 516–521.

Frost S (1998) Perspectives in advanced practice. In: Rolfe G, Fulbrook P (eds), Advanced Nursing Practice. Oxford: Butterworth-Heinemann, pp. 33–42.

Gibson F, Horsford J, Nelson W (1997) Oral care: practice reconsidered within a framework of action research. Journal of Cancer Nursing 1: 183–190.

Glen S (1996) Advanced clinical nursing roles in UCLH NHS Trust and the Hospital for Children Trust, unpublished report.

Greenhalgh & Co. (1994) The Interface between Junior Doctors and Nurses. Macclesfield: Greenhalgh & Co.

Greenwood J (1994) Action research: a few details, a caution and something new. Journal of Advanced Nursing 20: 13–18.

Hamric A (1998) Historical and current developments in specialist and advanced practice in North America. In: Castledine G, McGee P (eds), Advanced and Specialist Nursing Practice. Oxford: Blackwell Science, pp. 55–70.

Hamric A, Spross J, Hanson C M (1996) Advanced Nursing Practice: An integrative approach. London: Saunders & Co.

Hart E, Bond M (1995a) Action Research for Health and Social Care: A guide to practice. Buckingham: Open University Press.

Hart E, Bond M (1995b) Developing action research in nursing. Nurse Researcher 2: 4-14.

Hicks C, Hennessey D (1999) A task based approach to defining the role of the nurse practitioner: the views of UK acute and primary sector nurses. Journal of Advanced Nursing 29: 666-673.

Hodgkiss-Lagan S (1996) The advanced nurse practitioner in the ITU. Nursing in Critical Care 1: 225-229.

Holter M, Schwartz-Barcott D (1993) Action research: what is it? How long has it been used and how can it be used in nursing? Journal of Advanced Nursing 18: 298-304.

Hunt M (1987) The process of translating research findings into nursing practice. Journal of Advanced Nursing 12: 101-110.

Jones S (1996) An action research investigation into the feasibility of experienced registered sick children's nurses (RSCNs) becoming children's emergency nurse practitioners (ENPs). Journal of Clinical Nursing 5: 13-21.

Jones S, Smith J (1998) Expanding roles and practice within paediatric A/E departments: The children's nurse practitioner. In: Glasper E, Lowson S (eds), Innovations in Paediatric Ambulatory Care. Hampshire: Macmillan Press, pp. 1-13.

Kaufmann G (1996) Nurse practitioners in general practice: an expanding role. Nursing Standard 11(8): 44-47.

Kendall S, Latter S, Rycroft-Malone J (1997) Nursing's hand in the new deal: nurse practitioners and secondary health care in North Thames. Buckingham: Buckinghamshire College.

Kobryn M, Pearce S (1991) The paediatric nurse practitioner. Paediatric Nursing 3(5): 11-14.

Lathlean J (1996) Ethical dimensions of action research. In: De Raeve L (ed.), Nursing Research: An ethical and legal approach. London: Baillière Tindall, pp. 32-41.

Lauri S (1982) Development of the nursing process through action research. Journal of Advanced Nursing 7: 301-307.

Levenson R, Vaughan B (1999) Developing New Roles in Practice: An evidence based guide London: King's Fund.

Manley K (1996) Advanced practice is not about medicalising nursing roles. Nursing in Critical Care 1: 56-57.

Mayled A (1998) Medical admissions units: the role of the nurse practitioner. Nursing Standard 12: 44-47.

Meyer J (1992) New paradigm research in practice: the trials and tribulations of action research. Journal of Advanced Nursing 18: 1066-1072.

Meyer J, Batehup L (1997) Action research in health-care practice: nature, present concerns and future possibilities. Nursing Times Research 2: 175-184.

National Health Service Management Executive (1991) Junior Doctors: The new deal. London: NHSME.

Nichols R, Meyer J, Batehup L, Waterman H (1997) Promoting action research in healthcare settings. Nursing Standard 11(40): 36-38.

Nursing and Midwifery Staff's Negotiating Council (1988) A Guide to the Clinical Grading Structure. London: Macdermott & Chant.

Owen S (1993) Identifying a role for the nurse teacher in the clinical area. Journal of Advanced Nursing 18: 816-825.

Paediatric Oncology Nurses Forum (2000) A Framework for Developing Practice in Paediatric Oncology. London: Royal College of Nursing.

Pitts J, Seimer B (1998) The use of nurse practitioners in pediatric institutions. Journal of Pediatric Health Care 12: 67-72

Read S, Graves K (1994) Reduction in Junior Doctors' Hours in Trent Region: The nursing contribution. Sheffield: Trent: RHA/NHS Executive Trent.

Read SM, George S (1994) Nurse practitioners in accident and emergency departments: reflections on a pilot study. Journal of Advanced Nursing 19: 705-716.

Redshaw M, Harris A (1995) Breaking New Ground: An exploratory study of the role and education of the advanced neonatal nurse practitioner. London: English National Board for Nursing, Midwifery and Health Visiting.

Robson C (1993) Real World Research. Oxford: Blackwell.

Rogers M (1972) Nursing: to be or not to be? Nursing Outlook 20(1): 42-46.

Rolfe G, Phillips LM (1995) An action research project to develop and evaluate the role of an advanced nurse practitioner in dementia. Journal of Clinical Nursing 4: 289-293.

Romaine-Davies A (1997) Advanced Practice Nurses. London: Jones & Bartlett.

Royal College of Nursing (1975) New Horizons in Clinical Nursing. London: RCN.

Royal College of Nursing, Nurse Practitioners Association (1997) Nurse Practitioners: Your questions answered. London: RCN.

Royal College of Paediatrics and Child Health (1996) Developing Roles of Nurses in Clinical Child Health. London: RCPCH.

Salvage J (1991) Nurse Practitioners: Working for change in primary care. London: King's Fund.

Senior Nurse Workforce Planning (1996) Staff activity analysis: elephant day care, Unpublished report.

Shewan JA, Read S M (1999) Changing roles in nursing: a literature review of influences and innovations. Clinical Effectiveness in Nursing 3: 75-82.

Sparrow S (1997) Advanced nursing practice: changing roles, changing power relations. Managing Clinical Nursing 1: 63-67.

Stilwell B (1983) The nurse in practice. Nursing Mirror 158: 17-22.

Strauss A, Corbin J (1998) Basics of Qualitative Research, 2nd edn. Thousand Oaks, CA: Sage Publications.

Street A (1995) Nursing Replay, Researching Nursing Culture Together. Melbourne: Churchill Livingstone.

Titchen A, Binnie A (1993a) Research partnerships; collaborative action research in nursing. Journal of Advanced Nursing 18: 858-865.

Titchen A, Binnie A (1993b) Changing power relationships between nurses: a case study of early changes towards patient-centred nursing. Journal of Clinical Nursing 2: 219-229.

Touche Ross & Co. (1994) Evaluation of Nurse Practitioner Pilot Projects. London: South Thames RHA/NHS Executive.

United Kingdom Central Council For Nursing, Midwifery and Health Visiting (1992) Code of Professional Conduct for the Nurse, Midwives and Health Visitors. London: UKCC.

United Kingdom Central Council For Nursing, Midwifery and Health Visiting (1994) Final Report on the Future of Professional Education and Practice. London: UKCC.

United Kingdom Central Council For Nursing, Midwifery and Health Visiting (1999) A Higher Level of Practice: Report on the consultation on the UKCC's proposals for a revised regulatory framework for post-registration clinical practice. London: UKCC.

Waterman H (1995) Distinguishing between traditional and action research. Nurse Researcher 2: 15-23.

Webb C (1990) Partners in research. Nursing Times 86: 40-44.

Webb C (1996) Action research. In: Cormack D (ed.), The Research Process in Nursing, 3rd edn. Oxford: Blackwell Science, pp. 155-165.

Williams A (1995) Ethics and action research. Nurse Researcher 2: 49-59.

Yin RK (1994) Case Study Research, Design and Methods, 2nd edn. Thousand Oaks, CA: Sage.

Chapter 4

Developing clinical competencies

Faith Gibson and Louise Soanes

It has been argued (Carr-Saunders and Wilson, 1933, as cited in Eraut, 1994) that the formation of the professions in the nineteenth century began when groups of people doing the same type of work gathered together to discuss and exchange ideas. These discussions raised concerns that those practising the profession without the necessary competence to do so were undermining the public reputation of some of these occupations. This threat to public confidence led to the introduction of professional education and qualifying examinations to ensure that capability to practise was assessed and universally acknowledged. Likewise codes of conducts were developed to give assurance of honesty as well as competence (Eraut, 1994). In the last 100 years nursing has seen similar performance-based criteria developed and applied to it, although the status of the profession appears to remain elusive.

The issue that is presumed but not made explicit is what makes this standard of competence: how is nursing competency judged (Bradshaw, 1997a)? Reflecting on her own return to nursing, Bradshaw (2000) writes: 'I had no objective measures or standards by which to judge what I knew, what I should know, and most importantly, what I did not know' (p. 319). She argues that difficulties must therefore arise for nurses in accepting responsibility for their own competence when the meaning and nature of professional competence are still being debated. This chapter introduces the notion of clinical assessment using competencies, and then details the development and evaluation of clinical competencies in paediatric oncology nursing.

Competence and nursing

The apprentice model, as advocated by Florence Nightingale, was the foundation of nurse training for nearly 100 years. This changed in 1986 when the United Kingdom Central Council for Nursing, Midwifery and Health Visiting (UKCC) introduced *Project 2000: A new preparation for practice* (UKCC, 1986), with a resulting shift towards an education-focused student experience (Watkins, 2000). However, in recent years this has led to criticism, recognition of a theory–practice gap and doubts about fitness for practice in nurses completing this pathway of pre-registration education (UKCC, 1999). In answer to these points a commission was asked to look at these issues. Recommendations from this commission concluded that, although pre-registration nurse education should retain its education focus, this should be tempered with clinical placements suitable as arenas to ensure that nurses at the end of their programme were 'fit for purpose' and 'competent to practise' (UKCC, 1999, p. 34). To ensure that the latter two objectives were achieved, the UKCC has produced predetermined competencies within an outcomes-based approach to pre-registration education.

It was proposed that this new pre-registration nursing programme would be implemented across the UK by late 2002 (UKCC, 2001). But what of post-registration education? This appears to be in a greater state of flux with the demise of the English National Board (ENB) and the UKCC, and the amorphous implementation of the Nursing and Midwifery Council (NMC).

There also appears to be little recent evidence from the literature as to the agreed clinical outcomes for nurses completing post-registration education in specialist practice. Again with the demise of the so-called 'ENB long courses' outcome criteria are likely to become more fragmented and thus impede transferability of clinical assessment of practice from one trust to another for nurses following post-registration education. As competency seems primarily to be concerned with the affirmation of the individual's effectiveness in a specific area (While, 1994), nursing as a practice-based discipline needs to gain consensus on which skills, knowledge and attitudes are required by the nurse, the expected level of competence and whether, and if so in what way, performance should be classified (Woolley, 1977; Nicol et al., 1996). The next logical step is to ask: 'How is such effectiveness determined?' The answer to this question is less than straightforward.

Assessing clinical competence

From pragmatic and theoretical viewpoints there is no doubt that the assessment of clinical competence is a difficult and tenacious concern for nurses in education and clinical practice (Squier, 1981; Coates and Chambers, 1992; Chambers, 1994, 1998; Bradshaw, 1997a, 1997b; Clafin, 1997). Nevertheless, clinical assessment is required to provide effective and detailed feedback to students on their level of competence, achievement or performance, and contributes to the overall academic award. As previously discussed marrying the two concerns of academic award with a practitioner's competence to practise has presented a challenge to nurses in education for some time, thus resulting in a growing awareness of the contribution that practice-based learning makes to an academic award (Gerrish et al., 1997; UKCC, 1999, 2001). A clear understanding of the concept of competence has proved to be problematic (Coit Butler, 1978; Alspach, 1992; Ashworth, 1992; Nagelsmith, 1995; Bradshaw, 1997a, 1997b; Eraut, 1998; Lillyman, 1998). Short (1984, p. 207) concluded: 'the notion of competence itself is not a very useful conceptual tool for the task for which it has been intended.' The debates highlight that the concept of competence has been given several meanings, made even more complex by the fact that the UK and the USA movements spell the words differently: the UK's competence and competences are the North American competency and competencies (Wilson, 1997–98). These terms are often used interchangeably in the UK without explanation.

Despite these difficulties central to the discussion is the definition of the purpose of assessment, because the outcome of assessing the competency of nurses has local and national implications. In detailing the national implications of competency, Bradshaw (1997a) discusses the policy change and historical roles of the UKCC and other professional bodies in interpreting and influencing agreed levels of competence to ensure safe practice and the delineation of professional practice. The UKCC interprets the purpose of the assessment of competence as the identification of the nurse's fitness to practise (UKCC, 1989, 1992, 1996, 1998, 1999, 2001). However, fitness to practise goes beyond the adequacy of determining knowledge and skill acquisition (Sharp et al., 1995), reducing an occupation to a series of tasks ticked off a checklist, which provides a superficial representation of practice in any occupation. Nor can competence be thought of as a collection of advantageous attributes if these are taken out of the context of the clinical environment (Hager et al., 1994). Thus, it includes finding ways to make sense of the uncertainty and complexity of practice – the art of professional practice (Carper, 1978;

Benner, 1984; Schon, 1991). To fulfil this holistic remit to assess nurses' individual performance, a broader approach to assessing competency is called for, where the chosen knowledge, skills and attributes are set in the context of professional practice and clearly identified in performance criteria central to the assessment of competence within the profession (Hager et al., 1994).

Consistent with the holistic conceptualization of competence (Short, 1984; Le Var, 1996; Milligan, 1998) assessment should be based 'on a cluster of evidence' (Milligan, 1998, p. 278) gathered to facilitate the consideration of the elements of practice such as attitudes, behaviour and values.

Hence, according to Ross et al. (1988), the chosen method of assessing clinical competence needs to be objective, valid, reliable and practical, with the capacity to test a wide range of knowledge and skills while accommodating a number of assessors. It should also be dynamic, enable the student to reflect on performance and develop skills of self-assessment. This last component is congruent with the facilitation of individualized learning and the ethos of life-long learning (Henfield and Waldron, 1988).

Assessment using competence statements

The competence model is used as a vehicle in which to describe the nursing role in terms of discrete, assessable elements of behaviour or outcomes performed by an individual (Lillyman, 1998). Both advantages and disadvantages of such a model have been described. Boak (1997–98) identifies competency models as having the potential to provide guidance for all who are involved in staff development, recruitment, training, appraisal, promotion and succession planning. Specific to nursing Morin Robinson and Barberis-Ryan (1995) describe the benefits derived from using competency assessment to include: the ability to identify learning needs of individuals, to provide insight into areas of professional practice that can be implemented given the skill level of nursing staff, and to clarify allocation of educational resources for training and development needs. The use of competency statements can also facilitate individualized learning by enabling practitioners to reflect on their current practice and become self-directing (Henfield and Waldron, 1988). Concluding the advantages, the competence-based approach to education has been heralded as an objective assessment method, facilitating distinctions to be made in levels of competence when a variety of sources of evidence is used to support judgements concerning performance (Percival et al., 1994).

These positive views are balanced against some concerns raised by Ashworth and Morrison (1991). Their main arguments opposing the competence model centre on the use of competence because it describes a technically oriented way of thinking that is inappropriate for the training of human beings. The potential weakness of the competence model is in dealing with skills and qualities needed in maturely, reflectively and expertly dealing with patients and their problems (Ashworth and Saxton, 1990; Ashworth and Morrison, 1991), thus often emphasizing a focus on technical skills at the expense of knowledge and understanding (Ashworth and Morrison, 1991). Added to these concerns is the notion that the use of such a model also fails to analyse and assess critical thinking (Lillyman, 1998). In addition, it appears that using a competency model fails to bring objectivity to the process; Girot (1993) identifies that clinical assessors of practice use abstract concepts such as clinical judgement, intuition and a 'state of being', as well as concrete evidence, to judge whether a practitioner is competent.

An opportunity to re-visit the clinical assessment for a paediatric oncology nursing course arose with an impending re-validation of the course. The remainder of this chapter details the steps taken in the development of a competency-based clinical assessment of a practice tool (for a more detailed account, see Gibson and Soanes 2000), including a number of stages of evaluation. On balancing the choice of approach to this method of assessment, two factors influenced our choice: first, a competency model had the potential to assess theory and practice as an integral whole; and, second, developing competence statements would begin to define and describe the specialty of paediatric oncology nursing.

Creating the competencies

To ensure that the competencies produced were meaningful and appropriate to those who would be assessors and assessees, it was felt to be crucial to involve as many staff as possible. Two key practical issues were taken into consideration before deciding on the most appropriate technique to use. First, although the approach was required not to be too time-consuming, it needed to be comprehensive with quick results. Second, there was no financial support for the work, so the chosen tool needed to be cheap. A decision was consequently made to use a nominal group technique, because this would resolve all of the practical issues while achieving consultation and consensus with the professional group.

The nominal group process is 'a structured meeting which seeks to provide an orderly procedure for obtaining qualitative information from target groups who are most closely associated with a problem area' (Van de Ven and Delbecq, 1972, p. 338). As a planning and problem-solving process (Hall, 1983), it has been used previously in curriculum planning (O'Neil and Jackson, 1983). In addition, the technique has been found to be useful to identify researchable problems (Thomas, 1983; Gallagher et al., 1993; Carney et al., 1996), training needs assessment (Scott and Deadrick, 1982) and programme evaluation (O'Neil, 1981), and has been helpful to structure meetings and conferences (Butterfield, 1988).

The purpose of the nominal group process is to generate ideas, which are then discussed and ranked by the group (Moore, 1987). The group is highly controlled with discussion occurring only in the later stages of the group process (Gallagher et al., 1993). The group is guided by a facilitator who controls the group process through the management of information flow, acting essentially as a collector of ideas (O'Neil and Jackson, 1983) as opposed to leading the discussion. The work of the facilitator is complemented with usually one or two other individual(s) acting as note-taker, coordinating activities with the flipchart/whiteboard. The technique aims to avoid the known pitfalls of group interviews. Where some participants can be silent or overridden in the presence of more articulate and dominant personalities, particularly when perceived to be in a different position in the hierarchy, all its members have an equal opportunity to contribute (Carney et al., 1996). This equity and structuring for obtaining qualitative information is achieved through the steps identified in Table 4.1. The reasons for choosing the nominal group technique are justified using a structure provided by McMurray (1994) in Table 4.2.

Table 4.1 Nominal group process step by step (Butterfield, 1988)

Steps

1	Introduce nominal group process to the group
2	Silent generation of ideas in writing
3	Round-robin listing of ideas
4	Discussion of ideas on to a flip chart
5	Rank ordering ideas
6	Total rankings
7	Discussion
8	Conclusion

Table 4.2 Justification for using the nominal group technique in this work

McMurray (1994)	Justification for use in this work
Group activity: initial silent interaction with later discussion	The democratic style allows all members to have an equal opportunity to contribute through initial independent generation of ideas, avoiding the potential problems associated with discussion being dominated by more gregarious and articulate participants. The silent generation of ideas encourages independent creativity, enabling different perspectives to be revealed
Can be conducted in one session	This was particularly appealing when inviting practitioners to contribute and participate. Another factor in its favour was the fact that there was no need for any preliminary discussion or lengthy preparation and yet a substantial amount of work could be generated in a relatively short space of time (Carney et al., 1996)
Non-critical atmosphere desirable in discussion stage	The deliberate avoidance of interference or interpretation by the facilitator was considered to be important. Recognizing the experience of the nurse academics in undertaking group work, they would be skilled in managing the discussion and creating a non-threatening atmosphere. The overall aim was to encourage individuals to explore their ideas further, value their own contribution while listening and commenting appropriately on the ideas generated by other participants
Structured format: sequential steps or stages to be followed	This was useful, as neither of the two nurse academics had used this technique before, although Moore (1987) states that to undertake a nominal group technique there is a requirement that a group leader has mastered the process. As nurse academics with significant experience in undertaking group work, it was felt that these skills, facilitated by the clearly identified steps in the process, would be sufficient to ensure success. The sequential steps, shared with participants before the meeting, provided a structure that was easily understood, easy to follow and had the potential to allow the facilitator to keep the session on course
Promotes more and better quality ideas than brainstorming	The notion of initial independent generation of ideas was the deciding factor in not using brainstorming. In addition McMurray (1994) identifies that, although brainstorming is easy to conceptualize, it can prove difficult in undertaking because the free flow of ideas, fundamental to the technique, can be hampered by critical comments from other group members. Factors such as fear related to failure, criticism and ridicule, which could so easily intimidate group members, would be avoided by using the nominal group technique. The technique would also provide more ideas than individuals working alone
Peer influence likely only in discussion phase	This factor alone had the potential to ensure greater individual and group productivity (O'Neil and Jackson, 1983). This would also allow participants to pool individual judgements and arrive at desirable group decisions, through the process of voting and ranking, achieving a sense of completion and satisfaction (Hall, 1983)

Steps in the development process

Step 1: the nominal group technique

At the start of developing the competencies the plan had been to undertake three nominal group techniques (NGTs): one with senior staff/ward sisters on a haematology/oncology unit (group 1), one with course members currently undertaking the paediatric oncology nursing course (group 2), and a final group with previous course members. Only the first two groups were possible; as a result of work commitments the third group proved to be impossible. Group 1 consisted of seven members, and group 2 of twelve.

In both groups the steps of the process identified by Butterfield (1988) were followed. The nominal group task statement handed out to both groups asked the following question: Can you identify the knowledge, decision-making skills, and clinical attributes essential for successful performance as a paediatric oncology nurse? Although 90 minutes were allocated for each group the second group found it extremely difficult to make a final decision, and found the process of ranking almost impossible. A decision was made by the group and facilitators to conclude the discussion and ask members independently to vote at a later date after personal reflection and consideration of the ideas generated and the group discussion.

Group 1 generated 46 ideas, and group 2 66, out of which they awarded their eight votes to the most important ideas: eight being the most important, seven the next, and so on. Table 4.3 presents the ideas awarded the highest votes by both groups.

Step 2: refining process

It was envisaged that clinical nurses would be involved in the refining process. However, at the time the work was being undertaken, the clinical areas were very busy, negating the potential for nurses to give much more of their time. A decision was made by the nurse academics to undertake the refining process; this decision was shared with members of both groups. The nurse academics had almost 25 years of clinical experience between them, with strong clinical links in paediatric oncology nursing. This was considered to be sufficient experience to refine the statements from the NGT, ensuring that the essence of their meaning was not lost while maintaining the balance between the needs of education and practice in the assessment of competence to practise. The refining process consisted of shaping the ideas from the two NGTs into comprehensive competency statements. This process resulted in 17 competencies.

For each competency statement performance criteria were then identified. When developing the criteria the following points from Gurvis and Grey (1995) were taken into consideration: to ensure that criteria are focused on the learner, that they are measurable and achievable, and that they are relevant to the competency. In addition, the criteria needed to

Table 4.3 Ranked order of eight critical ideas by both groups

Votes awarded	Group 1	Votes awarded	Group 2
40	Indepth knowledge of symptom control	85	Knowledge of haematology and oncology
33	Understanding the basic principles of chemotherapy	80	Good basic paediatric nursing care
29	Understands how a diagnosis of cancer affects the family and friends	54	Good understanding of treatments
23	Care of the newly diagnosed child	36	Knowledge and understanding of symptom care
21	Knowledge of the cancer process	28	Communication skills
13	Knowledge and understanding of how to break bad news	25	Ability to give intravenous medications and deliver central line care
10	Prioritizing care of a sick child	24	Family-centred care, involvement of siblings
10	To have an understanding of taking on extended roles and the impact on nursing and the child	22	Counselling and supportive skills
10	Knowledge of research-based practice		
9	Knowledge of distraction and other ways of carrying out procedures other than ketamine		

facilitate the use of multiple sources of evidence to assess knowledge and understanding, and application of theory to practice, and to reflect on their caring role.

The competency statements and performance criteria were collated into an assessment document with space to record pass/refer/fail, and any comments. Guidelines for successful completion were also produced. As the piloting of the new assessment process was to run in tandem with the current assessment process, discrimination between satisfactory and unsatisfactory other than pass/refer/fail was not a requirement. The current assessment process in use incorporated the work of Benner (1984), providing descriptions of practice to distinguish the levels of advanced beginner through to expert.

Step 3: consultation process

An extensive consultation process was seen as a crucial part of the development of the competencies. Copies of the assessment document were circulated to members of both NGT groups and nurse academics. The consultation process asked participants to comment freely, making sure that the competency statements and performance criteria were clear and easily understood, jargon free, realistic and achievable. More importantly, they needed to guarantee that the competency statements and performance criteria truly reflected the nature of the specialty of paediatric oncology nursing.

Comments received reflected some general confusion and poor wording, with requests for examples to be included with some performance criteria. Although the document was felt to be too long, no competencies were identified at this time for removal. However, some performance criteria were linked, and thus the overall number reduced. Clarification and rewording were undertaken.

Step 4: pilot

The assessment document encompassing 17 clinical competencies was piloted with course members on a paediatric oncology nursing course that began in June 1998. There were 11 paediatric nurses on the course. The assessment was used in addition to the current validated document. This doubling of their workload was explained and participation agreed at the start of the course. For clinical assessors an incentive was the suggestion of a future assessment process that was less time-consuming to complete, retaining its roots in the specialty, while also focusing on the development of paediatric oncology nurses in the context of holistic care.

Time was spent before the course started preparing assessors for the new assessment process and documentation. Course members were prepared at the beginning of the course.

Step 5: evaluation

Informal evaluation was undertaken at 3 months and at the end of the course at 6 months with course members. In addition, evaluation undertaken at the end of the course included a sample of clinical assessors. A competency checklist to evaluate the competency model was produced, adapted from one described by Gurvis and Grey (1995). The checklist asked for comments on each of the 17 competency statements, performance criteria, learning options and evaluation methods.

As a result of this process the following changes were made:

- The 17 competencies were reduced to 14; reduction was made possible through a combination of some competencies and removal of one that was felt to be covered elsewhere as part of intravenous assessment.
- The wording of some performance criteria was changed; some wording was felt to be unclear and ambiguous, with clinical assessors not being totally sure what they were meant to be assessing.
- Core and specialty focus were indicated for all performance criteria, indicating which criteria were more reflective of core paediatric skills, and which specialty nursing skills were considered to be helpful, although there were some inconsistencies between the clinical assessors and the course members about the appropriateness of some of the criteria.
- The competency relating to bone marrow transplantation was made more expansive; additional performance criteria were added and thus clarified, making the assessment more realistic.

Step 6: implementation with a new course

Following consultation, changes were made and Benner's (1984) descriptors of novice to expert were incorporated as level indicators against which students would be assessed. The new approach to assessment was approved as part of a re-validation of the course, to be used with students undertaking the course at both diploma and degree levels. The new approach to clinical assessment thus encompassed the competency tool and a learning contract, with a portfolio being introduced as part of the formative assessment at the end of the 6-month course, in anticipation of students completing their diploma or degree pathway.

Step 7: return to Step 5 and continue evaluation

The competence approach to clinical assessment has been applied to a further five courses. Evaluation and consultation have continued, involving both paediatric nurses undertaking the course and clinical assessors.

Both positive and negative comments have been received. On the one hand, the competencies are clearly time-consuming to complete; they rely on an element of subjectivity and were difficult to achieve in a 6-month course. Extension of the course to one full academic year (9 months) since September 2000 appears to have helped to resolve this problem. On the other hand, the competencies identify learning related to theory and practice, and make explicit the knowledge, skills and attributes required by a paediatric oncology nurse. The element of subjectivity and the role of the clinical assessors are important. Any assessment involves an element of subjectivity (Gerrish et al., 1997). However, the use of a variety of approaches, which reveal a more complete picture and do not rely solely on inferring competence from performance, offsets the potential bias (Percival et al., 1994). Training of assessors, providing an opportunity to share views and perceptions about levels of expertise and the developing professional role of the paediatric oncology nurse, is one approach that must be part of the dynamic process of developing the competency model and must continue. The role and development of clinical assessors are an ongoing point of interest raised by both course members and the clinical assessors themselves; practical methods to support assessors include individual induction to the role and an annual workshop facilitated by the course leader.

Since the completion of this work, the competencies have been evaluated at the end of each course with both clinical assessors and course members. Feedback tends to reflect the practical issues surrounding the growing pressures in practice areas to provide teaching, learning and assessment to an increasing number of students, as well as balancing patient care. Despite these challenges, the ethos and framework of the competencies described in this chapter remain apparent in the current document. Although any assessment of practice seems to be a chore at the time for many course members, the emphasis on life-long learning, new knowledge and evidence-based care subsumed in the competencies do seem (anecdotally) to play a part in the development of course members' critical appraisal and personal development skills as they complete their degree/diploma pathway.

Formal evaluation

An opportunity arose to undertake a more formal evaluation of the competencies. This involved a longitudinal design using semi-structured interviews in order to examine changes over an extended period of time (Burns and Grove, 1997). This approach was taken to refine and test the list of competencies with paediatric oncology nurses who were using the document as part of an assessment on the paediatric oncology course. The sample targeted was purposeful, with course members undertaking the course that started in January 1999 being approached and invited to participate. The total population of nurses on the course was 13, of whom 6 agreed to participate in the study.

The interview schedule was developed from a competency checklist devised by Gurvis and Grey (1995), which had been used previously for the informal evaluation of the competencies. The main aim of the interview was to refine the list of competencies, so the questions sought to find out whether the competency document was comprehensive and reflective of the role of a paediatric oncology nurse, while providing participants an opportunity to comment on any aspect from their personal experience. The schedule also included a Likert scale in order to determine participants' overall opinion of the use of competencies in clinical assessment. The interview schedule was piloted for content with the course leader and other nurse academics. This interview schedule was used twice while nurses were on the course. By asking the same questions on repeated occasions the study aimed to identify whether the views of nurses altered in any way after consistent use of the assessment document. The third interview took place 6 months after the course was completed.

The interviews culminated in a collection of transcripts: 3 for each participant – 18 in total. The primary purpose of the interviews was to refine the competencies and to obtain perceptions and views from paediatric oncology nurses about their use and relevance in clinical practice. Descriptive analysis was undertaken to identify consistency of comments and the data were displayed in a time-ordered matrix (Miles and Huberman, 1994). A time-ordered matrix uses chronology as its basic principle. The display uses columns to show time-linked data referring to particular phenomena – in this case change in perception of clinical competencies. By use of this type of display, the rows will depend on what else is being studied. In this case the rows of the matrix were aspects or components of exclusivity of the competency statements and their relevance to clinical practice, making transparent the following:

- Are any competencies missing?
- Do the competencies reflect their role?
- Is there repetition of performance criteria?
- Do they understand the meaning of the core and specialty focus?
- Would they use them for personal/professional development?
- What is the overall usefulness of the assessment tool?

Transcripts were read and a highlighter pen was used to indicate comments that reflected all of the above areas. Notes were made in the margin of the transcripts with a summary detailed in the researcher's notebook. Data reduction and display are presented in Table 4.4, with a written summary of the data in Table 4.5.

The respondent's comments indicated that there was a level of consensus regarding the competency statements, in that they did reflect the knowledge and skills of a paediatric oncology nurse. Overall, it was felt that no additions were necessary; however, this must be balanced with a view shared by all respondents that 14 competencies were more than enough to complete during a course. Two respondents did identify

Table 4.4 Time-ordered matrix: changes in the perception of clinical competencies

	Interviewee a			Interviewee b			Interviewee c			Interviewee d			Interviewee e			Interviewee f		
1	N	N	Y	N	N	N	N	N	N	Y	Y	Y	N	N	N	N	N	N
2	P	P	Y	Y	Y	Y	Y	Y	P	P	P	Y	Y	Y	Y	P	Y	Y
3	N	N	N	N	N	N	N	N	N	Y	Y	Y	N	N	N	Y	Y	Y
4	N	Y	Y	Y	Y	Y	Y	Y	Y	Y	Y	Y	N	N	N	Y	Y	Y
5	Y	Y	Y	Y	Y	Y	Y	Y	Y	Y	Y	Y	Y	Y	N	Y	Y	Y
6	1	3	3	4	4	4	4	4	3	4	4	4	4	4	3	4	4

Legend for source of data:

Responses	Questions asked	Timing of interview shaded
Y (yes) N (no) P (partly)	1. Are there any competencies missing?	3/12
Likert 1-4:	2. Are the competencies reflective of their role?	6/12
1 not useful	3. Is there any repetition of performance criteria?	9/12
2 uncertain	4. Do they understand the core and specialty focus?	
3 useful	5. Would they use them for personal/professional development?	
4 very useful	6. What is the overall usefulness of the assessment tool?	

competencies to add. One respondent identified that, following the end of the course, knowledge was lacking in some aspects of symptom management. A competency specific to neutropenia, infection control and nursing management of the immunosuppressed child was considered to fill that gap. A second respondent, reflecting on her own role, identified gaps in relation to caring for children in the community and those requiring neuro-oncology nursing. On completion of the course this respondent commented that being creative with the assessment document and encouraging course members to reflect on their personal needs may fill this gap. However, she still felt that a focus on palliative care was lacking.

The competencies were considered to be reflective of the role of a paediatric oncology nurse; however, respondents consistently described a number of the competencies as being 'too broad', 'not specific to the specialty', and 'not accommodating of previous experience'. Comments reflected previous clinical experience, as well as the respondents' expressed need for specialist cancer knowledge. This perception did change over time with two respondents describing the benefit and application of core children's nursing knowledge to specialist practice. In contrast, one respondent found the core children's nursing competencies of less relevance on completion of the course. It was the timing that seemed to cause the most concern, particularly where previous knowledge and experience of an area were minimal for some, such as in the

Table 4.5 Summary table verifying and interpreting time-ordered matrix: changes in the perception of clinical competencies

	Interviewee a	Interviewee b	Interviewee c	Interviewee d	Interviewee e	Interviewee f
Competencies missing	At the start no, final interview perceived gaps in relation to symptom management	No	No	Start wanted more on community and neuro-oncology, end requested more on palliative care	No	No
Competencies reflect role	Only partly until final interview. At the start found them too general and broad, but found this useful later. Throughout felt they did not accommodate previous experience	Found some very general but understood why they were there. Bone marrow transplantation (BMT) and radiotherapy – small part of role, difficult to achieve	Some too broad and not reflective of previous experience, post-course even more difficult to see the relevance, e.g. prioritizing care of an acutely ill child	Partly, not able to personalize and reflect previous experience. Questioned relevance of some but in final interview understood why all there. BMT and radiotherapy difficult to achieve	Yes. Depended on starting point, e.g. giving chemotherapy. Some too theoretical, wanted more practice based. BMT and radiotherapy difficult to achieve	Some too broad and basic, insulted by wording of some, e.g. provide safe environment. Changed over time, could see importance of all of them. Radiotherapy difficult to achieve
Repetition of performance criteria	No	No. Some wording difficult	No. Some wording difficult	Yes. Overlap in relation to communication, breaking bad news. Expanded role too vague	No. Some wording difficult	Yes. Overlap in relation to communication, breaking bad news, providing holistic care
Understand core and specialty focus	First interview no. Developed understanding through the course	Clear from the start, core gave confidence in role at the start	Clear throughout	Clear throughout. Saw both developing in tandem	No, and no change over time	Clear throughout, but wanted more specialty focus
Use for personal and professional development	Yes, but not if time-consuming	Yes. Helpful guidelines and a resource	Yes, but levels difficult to interpret	Yes, but levels difficult to interpret and apply to own experience	During the course, yes but later no as too time-consuming. Wanted more of specialty focus	Yes, but would need to reflect BMT more
Were they useful	Changed over time, found levels unhelpful throughout	Initially daunting but always very useful	Always very useful, provides goals but not sure everything needed to be assessed	Always, offers guide and a framework	Always, gave confidence but time-consuming	Difficult to self-assess. View changed over time, doubted relevance of core focus at the start

specialty of bone marrow transplantation and radiotherapy, where these competencies were difficult to achieve.

Respondents identified some overlap of performance criteria, some appearing to be repeated in a number of competencies, e.g. criteria addressing communication needs appeared in two competencies. Some difficulties with wording were noted, with respondents describing the problems that this caused for them and their assessors. Wording in some was considered too vague, whereas in others it was described as verbose. One respondent suggested leaving gaps in the list of criteria where course members could add the evidence that they had used to achieve a competency.

The focus of the performance criteria to reflect core and specialist knowledge and skills failed to be considered relevant by a number of respondents. One respondent failed to grasp the difference throughout the whole assessment process, and even on completion of the course was unable to express a level of understanding. All respondents distinguished between general and specialist knowledge in their quest during the course for specialist knowledge. For some this did change, and respondents described the need to develop general and specialist knowledge and skills in tandem.

Comments that reflected on omissions or duplication of competency statements and performance criteria were considered. Professional judgement was used to decide whether the current list warranted changing. Some of the comments reflected content that was already present. Where this was the case words were altered to be more explicit. Where there was clear duplication of performance criteria some were removed. Some competencies were combined where there was overlap, and some were divided to retain and increase focus on that aspect of care. Some wording was altered to be more specific about the intended outcome. As a live document, the competencies continue to develop, reflecting the field of practice and the required learning outcomes for current post-registration nurse education. Currently, there are 11 competencies assessing both the knowledge base of contemporary paediatric oncology nursing and also the student's application of this to practice. With further proposed changes to the curriculum this development looks likely to continue, although the fundamental principles and ethos described in this chapter remain central to the competencies and the process of assessment.

Conclusion

There can be no doubt that professional competence is an issue that continues to dominate the nursing profession today (Hogston, 1993).

An emphasis on quality assurance in health and other caring professions, together with a national investigation into vocational education and training, has maintained a focus on the nature of professional competence as a key factor in the production of a quality service (Ellis, 1988). Although the importance of clinical competence is reasserted by the professional organizations and in many professional publications, the notion of what competence is in terms of judging someone as competent to practise is recognized to be difficult to define (Ashworth, 1992; While, 1994; Bradshaw, 1997a; Flintham, 1997). Bradshaw (1997a) states, however, that a universal agreement of the notion of competence is essential for determining advanced practice, extended practice and specialist practice in nursing.

Nevertheless, this chapter has presented one example where nurse academics and clinical practitioners have begun to address these issues. The development of an assessment tool that has the potential to assess clinical competence while also facilitating personal and professional development in a cyclical rather than a linear model of progression has been described. Other examples have yet to be revealed through the ENB project currently under way (Long et al., 2001). Clearly, there is still some way to go with a number of issues yet to be addressed, particularly about validity and reliability. However, the notion of face validity inferred from ongoing evaluation and feedback is considered to be sufficient to continue to use the competency model of assessment unchanged for the time being, thus providing stability for clinical assessors to develop their role and allow time for them to develop their thinking around the notion of competency and competence.

Acknowledgements

Thanks to the paediatric oncology students, past and present, who have contributed towards our thinking.

References

Alspach JG (1992) Concern and confusion over competence. Critical Care Nurse 12: 9-11.
Ashworth J, Saxton J (1990) On competence. Journal Further and Higher Education 14: 3-25.
Ashworth P (1992) Being competent and having 'competencies'. Journal of Further and Higher Education 16: 8-17.
Ashworth PD, Morrison P (1991) Some problems of competence-based nurse education. Nurse Education Today 11: 25-260.
Benner P (1984) From Novice to Expert: Excellence and power in clinical nursing. Menlo Park, CA: Addison Wesley.

Boak G (1997–98) Benchmarks for competency models. Competency 5: 24–28.

Bradshaw A (1997a) Defining 'competency' in nursing (Part I): a policy review. Journal of Clinical Nursing 6: 347–354.

Bradshaw A (1997b) Defining 'competency' in nursing (Part II): an analytical review. Journal of Clinical Nursing 7: 103–111.

Bradshaw A (2000) Editorial. Journal of Clinical Nursing 9: 319–20.

Burns N, Grove SK (1997) The Practice of Nursing Research: Conduct, critique and utilisation, 3rd edn. Philadelphia: WB Saunders.

Butterfield PG (1988) Nominal group process as an instructional method with novice community health nursing students. Public Health Nursing 5: 12–15.

Carper B (1978) Fundamental patterns of knowing in nursing. Advances in Nursing Science 1: 13–33.

Carney O, McIntosh J, Worth A (1996) The use of the nominal group technique in research with community nurses. Journal of Advanced Nursing 23: 1024–1029.

Chambers M (1994) Information technology in the curriculum. In: Wainwright P (ed.), Nursing Informatics. Edinburgh: Churchill Livingstone, pp. 139–158.

Chambers M (1998) Some issues in the assessment of clinical practice: a review of the literature. Journal of Clinical Nursing 7: 201–208.

Clafin N (1997) A practical approach to competency assessment. Journal for Healthcare Quality 19(6): 12–18.

Coates O, Chambers M (1992) Evaluation tools to assess clinical competence. Nurse Education Today 12: 122–129.

Coit Butler FC (1978) The concept of competence: an operational definition. Educational Technology 18: 7–18.

Ellis R (1988) Professional Competence and Quality Assurance in the Caring Professions. London: Chapman & Hall.

Eraut M (1994) Concepts of competence and their implications In: Eraut M (ed.), Developing Professional Knowledge and Competence. London: The Falmer Press, pp. 163–198.

Eraut M (1998) Concepts of competence. Journal of Interprofessional Care 12: 127–139.

Flintman V (1997) Competencies – or is it competences? British Journal of Health Care Management 3: 228.

Gallagher M, Hares T, Spencer J, Bradshaw C, Webb I (1993) The nominal group technique: a research tool for general practice. Family Practice 10: 76–81.

Gerrish K, McManus M, Ashworth P (1997) Levels of Achievement: A review of the assessment of practice. London: English National Board for Nursing, Midwifery and Health Visiting.

Gibson F, Soanes L (2000) The development of clinical competencies for use on a paediatric oncology nursing course using a Nominal Group Technique. Journal of Clinical Nursing 9: 459–469.

Girot EA (1993) Assessment of competence in clinical practice: a phenomenological approach. Journal of Advanced Nursing 18: 114–119.

Gurvis JP, Grey MT (1995) The anatomy of competency. Journal of Nursing Staff Development 11: 247–252.

Hager P, Gonczi A, Athanasou J (1994) General issues about assessment of competence. Assessment and Evaluation in Higher Education 19: 3–16.

Hall RS (1983) The nominal group technique for planning and problem solving. Journal of Biocommunication 10: 24–27.

Henfield V, Waldron R (1988) The use of competency statements to facilitate individualised learning. Nurse Education Today 8: 205–211.

Hogston R (1993) From competent novice to competent expert: a discussion of competence in the light of the post registration and practice project [PREPP]. (Some reference to work of Patricia Benner and use of professional portfolios.) Nurse Education Today 13: 167–171.

Le Var RMH (1996) NVQs in nursing, midwifery and health visiting: a question of assessment and learning. Nurse Education Today 16: 85–93.

Long T, Hale C, Sanderson L, Tomlinson P, Tovey P (2001) An evaluation of educational preparation for cancer and palliative care nursing for children and adolescents. Research report to the DoH.

Lillyman S (1998) Assessing competence. In: Castledine G, McGee P (eds), Advanced and Specialist Nursing Practice. Oxford: Blackwell Science, pp. 119–131.

McMurray AR (1994) Three decision-making aids: Brainstorming, nominal group technique and Delphi technique. Journal of Nursing Staff Development 10: 62–65.

Miles MB, Huberman AM (1994) Qualitative Data Analysis, 2nd edn. Thousand Oaks, CA: Sage Publications.

Milligan F (1998) Defining and assessing competence: the distraction of outcomes and the importance of educational process. Nurse Education Today 18: 273–280.

Moore CM (1987) Nominal group technique. In: Group Techniques for Idea Building. Newbury Park: Sage, pp. 24–38.

Morin Robinson S, Barberis-Ryan C (1995) Competency assessment: a systematic approach. Nursing Management 26: 40–44.

Nagelsmith L (1995) Competence: an evolving concept. Journal of Continuing Education in Nursing 26: 245–248.

Nicol MJ, Fox-Hiley A, Bavin CJ, Sheng R (1996) Assessment of clinical and communication skills: operationalizing Benner's model. Nurse Education Today 16: 175–179.

O'Neil M (1981) Nominal group technique: an evaluation data collection process. Evaluation Newsletter 5: 44–60.

O'Neil MJ, Jackson L (1983) Nominal group technique: a process for initiating curriculum development in higher education. Studies in Higher Education 8: 129–138.

Percival E, Anderson M, Lawson D (1994) Assessing beginning level competencies: the first step in continuing education. Journal of Continuing Education in Nursing 25: 139–142.

Ross M, Carroll G, Knight J (1988) Using the OSCE to measure clinical skills performance in nursing. Journal of Advanced Nursing 13: 45–56.

Schon, DA (1991) The Reflective Practitioner: How professionals think in action. Aldershot: Arena.

Scott D, Deadrick D (1982) The nominal group technique: applications for training needs assessment. Training and Development Journal June: 26–33.

Sharp KJ, Wilcock SE, Sharp DMM, MacDonald H (1995) A Literature Review on Competence to Practise. Scotland: National Board for Nursing, Midwifery and Health Visiting for Scotland.

Short EC (1984) Competence re-examined. Educational Theory 34: 201–207.

Squier RW (1981) The reliability and validity of rating scales in assessing the clinical progress of psychiatric nursing students. International Journal of Nursing Studies 18: 157–169.

Thomas B (1983) Using nominal group technique to identify researchable problems. Journal of Nursing Education 22: 335–337.

United Kingdom Central Council for Nursing, Midwifery and Health Visiting (1986) Project 2000: A new preparation for practice. London: UKCC.

United Kingdom Central Council for Nursing, Midwifery and Health Visiting (1989) Exercising Accountability. London: UKCC.

United Kingdom Central Council for Nursing, Midwifery and Health Visiting (1992) Code of professional Conduct for the Nurse, Midwife and Health Visitor. London: UKCC.

United Kingdom Central Council for Nursing, Midwifery and Health Visiting (1996) Guidelines for Professional Practice. London: UKCC.

United Kingdom Central Council for Nursing, Midwifery and Health Visiting (1998) The Scope of Professional Practice. London: UKCC.

United Kingdom Central Council for Nursing, Midwifery and Health Visiting (1999) Fitness for Practice: The UKCC Commission for Nursing and Midwifery Education. London: UKCC.

United Kingdom Central Council for Nursing, Midwifery and Health Visiting (2001) Fitness for Practice and Purpose; The report of the UKCC's Post-Commission Development Group. London: UKCC.

Van de Ven AH, Delbecq AL (1972) The nominal group as a research instrument for exploratory health studies. American Journal of Public Health 69: 337-342.

Watkins MJ (2000) Competency for nursing practice. Journal of Advanced Nursing 9: 338-346.

While A (1994) Competence versus performance: which is more important? Journal of Advanced Nursing 20: 525-531.

Wilson J (1997-98) National standards and qualifications - 'the failure of a revolution'? Competency 5: 31-36.

Wooley AS (1977) The long and tortured history of clinical evaluation. Nursing Outlook 25: 308-315.

Chapter 5

PEACE: paediatric education, active contribution, evolution

Julianne Hall, Wilma Stuart and Louise Soanes

The purpose of this chapter is to share the development and evaluation of the Graduate Certificate in Paediatric Palliative Care (GCPPC) developed at Auckland University of Technology, Auckland, New Zealand. At the time this programme was developed it was the only post-registration programme specifically providing education for paediatric palliative care nurses in the world.

About 30% of all children diagnosed with cancer in New Zealand will die of their disease, accounting for 40% of all non-accidental and sudden paediatric deaths (Horsburgh et al., 2002). The remaining numbers are the result of neonatal deaths and children dying from neurodegenerative disorders. Statistics indicate that the number of children requiring paediatric palliative care is approximately 6 children per 50 000 (Ministry of Health, 1997) similar to figures in the United Kingdom (Association for Children with Life-Threatening or Terminal Conditions and Royal College of Paediatrics and Child Health, 1997). This small population, in a country of similar size to the UK, means that the lived experience of nurses caring for children in the palliative phase of cancer or other chronic illnesses is limited and infrequent. Research outlining families' experiences of caring for their dying child at home does not exist in New Zealand so, during the programme, parents were invited to tell their story to the students. This forum exposed students to the expert knowledge of parents and, in hearing their stories first hand, this had an impact on the developing practice of the students. The challenge to provide a paediatric palliative care education programme in New Zealand relates to the sparseness of the population. Four million people live in New Zealand, 35% of whom live in Auckland; many of the remaining population live in isolated rural of parts of the country.

New Zealand has similar health-funding issues as countries in the Western World. Professional bodies and consumers now demand that healthcare providers demonstrate competence and accountability in service delivery. This includes those nurses providing paediatric palliative care, particularly in the home setting, and those providing respite care. The aim of the programme was to develop a group of nurses with the ability to provide care based on evidence and justify their decisions based on knowledge, skill, clinical reasoning and problem-solving. The development of these skills was measured through assessment points in both the theoretical and practice papers of the programme, in which students were obliged to demonstrate reflective and critical thinking in the analysis of their practice, with the aim of encouraging the application of evidence-based care.

The development of this education programme was timely with the New Zealand's specialist paediatric services review being published shortly before the programme began. This review identified the need to provide a paediatric palliative care service in New Zealand. Paediatric palliative care contracts existed in Auckland, Otago and Dunedin (Horsburgh et al., 2000), providing a service for each of the islands. The regional oncology units in Auckland, Wellington and Christchurch also delivered some palliative care locally. The proposed national model of paediatric palliative care to be developed in negotiation with primary paediatric providers saw paediatric community nurses, working alongside general practitioners, providing a home-based service for children and their families; such a service had already been established in both Dunedin and Northland before the development of a national service in Auckland. Although still in its embryonic phase, the GCPPC programme has given students insight and the opportunity to be proactive in the development of a service to meet the needs of children and families living in New Zealand.

The philosophy underpinning the development of this programme was the child's continued presence with the family in the home, who with the support and assistance from appropriately educated and skilled health professionals could primarily care for the child, acknowledging that there are occasions when time away from home is preferable for either the child or family. Ultimately it remains the decision of the child and the family as to where the child is cared for in the final months, weeks, days or hours of his or her life, and the family must not be judged for their choice (Goldman and Baum, 1998). Some families in New Zealand choose to return to a familiar hospital ward where they feel confident and secure in the terminal stage. Hospital protocols should be flexible enough to allow prompt readmission and support of all the members of the family who want to stay with the child, although in practice this may at times be challenging to achieve in acute areas.

Resources to develop this programme were available as a result of the foresight of the National Executive of the Child Cancer Foundation (NZ),

Inc., New Zealand and the commitment to the programme from the School of Nursing and Midwifery, Auckland University of Technology. The Child Cancer Foundation (NZ), Inc. has a high profile in New Zealand; this organization raises substantial amounts of money for children with cancer and their families, although previously only a minimal amount of these funds had been used to support children dying from cancer. In financially supporting the development of the GCPPC, the Child Cancer Foundation (NZ), Inc. was able to promote the opportunity for New Zealand children to die at home, with care provided by specialty-educated nurses. The programme attracted 15 students who were scattered between Otago and Northland, the two extremes of New Zealand. Long distance learning, block courses on campus and self-directed learning were used to limit the costs of more frequent travel to Auckland, and to ensure that the programme was financially possible for prospective students.

The lack of an identified nursing or medical specialist in paediatric palliative care in New Zealand meant that advice and support in the initial stages of the programme was sought from abroad. Anne Goldman, Consultant in Paediatric Palliative Care, Great Ormond Street Hospital for Children NHS Trust, London was invited to facilitate a series of lectures and workshops on the first block course. She was quickly able to identify the experience within the group and promoted an environment of shared learning in partnership with the students to ensure that their needs were met. Although enabled by Anne's expertise and the students' motivation, this was challenging at times because the student's individual areas of nursing practice varied.

Theoretical assessment of the programme involved three papers: two theoretical papers on the bioscience and nursing knowledge to support the development of paediatric palliative care practitioners and a final paper, the specialty practice paper, which included content identified by the students during their first semester. Pain management, alternative therapies and supervisory counselling were the main threads. Skills incorporating imagery, massage, art therapy, and group supervision were also introduced. Self-reflection and professional reflection were encouraged as a process of learning. The students were also required to develop an educational package focused on palliative care which they designed to be used in their area of practice. Students shared these and they were encouraged to use each other's packages in their own areas of clinical practice if and when appropriate. These packages varied and included brochures, referral data for units and the development of protocols for practice. The students themselves had mastered a variety of clinical skills in their own fields of practice, which they presented to others; this extended their confidence in teaching and extended their colleagues' exposure to interventions available in paediatric palliative care.

At the completion of the programme the programme coordinators informally interviewed the students. Two questions were used to focus the interviews, these were:

1. Had learning gained on the programme altered their practice?
2. Did they now view caring for a dying child differently?

Analysis of the data from the taped interviews identified some common themes from the students' experience of the course:

- Students now have a greater understanding of the theory underlying paediatric palliative care nursing practice.
- A greater understanding of the rationale behind paediatric palliative nursing care has allowed some students to develop guidelines and operational standards back in their working environment.
- Adult nurses caring for children have increased their understanding of a child's cognitive development of health, illness, dying and death; this has had an impact not only on the care provided to the affected child but also on their well brothers and sisters.
- Learning from the programme has given students the confidence to share new knowledge with others, in both formal and informal educational settings, to educate and support different units in providing appropriate care to the child and his or her family.
- It was important to maintain a national programme for the discipline of nursing, and to incorporate the interdisciplinary health professionals into the learning rather than an interdisciplinary programme. This provided the opportunity to develop and refine their role in paediatric palliative care.
- Nurses report greater confidence in working with the multiprofessional team since completing the programme; again this was reported to reflect greater understanding of paediatric palliative care and the rationale behind it.
- Principles of practice gained on the programme have been extended to other areas of practice, namely children and families at the time of relapse, during bone marrow transplantation, respite care and for children of adults with cancer.
- Universally the nurses agree that the programme has given them the confidence to advocate for families to ensure that their children receive palliative care appropriate to their individual needs using a family-centred approach.

The benefits of the programme to nurses remain evident through feedback from nurses who undertook the programme; this is illustrated by the following two case studies.

One nurse working in a geographically isolated area of the country, often travelling great distances to see each patient, was primarily employed as an adult oncology/palliative care nurse but had sporadic numbers of children in her caseload. She is now used as a resource in paediatric palliative care for the paediatric ward in the hospital as well as coordinating and providing comprehensive, developmentally appropriate palliative care for children with varying conditions.

Another nurse, working in a recently opened paediatric neurological services unit, gained confidence in advocating for palliative care based on principles taught in the programme within a busy acute setting. Although acknowledging that ideally some of these children could be cared for at home, she has found it satisfying that through her efforts good palliative care has been provided in the hospital setting. In turn, as a result of her efforts, this has led to other nurses in the unit giving more thought to providing palliative care within the paediatric hospital setting and how the principles of paediatric palliative care can be applied.

Although the focus and belief is that dying children should be cared for at home, it remains clear that a hospice, in its broadest sense, can have an important role to play in the provision of shared care with community-based paediatric nurses. The programme has sought to build bridges between the two providers of care through the sharing of knowledge and expertise, each building on each other's strengths with the development of a strong bond and a resulting network of those who completed the GCPPC. Hospice services were identified as important providers of care for children, but within these organizations there needed to be development of the knowledge required to nurse children. A nurse employed by a hospice service found that the programme gave her insight into the behaviours of the child and siblings' concepts of illness and death, and was further able to use this when caring for children who have a dying parent. She also valued the inclusion of the concept of family-centred care new to her as an adult nurse – which further built on the philosophies of care within the hospice service. She came to appreciate that children were not just miniature adults and, as a result of undertaking the programme, was instrumental in the advent of a child-friendly room within the hospice for siblings and visiting children. The main reason that children are admitted to hospices or hospice programmes tends to be to offer respite care to families caring for children with ongoing deteriorating neurological conditions, rather than children dying of cancer (Herd, 1990; Hill, 1990; Hunt, 1990). Belasco et al. (2000) support the view of the Child Cancer Foundation (NZ), Inc. in their belief that that there is no need for children to be nursed in the palliative phase of their disease anywhere other than home. Both acknowledge that the partnership between health professionals and family to provide technological interventions in the home assures a quality of life for the child in the palliative phase. The development of nursing knowledge and skills is recognized as a need to support and acknowledge the preference of families.

The special needs of adolescents were also addressed and debated within the programme. The nurses recognized that adolescents were no longer children but were struggling to gain independence at a time when they often needed more help than they would care to admit to. Adolescents were usually cared for within paediatric units and by paediatric nurses in the community, but sometimes in adult wards or by adult-focused district nurses in the community, with little recognition given to their special needs. Each of the students agreed that little was being done for dying teenagers and they tended to fall between services, but that they deserved recognition of their individual status as adolescents; as a result of the programme the students were more aware of their needs. This would appear to be an area for development in future programmes.

Conclusion

Nursing the child at home was the focus of the programme; however, it was acknowledged that for some families the need to be within a supportive hospital or hospice environment was inevitable. New Zealand, to our knowledge, is one of the few countries to provide a programme to educate only nurses in paediatric palliative care; others are multidisciplinary. Those nurses who participated in the programme later supported this decision.

The philosophy of family-centred care underpinned the programme which had been developed to enhance the provision of care when a child is dying. The expertise of Anne Goldman provided benefits to both the medical and the nursing professions in New Zealand, as we developed a paediatric focus to provide the expert knowledge and define the differences in caring for children compared with adults in the palliative phase of their illness. The other experts in paediatric palliative care, without whom this programme would not have been such a success, were the parents who told their stories.

The students' evaluation of the programme, and how the programme has supported their ongoing practice, have highlighted that nursing a dying child requires an experienced educated practitioner to cope with the complexities that occur. Fifteen nurses with this ability may not seem to be many, but in New Zealand these nurses now have the power to work with families and be an advocate for them in the provision of healthcare that meets the family's individual needs.

The insight and drive of the Child Cancer Foundation (NZ), Inc., led by Kay Morris, has been proactive in promoting the education and service needs of nurses and families in New Zealand, for some time now. As a result competent palliative care for the child is now available in many areas of the country. The provision of further education in this specialty area relies on the response of healthcare services and the drive of paediatric and community nurse practitioners to participate in the programme.

References

Association for Children with Life-Threatening or Terminal Conditions and Royal College of Paediatrics and Child Health (1997) A Guide to the Development of Children's Palliative Care Services. Royal College of Paediatrics and Child Health.

Belasco J ,Danz P, Drill A, Schmid W, Burkey E (2000) Supportive care: palliative care in children, adolescents and young adults- model of care interventions and cost of care: a retrospective view. Journal of Palliative Care 16: 39-48.

Goldman A, Baum D (1998) Care of the dying child. In: Goldman A (ed.), Provision of Care, 2nd edn. Oxford: Oxford Medical Publications, pp. 107-114.

Herd E (1990) Helen house. In: Baum J, Dominica F, Woodward R (eds), Listen My Child has a Lot of Living to Do. Oxford: Oxford University Press, pp 49-54.

Horsburgh M, Trenholme A, Huckle T (2002) Paediatric Respite Care: a literature review from New Zealand. Palliative Medicine 16: 99-105.

Horsburgh M, Trenholme A, Nichols J, Noonan M, Bycroft K, Fa'alau F (2000) Respite Provision for Children Who are Dying and Their Families. Auckland, New Zealand: Division of Nursing, University of Auckland.

Hill L (1990) Martin house. In: Baum J, Dominica F, Woodward R (eds), Listen My Child has a Lot of Living to Do. Oxford: Oxford University Press, pp. 55-60.

Hunt A (1990) A survey of signs, symptoms and symptom control in thirty terminally ill children. Developmental Medicine and Child Neurology 32: 222-226.

Ministry of Health (1997) Morbidity and Mortality Data. Auckland: Ministry of Health.

Chapter 6

Developing roles in paediatric oncology: a case study

Monica Hopkins and Karen Selwood

A document of the United Kingdom Central Council for Nursing, Midwifery and Health Visiting (UKCC, 1994) supports the idea of advancement of nursing practice through narrowing the field of expertise in order to refine the quality of nursing care. Authors such as Autar (1996) advocated a ground-breaking practitioner who would push back the boundaries of practice, especially in a climate where medical nursing boundaries are blurring. However, Smith (1995) strongly asserts that advanced practice has not been developed to fill a gap in medical care, which is a common fear in the UK with the reduction in junior doctors' hours (Bull and Anderson, 1991; Gee, 1996). Rather advanced practice will fulfil an unmet need in healthcare of a nursing practice that medicine will not and cannot ever meet with its philosophy. This gap should be the holistic assessment of patient experience, knowledgeable advocacy and the seeking of patient-controlled measures of health maintenance (Smith, 1995). This chapter examines the development of advanced nursing practice in paediatric oncology within a regional unit.

National perspective

The development of expert clinical nursing roles has been a topic for debate over the last 10 years. In many areas of nursing they have evolved in a haphazard fashion (Gibson and Hooker, 1999), often reflecting the needs of the local service with little guidance from a national perspective.

The actual concept of advanced nursing practice is increasingly debated at all levels of the health service in the drive to encourage expert nurses to remain at the bedside and promote evidence-based and coordinated care (Castledine, 1991; Manley, 1993). The central principle of advanced nursing practice is to enhance the quality and effectiveness of care, by using expert nursing skills to assess, plan and initiate a whole programme of multidisciplinary care for a defined patient population (Sutton and Smith, 1995).

At the time of our appointment there was indeed growing concern within the literature that so-called advanced practice roles were developing nationally in no fixed context, with little parity across roles, education or responsibilities (Cahill, 1996; Ashburner et al., 1997; Hicks and Hennesey, 1999). Indeed Ashburner et al. (1997) demonstrated that there appeared to be little or no common understanding of the role requirements, and in consequence roles were emerging with no prerequisite qualification or skills for holders.

The educational response was equally as haphazard. The Royal College of Nursing in 1990, had begun the development of a course that followed the model espoused by Barbara Stillwell (1982), i.e. focusing on primary care and firmly in the adult field of practice. Alternative courses were being developed, however, with the acute sector care in mind and, in some cases, a paediatric focus (Brown, 1995). Unfortunately, with little guidance or leadership from the UK professional bodies, courses were often a loose amalgamation of an American model adapted to fit a local services management wish list for a single practitioner to meet the ever-present gaping holes in a so-called effective service (Gibson and Hooker, 1999).

In addition to these problems there was great confusion with respect to the difference between advanced nurse practitioners (ANPs) and clinical nurse specialists (CNSs). The situation is still perplexing; however, levels of educational preparation may now reflect some of the differences in the ANP and CNS roles. The CNS will in future be required to hold a first degree to demonstrate analytical thinking, and it is hoped to facilitate research skills and analysis of evidence to determine good practice (Brown, 1995; Fulbrook, 1996; McGee et al., 1996; UKCC, 1996). It is argued that the ANP requires preparation to Masters level to synthesize new nursing knowledge, to increase expertise in research, and to facilitate the utilization of theory to guide practice in the absence of scientific fact (UKCC, 1994; Fulbrook, 1996).

With specific regard to advanced nursing practice in paediatric oncology, even in the USA limited literature on the concept is available. Indeed advanced practice is considered to be an umbrella term given to a registered nurse who has met advanced educational and practice requirements, usually at the Master's level (American Nurses Association, 1993). Possible advantages and political implications of advanced practice roles are documented (Ackerman et al., 1996). The recurring themes in descriptions of such roles are: independent research, advanced autonomous clinical practice, education and case management with an emphasis on pioneering and innovative practice (Elliott, 1995; Gaedeke and Blount, 1995; Berger et al., 1996; Castledine, 1996). Literature on the scope and levels of practice evident in the UK is increasing (Manley, 1997; Torn and McNichol, 1998); however, paediatric practice is as yet under-defined and under-developed.

UKCC response

In 1992, the UKCC released the *Scope of Professional Practice*, which was intended to pave the way for advanced practice but failed in the clarification of such roles and requisite education for them. A year later, the UKCC (1993) maintained that advanced practice should demonstrate higher levels of judgement using a more extensive and varied knowledge base for practice. These judgements should be made to improve patient outcome even when at variance with current practice.

However, in 1994, they produced a document of post-registration and practice, which appeared to be a U-turn in policy because it seemed to reject the nurse practitioner title as ambiguous and even misleading. Although the desire for registration of such roles was dwindling, perhaps in realization of the difficulties inherent in developing a robust assessment strategy, there was still a move for academic preparation to Master's level to define advanced nursing practice. However, indicative content for such courses was not forthcoming (Salussolia, 1997). There is no national framework for course validation and as yet no formalized criteria for evaluation of educational outcomes.

In 1995, the UKCC admitted that there were grave reservations about ascribing a nurse an advanced practitioner based on an academic course alone, so evidence of clinical expertise to an advanced level would have to be ascertained. This was perhaps the prompt for the consultation and final pilot project to develop a structure for a registrable higher level of practice accreditation (UKCC, 1998). There was, and unfortunately still is, no regulation of practice and therefore little public or indeed professional protection.

In such a climate, practitioners must strive to demonstrate clearly their philosophy, preparation, objectives and fitness for practice, in the absence of professional frameworks, or risk losing the momentum on this valuable opportunity. Perhaps it could be proposed that advanced practice should be the response of nursing to meet and collaborate with medicine in order to breech the gap in healthcare; by seeking to meet medicine, however, there is inevitably going to be an overlap in skills and knowledge. This sounds extremely risky in such a previously tightly regulated profession, with grading often closely defining responsibilities and practice, and indeed the recent foray into graded competencies.

Patterson and Haddad (1992) describe the ANPs as visionaries who push the boundaries of practice. These boundaries are the professionally agreed nursing interventions, which have become increasingly vague as nursing responds to service need. This has made national professional agreement almost impossible, so locally agreed competencies for nurses have become more and more prevalent. They propose that uncertainties and new experiences embraced by these practitioners are excellent opportunities for growth and development. They are not advocating that all practice be based on intuition, but rather on the use of experience, knowledge of the client and understanding of the client experience in total, as well as fundamental knowledge about the biological, social and psychological aspects of care and health. This would allow knowledgeable decisions to be made in the best interests of the client, and not unfounded risks, but calculated ones, similar to those taken in medicine. Davies and Hughes (1995) argue that breaking down the advanced practice role into skills and responsibilities for analysis loses the essence of the role that is more than the sum of the parts, i.e. the practitioners' philosophy is the essence that binds all subroles together and enhances it. Therefore, discussion on the overlap or poaching of skills is inappropriate because the role is so diverse in skills and indeed the role is so much more than the sum of the skills.

For all those who regard advanced nursing practice as an exciting development, however, criticism also abounds. In particular there is a repeated suggestion that ANPs are in danger of becoming pseudo-medics and that this role may aim to replace junior doctors (Castledine, 1995; Dowling et al., 1995). The description favoured by this Trust is that of practitioners performing complementary roles to solve complex patient-care issues (Ludder Jackson, 1995). However, it is conceded that the foreseen implication of changes in junior doctors' training, as outlined in the Calman report, did have a major part in raising the issue of an expert nurse managing care in the oncology setting (Department of Health, 1993).

Why these roles were wanted/needed in Alder Hey Hospital, Liverpool

Continuity of care between caring disciplines has long been recognized as being pivotal in the care of many diseases that have a chronic element (Beddar and Aikin, 1994; Lipman and Deatrick, 1994). However, as a result of increasingly complex treatment protocols and changes in medical staff working practices, this concept as a standard of care had been eroded and a gap in the service had developed for several reasons. National protocols form the basis of the management of children with a malignancy, but the 3- or 6-month rotation in which medical staff partake limits the depth of knowledge that they are able to gain. The production of the 'New Deal' hours of working for medical staff has further decreased their time for exposure to the clinical management of oncology patients (NHS Management Executive, 1991). In addition, oncology is one of the most unpopular rotations because trainee medical staff perceive it as having one of the heaviest workloads within the trust, and for some the experience can be very emotionally draining.

Communication between nursing and medical staff had also been limited as a result of the lack of experience that some of the medical staff had in such a multidisciplinary specialty. This, in turn, had repercussions on some aspects of the service for the child and family at this difficult time. Families were frequently seen by different junior medical staff at each visit to the unit, leading to repeated questioning about their past history, poor symptom management experience and lack of understanding of all their needs in the present admission. Experienced nurses were anxious to advocate for the children and families in their care, but unfortunately inexperienced medical staff were not always able to recognize the value of these opinions. Limited understanding of each other's roles and experiences also caused frustration and exacerbated the communication problems.

These difficulties led to a situation in which there was limited development of junior nursing staff, with the more experienced nurses using all their skills to maintain communication and advocate for the child and family. There was insufficient practice supervision and specialist education being led by the nursing team.

A feeling of frustration and anxiety had slowly suffused into the unit by 1995. This appeared to indicate that this highly specialized branch of paediatrics, which demands considerable background knowledge by all members of the caring team, was struggling through lack of interdisciplinary supervision, clinical support, practice development, and a coordinated approach to the long-term therapeutic care of complex child and family needs.

The need to address some of these issues quickly was fuelled by an ever-increasing demand on all disciplines, especially nursing, to produce a high standard of care with no increase in the resources. Mindful of risk management concerns, senior nurses felt that the situation was becoming unacceptable, and a proactive strategy was required.

By means of a focused group, including representatives of the main therapeutic disciplines, a detailed review of the service was conducted with training and practice needs for all staff included. A number of issues were identified as outlined above and discussion continued as to how they could be tackled. The need for experienced practitioners with the skills to address some of the most pressing problems was evident. When these needs and attendant skills were analysed further by nursing managers and the lead consultant, it was felt that senior oncology nurses could fulfil most of those required because they could offer the unit clinically expert practice and work towards enhancing communication between all disciplines and the child and family. It was also felt that, with the development of nurse practitioner/clinician courses in the UK, they could undertake the coordination and care of all children receiving chemotherapy. This would require the ability to conduct indepth health assessments before each admission and coordinate protocol investigations for effective side-effect surveillance.

It was therefore decided that the most appropriate professional to carry service demands forward would be an experienced paediatric oncology nurse who could enhance patient care. This could be achieved by case managing the predominantly protocol-driven treatment for these children and their families, and so unite fragmented elements of care and members of the team in one person, as a coordinator and manager (Campbell et al., 1995). This role outline fitted with the trust's burgeoning policy of the development of nursing roles for practice development.

The introduction of this nursing role would also help with the ongoing development of nursing staff by increasing support in practice, education and development of research or evidence-based practice, not just by the practitioners but by involving all members of the nursing team.

How the roles developed in Liverpool, including preparation

Once it was agreed that the gap in the service would best be filled by advanced nurse practitioners, a job description was established that would specifically address some of the issues in promoting evidence-based care for the child and family. The enhanced clinical skills that would be needed by such practitioners to fulfil this role were also identified, as were their education and training needs.

The resultant job description, developed by the senior nurse of the unit, the clinical directorate manager and the consultant medical team for oncology, reflected an expert nurse who could carry out many of the clinical roles of a pre-registration house officer, combined with their existent expert paediatric oncology nursing knowledge. The role would include some previously medically dominated skills, such as clinical examination skills to recognize normal physical status, empowerment to assess patients as to whether they were fit for treatment, writing clinical notes, and pre-scribing defined treatments according to clinical guidelines that were well established.

This development was always proposed to supplement existing nursing roles and not replace it. There was no role at this time within the UK that met these specifications and there was no guidance on how this could be achieved from the UKCC. To take this forward, a decision was made that the practitioners would attend and complete a clinically based Master's in Advanced Nursing Practice at the University of Central England, com-bined with an inhouse clinical skills training programme. This particular course was chosen on the premise that it was the only one of its kind in 1996 that proposed to maintain a paediatric focus. The practical educa-tion would culminate in a clinical examination at the end of the course by two clinicians unknown to the individuals. Two posts were set up under the title advanced nurse practitioner (ANP). Two nurses would allow con-tinuity of ANP activity when one post-holder was on holiday, and allow comprehensive cover on 5 days per week, when chemotherapy admissions are scheduled.

Both ANPs undertook the Masters in Advanced Nursing Practice to ensure adequate preparation academically and practically for the role. The modules included analysis and evaluation of advanced practice, ethics, economics of healthcare, management theory, advanced health assessment and research. During the course, they were extensively tutored by the oncology medical team in clinical examination, surveillance monitoring, and the relative importance of specific clinical findings. These skills were practised for several months under supervision in Liverpool, before the formal practical assessment, arranged by the trust, was undertaken.

On reflection there were some concerns expressed by these two candi-dates about being among the first cohort of this ground-breaking course. They suffered from being the cohort in which all curriculum issues underwent trials and were adjusted; it was overwhelmingly theory orient-ed although it was marketed as a practice-based course, and practical teaching was minimal and then only by medical personnel. There was only a small paediatric focus although most of the cohort was from a child health background and so allowed focused discussions. Although it provided invaluable networking with other practitioners, it soon became obvious that they were the only two students with a job description, defined roles to return to, and an organized and agreed clinical placement with excellent clinical skills training.

Reality of the role

This role presented an enormous challenge to the nurses employed. It has been established but has constantly changed over the last 5 years and continues to change. There are four main areas that the role can be divided into but as in all nursing roles these are interlinked.

Advanced autonomous clinical practice

All children who attend the unit for routine chemotherapy come under the ANPs' care. This includes performing an advanced health assessment, which includes a full physical, social and emotional history on admission highlighting any new or ongoing problems. It also includes ensuring that their admission runs smoothly, with the relevant investigations performed at the appropriate times, and that their follow-up is coordinated and communicated to all relevant personnel. The pre-chemotherapy assessment was developed from a template used on the course, which was discussed and modified with practitioners from all disciplines to identify pertinent family and child information that would indicate fitness for therapy – physically, psychologically and socially. It would include data that professional carers felt should be re-evaluated and documented on each admission.

Most of the children assessed are cared for within the guidelines of a clinical trial and it is imperative that their care is documented clearly. This can be difficult with complicated protocols in which dose escalations, pulsed medications and changing drug interactions demand a thorough knowledge of the background to the protocol. Accurate surveillance of physical status, disease response and drug toxicity are also demanded during treatment, and the continuity of care received by these children and their families through seeing the same person on each admission enhances this. This, in turn, has significant implications for the safe administration of therapy and advancement of research or evidence-based knowledge as a result of the accuracy of the data collected and their use in risk management and plans of care. To this end, a multidisciplinary proforma has been developed by the ANPs which includes a clinical assessment, family status review and psychosocial/developmental assessment, as well as a plan of continuing care completed on each admission. All information on the proforma is designed in layout to be accessible and informative for other personnel to use and document their interventions, e.g. discharge documentation.

Children who present to the unit with a fever and neutropenia can also be assessed and admitted by the ANPs. The unit policy is that the child is seen by the first available healthcare professional – ANP or doctor – to ensure prompt assessment and start of treatment. Limited prescribing according to a protocol has been established through liaison with the pharmacist and consultants to enhance the clinical care of these children. It must be argued that, when a health assessment has taken place that identifies a health need that can be met by a drug, the person assessing the child should be able to prescribe the treatment. ANPs identify appropriate situations within which they can use their prescribing skills, but refer to a member of the medical staff if it is beyond their remit.

Education and clinical resource

The clinical resource and educator roles can be linked. Acting as a resource involves being available to assist all oncology staff and hospital personnel with issues concerning the care of the child with cancer. This is achieved by working with or being available to answer questions with members of the oncology team on a daily basis. Collaboration on care issues on ward rounds and nursing conferences also takes up a substantial amount of time because the regular contact with the child and family can bring different assessments and knowledge to these situations. The ultimate aim is to facilitate the development of expert nursing practice of all staff and to push their abilities forward in the development of practice. Since starting in post there has been a development of the chemotherapy training programme to ensure that staff have adequate knowledge to deal with this aspect of their daily work – all staff have now been through this programme and it is now used to update staff on specific issues.

Educational intervention initially included an analysis of the learning needs of the nursing staff, with identification of areas of clinical practice or knowledge that could be enhanced by further individual education and/or a rolling teaching programme. The organization of the teaching programme has now been taken over by the ward staff with input from the ANPs as required. Ongoing education has been established into the working week on the unit and is now recognized as an important area by all staff to ensure continued development. The recognition by the nursing team that all members have something to offer in this area is important and has helped develop self-esteem and confidence in their educational ability. One-to-one tutorials and bedside clinical supervision support are available from the ANPs. Some of these needs are highlighted by staff through the practice development sister, possibly linked to objectives on their personal development plans, and they can then make specific appointments with the ANP to cover this.

As in all roles the education perspective does not just stop on the ward with nursing staff. A more indepth orientation to the ward for junior medical staff has been established to try to ensure that they have grounding in the day-to-day issues on the ward. Regular teaching sessions for any professionals in oncology or nursing issues are offered within the trust.

Facilitation and support of staff undergoing further education at various levels are an important educational area that can be used.

Independent researcher

As nurse researchers, the focus is on the validation of current nursing practice as a benchmark for care and on the further advancement of practice for the specialty as a whole. Active nursing research and audit are the primary aim. Each of the ANPs has personal research interests that has led to initiatives in the development of evidence- and research-based integrated care pathways for children with febrile neutropenia, care of children with brain tumours and the care of children undergoing radiotherapy. The lead in this part of the role is also to help develop and guide other members of the team in areas of specific interest to develop credible research or audit. This role also extends into the trust as part of the wider remit of the roles.

Professional development

Professional development is an important part of any role in nursing. This includes positive networking at a local, national and international level with other paediatric oncology units and paediatric advanced nurse practitioners. However, it is also important to be involved in the development of nursing and enhancing practice generally within the hospital and on a wider scale, to help nurses push back the boundaries in enhancement of their profession. Recognition of the importance of national initiatives to examine practice is vital. Involvement in the Higher Level Practice Pilot has allowed feedback to the UKCC on possible assessment of nurses working at a higher level (UKCC, 1998).

Literature does make mention of the already blurred professional boundaries between many of the caring disciplines, especially medicine and nursing (MacAlister and Chiam, 1995; Nolan, 1995; Salvage, 1995; Jackson, 1996). Much was made of the possible conflict that may ensue if this was taken further by the cause undertaken. However, we found this to be misguided. The boundaries between our practice and that of our colleagues interlocks our specialist knowledge and experience meshed with the wider paediatric acute care knowledge of the junior medical staff, especially specialist registrars. The unexpected challenge has been ensuring that our clinical practice does not supersede or overshadow that of senior oncology nurses/primary nurses on the unit. Our assessment and interventions should aim to 'glue' medical and primary nurse intervention together, enhancing the practice of both.

Conference presentations and publication are also opportunities for professional development. This also includes the support and development of other professionals within the team to take this step forward.

Audit and evaluation of the role

Ongoing evaluation of both the development of the advanced practice role and the audit of its impact on the oncology unit is vital. Martin and Coniglio (1996) identified increased compliance with treatment, increased patient satisfaction, fewer delays, earlier discharges and decreased unplanned readmissions for those using such collaborative practice. Many of the positive developments in our own unit involve qualitative aspects of care, which are hard to measure. However, parental response has been positive although this is anecdotal. Some families have unfortunately been to the unit both before and after the development of the ANP role. These parents particularly approve of continuity of care, with the predictable contact of familiar personnel for chemotherapy admissions. Advice is more consistent as a result, supplied by the expanded knowledge held by the ANPs and shared with the nursing staff.

The post-holders feel that their appointments have contributed to positive outcomes in many of these areas, although the data to indicate this are still being gathered. The febrile neutropenia care pathway has significantly contributed to evaluation of the antibiotic guidelines and has led to greater compliance with a systematic approach to care as shown in the variance analysis.

Coordination of the child's care ensures minimal attendance at hospital by arranging as many investigations for one visit and by planning ahead, allowing precious time to be spent at home. Close liaison with various members of the multidisciplinary team allows chemotherapy admissions to be more effective in meeting the needs of the families in one episode of care.

An audit has recently been undertaken by the ANPs into the effectiveness of liaison and communication of care needs for shared care centres. This is the second audit in 3 years and indicates significant improvements in communication, with recommendations employed from the first audit having a positive effect. Telephone enquiries have always been documented and have fallen dramatically over the last 18 months. Nursing staff have also been positive about improved access to education and expert knowledge about the oncology patients, and this is now reflected in their lead in the education programme and the development of staff.

We continue to identify areas within the service where development is required. Our most recent priority has been nurse prescribing. The recent publication of the Crown Report has given valuable guidance on prescribing within protocols or guidelines, e.g. first-line antibiotics and antiemetics (Crown, 1999). Both practitioners are now able to prescribe these medications within therapeutic guidelines. Each ANP is what is termed 'a dependent prescriber'. Using clinical assessment to establish that a child, on examination, fits the inclusion criteria for such protocols, the nurses are able to instigate early and possibly more effective interventions, such as antibiotics within 30 minutes of arrival of a febrile child with post-chemotherapy neutropenia. There has been an audit to compare discharge prescriptions pre-ANP prescribing and post-ANP prescribing, and this has shown that ANPs can prescribe safely and accurately.

Where are the roles going now?

There is still great discussion in the UK about the development of nursing roles. With the introduction of the nurse consultant post and the career framework for nurses, midwives and health visitors that reflects nurse specialist and then nurse consultant role development, the question arises of where advanced nurse practitioners will 'fit in' (Department of Health, 1999). It is important that we are part of ongoing discussions of nursing development both within the trust and nationally, in order to have input into what may happen to nursing in the UK.

Locally there are still exciting developments to be undertaken. These include: the extension of integrated care pathways in paediatric oncology, establishment of evidence-based practice in the preparation and aftercare of children receiving radiotherapy, and nurse-led day care within the oncology department, with satellite clinics in the local radiotherapy unit. The ongoing discussions on nurse prescribing are also moving forward and more freedom within this role for enhancing our practice within our own competence would be exciting. There is also the ongoing challenge of facilitating experienced oncology nurses to consolidate expert practice and provision of excellence in clinical care, with patient and family assessment.

Changing the past

During the 5 years in post, there has been a steep learning curve that could rival any roller coaster. There are definitely some things that we would do differently if we had the chance, but, by reflecting on these areas and our development, plans for the future can be made. First, when starting a new role with so much expectation of problem resolution, it is almost irresistible to try to match some of these expectations and become involved in every aspect of care from day 1. Retrospectively, we feel that we would have set a more realistic agenda for growth areas and indeed for outcome. We would not seek to be all things to all people, which in fact just creates an atmosphere of dependence; it is never useful for any role to be indispensable within a well-constructed team. Rather, we would hope to enhance the nursing contribution to the service and the service as a whole through coordination and communication. We would aim to spend more energy enabling others to develop themselves and those around them, so that the service benefits from good practice and optimal communication whichever team members are present in a care situation. Consultancy should never narrow the development of those around it.

Second, our goal initially was to address qualitative issues within oncology care, and having such proactive management support within the unit we really did not stray into the rest of the trust for the first 2 years in post. This was probably both naïve and short-sighted. Actively engaging with other trust professional and management teams to participate in the construction of a trust-wide climate in improved clinical care is essential in improving the service offered to children with cancer and their families, as well as promoting the value of nursing across the trust.

We have often wondered whether, if our specialist interest group for advanced paediatric nursing practice had been set up even a few months earlier as a forum, it would have been a more robust candidate for voting membership of the paediatric society as a whole during the RCN organizational shake-up of the late 1990s.

Finally, it is a source of concern to us that a more robust audit/evaluation of the service as a whole was not carried out before we entered into post. It would have been extremely useful to have such data now to compare and contrast aspects of the service for the evaluation of both qualitative and quantitative outcomes in the current climate of clinical effectiveness and governance.

Conclusion

The establishment of two advanced nurse practitioner posts within the oncology unit of the RLC NHS Trust has been an innovative and positive development for paediatric oncology nursing. It has offered an ever-expanding challenge and potential for development both locally and nationally. The primary objectives for establishing these posts are being fulfilled. As a result, further challenges have appeared. As Davies and Hughes (1995) have commented:

> . . . in the oncology setting the advanced practitioner can maintain the child and family as the primary focus. They can continue to excel in complex practice situations and articulate and demonstrate how advanced nursing practice can make a difference.

Above all the approach to care of children with a malignancy has profited in efficiency and enhanced quality of care with the establishment of these posts in advanced nursing practice.

References

Ackerman MH, Norsen L, Martin B, Wiedrich J, Kitzman HJ (1996) Development of a model of advanced practice. American Journal of Critical Care 5: 68-73.

American Nurses Association (1993) Working Definition: Nurses in advanced clinical practice. Washington DC: American Nurses Association.

Ashburner L, Birch K, Latimer J, Scrivens E (1997) Defining role. Health Services Journal 107: 32-33.

Autar R (1996) The scope of professional practice in specialist practice. British Journal of Nursing 5: 984-989.

Beddar SM, Aikin JL (1994) Continuity of care: a challenge for ambulatory oncology nursing. Seminars in Oncology Nursing 10: 254-263.

Berger AM, Eilers JG, Pattrin L et al. (1996) Advanced practice roles for nurses in tomorrow's healthcare systems. Clinical Nurse Specialist 10: 250-255.

Brown R (1995) Education for specialist and advanced practice. British Journal of Nursing 4: 266-268.

Bull A, Anderson N (1991) Entering junior doctors duties. Nursing Standard 5: 41.

Cahill H (1996) Focus on specialist nursing: Role definition, nurse practitioner or clinicians assistant. British Journal of Nursing 5: 1382-1386.

Campbell ML, Brandel SM, Daramola OI et al. (1995). An advanced practice model: Inpatient collaborative practices. Clinical Nurse Specialist 9: 175-179.

Castledine G (1991) The advanced nurse practitioner. Nursing Standard 5: 34-37.

Castledine G (1995) Will the nurse practitioner be mini doctor or maxi nurse? British Journal of Nursing 4: 938-939.

Castledine G (1996) The role and criteria of an advanced nurse practitioner. British Journal of Nursing 5: 288-289.

Crown J (1999) Review of Prescribing, Supply and Administration of Medicines – Final Report. London: Department of Health.

Davies B, Hughes AM (1995) Clarification of advanced nursing practice: characteristics and competencies. Clinical Nurse Specialist 9: 156-160, 166.

Department of Health (1993) Hospital Doctors: Training for the Future. The Report of the Working Group on Specialist Medical Training. London: Health Publication Unit.

Department of Health (1999) Making a Difference. Strengthening the nursing midwifery and health visiting contribution to health and health care. London: DoH.

Dowling J, Barrett S, West R (1995) With nurse practitioners who needs house officers? British Medical Journal 311: 309-313.

Elliott PA (1995) The development of advanced nursing practice: 1. British Journal of Nursing 4: 633-636.

Fulbrook P (1996) Advanced practice: do we really know what it is? Nursing in Critical Care 1: 9-12.

Gaedeke MK, Blount K (1995) Advanced practice nursing in pediatric acute care. Critical Care Nursing Clinics of North America 7: 61-70.

Gee K (1996) Competency through being: the enemy within. British Journal of Nursing 4: 537-540.

Gibson F, Hooker L (1999) Defining a framework for advancing clinical practice in paediatric oncology nursing. European Journal of Nursing 3: 232-239.

Hicks C, Hennessey D (1999) A task based approach to defining the role of the nurse practitioner: the views of UK acute and primary sector nurses. Journal of Advanced Nursing 29: 666-673.

Jackson S (1996) The case for shared training for nurses and doctors. Nursing Times 92(26): 40-41.

Lipman TH, Deatrick JA (1994) Enhancing specialist practice for the next century. Journal of Nursing Education 33: 53-58.

Ludder Jackson P (1995) Advanced practice nursing part 2 – opportunities and challenges for PNPs. Pediatric Nursing 21: 43-46.

MacAlister L, Chiam M (1995) Why do nurses agree to take on doctors' roles? British Journal of Nursing 4: 1238-1239.

McGee P, Castledine G, Brown R (1996). A survey of specialist and advanced nursing practice in England. British Journal of Nursing 5: 682-686.

Manley K (1993) The clinical nurse specialist. Surgical Nurse 7: 21-24.

Manley K (1997) A conceptual framework for advanced practice: an action research project operationalizing an advanced practitioner/consultant nurse role. Journal of Clinical Nursing 6: 179-190.

Martin B, Coniglio J (1996) The acute care nurse practitioner in collaborative practice. AACN Clinical Issues 7: 309-314.

NHS Management Executive (1991) Junior Doctors: The New Deal. London: NHS Management Executive.

Nolan M (1995) Towards an ethos of interdisciplinary practice. British Medical Journal 311: 305-307.

Patterson C, Haddad B (1992) The advanced nurse practitioner; common attributes. Canadian Journal of Nursing Administration Nov/Dec: 18-22.

Salussolia M (1997) Specialist nursing. Is advanced nursing practice a post or a person? British Journal of Nursing 6: 928, 930-933.

Salvage J (1995) What's happening to nursing? British Medical Journal 311: 274-275.

Smith M (1995) The core of advanced nursing practice. Nursing Science Quarterly 8: 2-4

Stillwell B (1982) The nurse practitioner at work in primary care. Nursing Times 78: 1799-1803.

Sutton F, Smith C (1995) Advanced nursing practice: new ideas and perspectives. Journal of Advanced Nursing 21: 1037-1043.

Torn A, McNichol E (1998) A qualitative study utilizing a focus group to explore the role and concept of the nurse practitioner. Journal of Advanced Nursing 27: 1202-1211.

United Kingdom Central Council for Nursing, Midwifery and Health Visiting (1992) The Scope of Professional Practice. London: UKCC.

United Kingdom Central Council for Nursing, Midwifery and Health Visiting (1993) Post-registration Education and Training Report. London: UKCC.

United Kingdom Central Council for Nursing, Midwifery and Health Visiting (1994) The Future of Professional Practice - the Council's Standards for Education and Practice Following registration. London: UKCC.

United Kingdom Central Council for Nursing, Midwifery and Health Visiting (1995) Implementation of the UKCC's Standard for Post-registration Education and Practice (PREP). London: UKCC.

United Kingdom Central Council for Nursing, Midwifery and Health Visiting (1996) Transitional Arrangements - Specialist practitioner title/specialist qualification. London: UKCC.

United Kingdom Central Council for Nursing, Midwifery and Health Visiting (1998) A Higher Level of Practice Consultation Document. London: UKCC.

Part 2

Perspectives on the service

Janet Williss

With increasing demands being made upon the health service to modernize and continually improve (Department of Health or DoH, 1998, 1999, 2000a), there is a need for all staff who provide healthcare to analyse current positions, share their experiences, and seek to further the knowledge base that provides the evidence for practice. By sharing their experiences and findings with a wider population, the authors who have contributed to this book are supporting the modernization and improvement agendas.

The first three chapters of Part 2 focus on issues dealing with young people, the often forgotten group that falls between childhood and adulthood. It is encouraging to see this focus on adolescents, and is perhaps indicative of the level of interest within paediatric oncology nursing in the distinct needs of this group of patients. Later chapters deal with the issues of parents' experiences of shared care, a previously unexplored area, and the complex issue of identifying appropriate nurse staffing levels for paediatric oncology units.

In Chapter 7, Morgan and Hubber present an honest and personal account of the complexity of introducing a new approach to service delivery. Their descriptive account of the trials and successes experienced in establishing a teenage cancer unit and adolescent service offers support and encouragement to others seeking to go along the same path. They also offer guidance in highlighting some of the pitfalls in the process of initiating and maintaining a change.

As Morgan and Hubber state it is over 40 years since Platt (Ministry of Health, 1959) recommended the need to care for young people in separate hospital accommodation. It is distressing to note that, although some progress has been made, the Royal College of Paediatrics and Child Health (RCPCH, 2002) state that the 'care of adolescents needs much more attention' and that 'adolescent services cannot continue to languish'. Despite there being national standards for cancer treatment (DoH, 2000a) and the Tri Regional Process of Peer Review for Paediatric/Adolescent Oncology Centres (2001), the specific needs of adolescents and young people with cancer are not clearly identified.

A key message from this development is the importance of involving users of the service. Patient and public involvement is a major theme within the Government's agenda (DoH, 2001) and is one of the seven pillars of clinical governance identified by the Commission for Health Improvement (CHI, 2002). It is significant that the authors achieved a 74% response rate to their postal questionnaire from present and past users of the service, although they do not report the total numbers involved. It is probable that involving the public in developments will become a key factor in achieving support from commissioners in the future.

In Chapter 8, Shaw et al. deal with the specific issue of semen collection. Following a very useful overview of relevant literature, they conclude that it is an area that is almost universally overlooked. The authors identify four key reports on cancer care from the past 8 years, all citing the importance of offering uniform standards of care, but only one of which specifically identifies the need to enable young males with cancer to be offered the opportunity to retain their ability to procreate.

Without national guidelines or standards to support sperm cryopreservation and the associated counselling for this group of young people, the authors sought to undertake a survey to determine why the number of adolescent males offered cryopreservation services was so low. The results, while far from offering a full picture, are an indictment of the level of service offered and are illustrative of the unacceptable variations in care for young people within the UK. 'The receipt of high-quality care should not depend on the geographical accident of where the young person lives (DoH, 1998).

It may be that the position has changed since 1995, when this survey was conducted, but this is a field that is open for benchmarking throughout the 22 UKCCSG centres. Ellis (2001) described benchmarking as a of 'way of universalizing the best'. Taking best practice from those centres providing that level of care and using this to develop guidelines to support practice is an urgent requirement. It is hoped that the authors will take this work forward, possibly under the auspices of the UKCCSG.

The ability to procreate is an area of key importance to young people and their families but is an area that many nursing staff are ill equipped to deal with. There is an urgent need for training for all staff working in this field, to support their ability to communicate and support young males in this area. It needs to be built in as a core competency for medical and nursing staff. The RCPCH (2002) report that this is a long-standing issue and recommend that it is a matter for basic training for all health professionals.

Hooker takes forward the theme of young people with cancer in Chapter 9, this time focusing on the information needs of this group. A clear overview of the issues related to the care of adolescents and young people with cancer is presented, together with a critical evaluation of the literature from which she identifies key themes.

Using a card-sort game, Hooker explores the information needs of a small, convenient sample of young people. She identifies sixteen themes, which she classifies into four categories. Although recognizing that the results are not generalizable to the wider population, Hooker demonstrates that young people are not different from adults in the nature of the information they seek. It is very telling how perceptive young people are of the needs of others and their very mature responses to consideration of the impact of knowing, before asking the question. Knowledge is power and young people in this study clearly demonstrate that they want knowledge of their illness and treatment to be able to exert some control over events and their lives. The young people also indicated that they were concerned about planning for the future, suggesting that professionals need to avoid making assumptions made about this age group.

The discussion has relevance to all staff dealing with young people in any healthcare setting not just those with cancer, especially others with chronic illnesses. It again raises the issue of the development of core competencies across professional groups relating to communication.

Shared care has been a key feature of children's cancer care in some parts of the UK, mainly in the London region, for over 20 years. 'It is recognized that malignant disease is best treated under the supervision of a paediatric oncologist based on an increasing use of "shared care"' and that 'results for some malignancies are known to be better when treated this way' (RCPCH, 2002). The Bristol Royal Infirmary Inquiry noted that 'the requirements of quality and safety should prevail over considerations of ease of access' (2001).

In Chapter 10 Sepion considers the shared care approach to care delivery from the perspective of the parents and seeks to gain an understanding of their experience of shared care. She uses a phenomenological approach to her study, again with a small convenient sample of parents. Drawing out 21 themes from the data, Sepion condenses these into three 'focal meaning units'. She identifies particular difficulties for parents when they become more knowledgeable about their child's care and treatment than the local shared care teams. She cites how staff at local units find it difficult to develop and maintain their skills and knowledge, a point reinforced by the findings of a recent report, which highlighted that only 36% of nurses working with children with cancer have relevant specialist qualifications (Elston and Thornes, 2002).

The importance of involving users of the service in decisions about how services are delivered cannot be understated (DoH, 2001; CHI,

2002). In the recent process undertaken by the four Thames Paediatric Oncology Centres and the Paediatric Oncology Shared Care Units to review and rationalize the network, parents and children were not given the opportunity to contribute to the process. Shared care may indeed be the best approach for management of childhood cancers, but collaboration with users in planning these services for the future may ensure that support is planned and provided for parents to enable them to take on the parental adaptive tasks cited by Sepion.

In Chapter 11, Hollis and colleagues present the results of a benchmarking exercise that they undertook to establish actual staffing levels, patterns and differences in the 22 UKCCSG centres. This is a very timely piece of work. With the increased pressure from trusts to examine staffing levels and skill mix critically, paediatric oncology nursing is vulnerable. Although there is an urgent need to identify appropriate staffing levels, the work undertaken by Hollis and colleagues clearly illustrates the complexity of establishing meaningful comparators.

Paediatric oncology nursing would benefit from having a national framework similar to the paediatric intensive care framework (DoH, 1997) which established nationally agreed levels of care and associated staffing levels. There is support for this approach, with the Royal College of Pathologists (Clinical Standards Advisory Group, 1996) and the Tri Regional Standards for Paediatric Oncology (2001) recommending that 'one third of all paediatric oncology beds should be staffed to support high dependency patients' but the latter goes further in giving a specific ratio of 4.2 nurses per high dependency bed.

One aspect of this survey that was very worrying was that nurses did not have, or did not know how to access, information about occupancy. There is a need for clinical staff to work more closely with managers and to ensure that IT systems are accessible and support clinicians in their work.

Hollis and colleagues have undertaken a preliminary study that has raised a significant number of questions requiring further work, particularly in relation to several key variables. The authors refer to subsequent work in this area and it is to be hoped that they will be able to follow up their recommendations with further joint working between the UKCCSG and PONF.

In conclusion, it is clear that there are a number of common themes that are raised by the work of these authors. The first is that of leadership. Nurses within cancer care need to take on leadership roles, especially where frontline clinical services are provided (DoH, 2000b). Leadership is key to the Government agenda to modernize the health service generally and cancer services specifically (DoH, 1999, 2000b). Nurses are central to this. Strong nursing leadership is needed to drive forward multidisciplinary working, to improve quality and practice, to plan and commission services locally, and to provide effective management of clinical services. As nurse leaders develop their strategic thinking, they are able to influence agendas internally within trusts, but also in the wider community. By asking big questions, using influence, negotiation and persuasion at local and national levels, and by working together, nurses can and do make a difference. Those who have shared their experiences and work in this book will have influenced services locally and nationally.

The second theme to emerge is the need to develop communication skills across the disciplines. In recognition of the importance of effective communication, the Department of Health has developed two further patient-focused benchmarks: 'communication between carers and healthcare personnel' and 'communication between patients and healthcare personnel' (DoH, 2003). These benchmarks clearly express what patients and families want from healthcare personnel and, if used together with children, young people and families, should help teams work out where they are succeeding and where they could improve practice.

The third theme is that of patient and public involvement. We do not always know what is best for our patients and their families, and need to challenge assumptions more and involve users of services increasingly in determining how these services are provided.

A final thought, however, is a plea to nurses within the 22 UKCCSG centres to work together. Some of the studies discussed in this section are examples of small-scale studies. There is a need to develop collaborative working among the UKCCSG centres for further development of the body of knowledge and development of guidelines to inform practice. Paediatric oncology nurses need to develop collaborative research and comparative benchmarking to seek for continual improvement in the service delivered to children and young people with cancer. It is hoped that readers will be stimulated to participate or lead future studies and share the outcomes of their work, as the authors here have done.

References

Bristol Royal Infirmary Inquiry (2001) Learning from Bristol: the report of the public inquiry into children's heart surgery at the Bristol Royal Infirmary 1984-1995. Command paper CM 5207. Bristol Royal Infirmary Inquiry.

Clinical Standards Advisory Group (1996) Standards of Care for Children with Leukaemia. London: Royal College of Pathologists.

Commission for Health Improvement (2002) A Guide to Clinical Governance Reviews. Acute Trusts at www.chi.nhs.uk

Department of Health (1997) Paediatric Intensive Care. A framework for the future. London: HMSO.

Department of Health (1998) A First Class Service. Quality in the new NHS. London: The Stationery Office.

Department of Health (1999) Making a Difference. London: HMSO.

Department of Health (2000a) Improving the Quality of Cancer Services. London: HMSO.

Department of Health (2000b) The Nursing Contribution to Cancer Care. London: HMSO.

Department of Health (2001) Involving Patients and the Public in Healthcare. A Discussion Document. London: HMSO. www.doh.gov.uk/involvingpatients

Department of Health (2003) Essence of Care - Consultation on communication benchmarks. London: HMSO - www.doh.gov.uk/essenceofcare

Ellis J (2001) Benchmarking: A way of universalizing the best? NTResearch 6: 566-567.

Elston S, Thornes R (2002) Children's Nursing Workforce July 2002. A report to the Royal College of Nursing and the Royal College of Paediatrics and Child Health. London: RCN/RCPCH.

Ministry of Health (1959) The Welfare of Children in Hospital (The Platt Report). London: HMSO.

Royal College of Paediatrics and Child Health (2002) The Next Ten Years - Educating paediatricians for new roles in the 21st century. London: RCPCH.

Tri Regional Process of Peer Review for Paediatric/Adolescent Oncology Centres (2001) Manual of Cancer Services Assessment Standards (Paediatric 2001). London: NHS Executive. Regional Offices.

Chapter 7
Setting up an adolescent service
Sue Morgan and Diane Hubber

Teenagers and young people with cancer have complex needs, which have become more widely recognized over recent years; however, they remain a low priority on the national agenda. Cure is often achieved in this group of patients, but often at considerable cost in terms of treatment toxicity and disruption to their lives. The need for dedicated services for this patient group has been accepted, but the resource to meet that need is rarely identified. Adolescence can be a time of tension and uncertainty as the individual strives to achieve independence, establish an identity and plan for the future. A diagnosis of cancer at this critical time is devastating, and brings with it many difficulties for the patient, family and friends, and for healthcare professionals (Hollis and Morgan, 2001).

It is over 40 years since the Platt Report (1959) first recommended separate hospital accommodation for teenagers. Later work by the Expert Advisory Group on Cancer (Department of Health or DoH, 1995) stated that 'purchasers should look for opportunities for developing the treatment of adolescents with cancer'. The Report recognized the 'special medical and psychological problems' of these patients. The general principles governing this report are:

- access to a uniformly high quality of care
- education to help early recognition of cancer
- clear information to patients
- patient-centred services
- involvement of all sectors of the primary healthcare team
- recognition of the importance of psychosocial aspects
- support for cancer registration and careful monitoring of treatment outcomes.

However, in the current National Health Service Cancer Plan (DoH, 2000), there is no reference to teenagers and young people, although the

National Institute for Clinical Excellence (NICE) has been charged to develop plans for future inclusion.

Definition of adolescence

Adolescence has been defined in many ways, and the literature certainly identifies many differing opinions. Barr (2001) stated that, in the context of cancer, adolescence is the period between 15 and 19 years. The World Health Organization (WHO, 2000) defines adolescents as those individuals aged between 10 and 20 years. Eiser (1996) states that adolescents may have an adult understanding of cancer, but the emotional resources of the child for coping; they want to be treated like an adult, and yet nurtured as a child. However, we believe that the most effective way of viewing adolescence is as the time between childhood and adulthood (Whyte and Smith, 1997). In essence, they are neither adults nor children (Lewis, 1996).

A nest

Before the development of adolescent units, young people aged from 13 to 25 years with cancer were cared for on either adult or paediatric oncology wards. These included paediatric wards, where their beds may have been next to babies and toddlers, or adult oncology wards, next to the older generations with whom they had little in common. Although both areas provided excellent care, the philosophies were very different in terms of addressing the needs and support of these young people. In Leeds we knew that neither was appropriate for them, and only had to listen to what they told us:

> I am writing to tell you of the very distressing experience, which my son had during his stay on the ward last weekend. [He] is 14 years of age and yet he was in a bay with two small toddlers and a baby. He was unable to sleep because the baby cried during the night and consequently spent a great deal of time in tears himself . . . . It is embarrassing and humiliating for a boy of his age to be in this position.

Adult cancer wards can be equally unsuitable in very different ways:

> I do not like [my daughter] to be on the open wards with older people who are often very ill. At the very least she should be in a single room. But, because it is of paramount importance to keep her spirits

high, at best she should be with other young people where there is a 'more fun' atmosphere.

Parents, through their writing, expressed their thoughts to us:

> ... the child is at a complex stage of achieving independence and self-reliance, laying the foundations of the future; the parent is learning to let go. Add cancer to the highly charged atmosphere of adolescence and the emotional effects are less predictable than the physical. Not only the patient, but the whole family need support .. . frequent visits to the Teenage Unit hold no dread and, as a result, there is little antagonism or resentment about treatment. The question 'Why me?' is less likely to be asked in such cheerful and positive surroundings.

The first adolescent oncology unit was formed in the Middlesex Hospital, London in 1990. Since then, several other Teenage Cancer Trust units have been developed around the country. Most of these units have evolved from paediatric oncology centres, although, more recently, some impetus has come from adult oncology units.

The development of these units has many benefits for the patients, their families and the staff. These young people need to have a 'nest' – a place where they can come without fear in times of illness and uncertainty. They also need one that is very easy to leave behind once they have learned the ropes, safe in the certainty that it will always be there!

The Teenage Cancer Trust

Background to development of the service

In the Leeds Cancer Centre the professionals working within the adult and paediatric oncology units, which included both medical and nursing personnel, realized that there was a need to develop a service for adolescents. This was ground-breaking development because it involved both of these disciplines working towards a common goal – that of creating a centre of excellence for the care of teenagers and young adults with cancer.

The Teenage Cancer Trust (TCT) Unit development (Table 7.1) has been ongoing since 1995 following the identification of the need by both the adult and paediatric oncologists in Leeds. This occurred in the following stages:

- A conference, sponsored by the TCT, was organized by adult and paediatric oncologists in Leeds. This helped to raise awareness, both nationally

Table 7.1 The Teenage Cancer Trust

- Since the opening of the first Teenage Cancer Trust Unit in 1990, the Teenage Cancer Trust (TCT) has opened a further five units around the UK, treating adolescents and young adults with cancer, leukaemia, Hodgkin's disease and other related malignancies. Two more units are currently being built and discussions are under way for the development of further units

- The charity has extended its activities to include support for their units in the provision of nurses, activity coordinators and medical staff

- They sponsor periodic international conferences and sponsor the TCT Multidisciplinary Forum. This Forum enables the participants to gain support and information from one another while working in this specialty. This Forum is, in turn, sponsored by the TCT to organize conferences for the teenagers themselves. This enables them to realize that they are not alone and that to share their experiences not only provides them with a back-up, but also gives them a voice

and internationally, and contributed to the further development of working relationships between the Leeds adult and paediatric oncologists.

- The TCT was approached for the funding of a 10-bedded unit identified for the proposed Children's Wing at Leeds.

- Paediatric oncology managers approached Macmillan Cancer Relief to fund a new post to explore the needs of patients and the requirements of a service tailored to adolescents.

- At this time there was also pressure on the Paediatric Oncology Unit to develop more beds that were separate from the main ward. This gave the opportunity to develop facilities for the older age group within paediatric oncology practice.

- Five extra beds were made available to paediatric oncology which provided the opportunity for the development of a fledgling adolescent unit. At this time it became apparent that the new Children's Wing would not happen.

- In 1997 a Macmillan Clinical Nurse Specialist (CNS) was appointed to take a lead in the development of a service tailored to the needs of teenagers and young adults with cancer.

- As part of the refurbishment of the Paediatric Oncology Unit (POU) the development of a discrete adolescent unit was undertaken. The TCT agreed to fund this work as an interim arrangement before a more permanent accommodation.

- No funding was available from the NHS Trust or purchasers for the revenue consequences of this development; therefore, the inpatient facility was designed to accommodate the 'historical older patient' from the patient population in the Paediatric Oncology and Haematology Unit. It was acknowledged at the time that such a unit might attract patients not previously referred to the team.

- 1997–1998: a 'core team' of staff was developing and the rudiments of a philosophy of care, clinical expertise and experience of caring for these patients were evolving.
- The Macmillan CNS, working across the city, developed links to promote the concept of a 'Virtual Adolescent Unit', and identify key players.
- In June 1998, the TCT Unit opened. The 'core team' continued to evolve; this was the beginning of a multiprofessional team who would work alongside the medical team and managers to steer the service development. These professionals were wholly committed to the vision of an Adolescent Service for these young people.

The following account describes some of the experiences of establishment of a TCT Unit and the subsequent development of an adolescent service for these young cancer patients.

The route

Six beds were opened in June 1998, born from the inevitable growth of the POU. However, before the unit opened to patients a lot of groundwork needed to be undertaken

The first priority was to define 'adolescence' for the working of the unit. The multidisciplinary perspective was that adolescence might most usefully be viewed as a continuum of development that encompasses patients within the age range 13–24 years. This would facilitate flexibility at either end of that range for any individual, taking into account his or her own needs and circumstances, the type of cancer and the developmental tasks required by the individual and by society (Hollis and Morgan, 2001), e.g. a mature 23 year old may not want to be cared for on the Adolescent Unit; however, requests have been received from the patients themselves who are over the age definition. Patients such as these, for medical and social reasons, are not able to be cared for on the Adolescent Unit, but can have access to the Adolescent Service.

Identifying the team

Young people with cancer require professionals who are wholly committed to the vision of improving services for these young people. It is an undertaking not to be taken lightly because it can be a very emotive place in which to work.

There is a requirement for a team of professionals who work well together and who provide a variety of professional skills such as enthusiasm,

compassion, a sense of humour, innovation and patience! It is also important that a multiprofessional perspective is adopted within an adaptable
team that copes with change. Representatives from nursing, medicine,
social work, dietetics, psychology, pharmacy, surgery, anaesthetics, activity
coordination and physiotherapy disciplines are required. Skilled leaders
from the fields of nursing and medicine who are adept at managing change
are also vital.

The team for this Unit all came from within the POU. The Macmillan
CNS became the Clinical Lead for Adolescents within the Leeds Cancer
Centre, and the other nurse members were those who had expressed an
interest in working with the older end of the paediatric range. Other
members of the multidisciplinary team, as identified above, were already
in post as members of the POU, and a social worker, liaison nurse and an
activity coordinator joined the team as the work increased. All patients
referred to the Unit are under the care of the paediatric consultant oncologists and haematologists.

Sharing experiences

At the time of setting up the Unit there was very little experience nationally on which to base practice. The team found that liaison with other
units and the sharing of ideas were a pivotal point in its development.
Visits to other units around the country were made, because it was identified as being important not to re-invent the wheel. Many vital links were
made and an invaluable group named the Teenage Cancer Trust
Multidisciplinary Forum (TCTMDF) was established. This group meets
regularly to exchange ideas and share difficulties and successes. A priority for the TCTMDF team was the willingness to share expertise and
experiences with others locally and nationally.

Asking the consumers

Following the liaisons and the networking, the multidisciplinary workers
identified that if the Unit were aiming to empower the young people, then
the young people themselves would need to be involved in its development.
To achieve this a postal questionnaire was sent to past and present
patients, aged 13 years and above, which they were asked to answer
anonymously (Table 7.2). The Unit was still in its planning phase and any
comments from the young people would, where possible, be incorporated
into the design and setting up.

Table 7.2 Questionnaire

- Age; sex; diagnosis
- Feelings around diagnosis
- Were you given a choice in where you were treated?
- If you had the choice, where would you choose?
- How much choice did you get in your care?
- Would you have liked more choice in your care and treatment?
- How much information were you given about your disease?
- Would you have liked more?
- If so, what additional information would you have wanted?
- How much information were you given about general 'teenage' issues?, i.e. diet, smoking, exercise, drugs, alcohol, sex, etc.
- Would you have liked more information about these issues?
- Would you have liked more contact with any of the following staff? [list]
- Did you feel that you had enough space on the ward to do the following: relaxing, studying, watching TV?
- How would you describe the way that the ward looks?
- Could we improve it and, if so, how?
- How would you describe the educational facilities on the ward?
- Could we improve them, and how?
- How would you rate the recreational facilities on the ward?
- Could we improve them and, if so, how?
- How would you describe the amount of privacy you get on the ward?
- Could we improve this. If so, how?
- Were you ever prevented from sleeping on the ward?
- If you were, what could we do to improve this?
- How often did your friends visit you on the ward?
- How did you feel when your friends came to visit you?
- Is there anything that we could have done to make these visits more enjoyable?
- Were you happy to express your feelings to the staff on the ward?
- On a young person's unit, what should the nurses wear? (Everyday clothes, informal uniform or formal uniform?)
- Why?
- Do you think that having a young person's unit is an excellent, good, poor or very bad idea? Give your reasons
- What should the unit be called? A teenage unit, adolescent unit or a young person's unit?
- Complete the following sentences.
  The things I like the MOST about the ward are _ _ _ _ _ _ _ _ _ _ _ _ _ _ _
  The things I DISLIKE the most about the ward are _ _ _ _ _ _ _ _ _ _ _ _ _ _
- In an ideal world, what changes would you make to the ward?

The response was an overwhelming 74% reply rate and yielded the following points. They wanted:

- a recreation room for their own use
- computers, videos, DVDs, etc. If it had a plug – they wanted it!
- a pool table
- the Unit to be bright and cheerful
- the Unit to be quiet at night
- facilities for their parents, relatives and visitors
- privacy
- information
- a choice in their care
- a voice in their care
- better educational facilities
- to see their consultant more
- to have a 'quiet' room
- nurses in uniform not everyday clothes
- they said that a separate Unit for them was a 'very good idea'
- they did not want to be known as an 'adolescent'; therefore they wanted the Unit to be called a 'Teenage Unit'.

Providing the goods!

In spite of the limited space and resources we were able to meet most of the above requirements. The 'comfort' items were provided through public donations. Curtains were made using double thicknesses of material to promote privacy; the areas around their beds had space for posters, cards, photos, etc. so as to promote individuality. The areas were bright and cheerful, the recreation room was created and televisions were supplied with headphones, Sky television and telephone handsets! Electric beds with comfortable mattresses were also installed, along with duvets.

The Recreation Room 'rules' were devised by the patients themselves. This room is for the sole use of the teenagers; visitors are allowed in at the patients' discretion and no one under the age of 13 years is allowed in. In this room they can make themselves and/or their visitors a drink or a snack, have a game of pool and so on. There is a table with chairs, which has been host to many 'take-away meals'! The young people wanted this room to be under their control. They wanted a space that would allow them to get away from everything, a place where medical or nursing procedures are banned. They also wanted to be able to 'invite' visitors/friends/relatives in and evict them if necessary. There was a general consensus that this room should not be used as a communal area for parents because, from experience, it made it difficult for young patients who wanted to go in, but were embarrassed by a room full of adults. This has mostly worked well, but has created some difficulties, which are described later.

They were also asked what they wanted to have in their Unit and how they wanted it to run, and to develop their own guidelines involving the day-to-day running of the ward. The replies were surprisingly realistic and reflected their morals. They did not want illegal drugs, alcohol, sex, swearing, smoking or nakedness. They wanted lights out by 10pm, unless a common consensus was obtained, and headphones were to be used if they were watching television in the bay. True to adolescent nature, they wanted to lie-in in the morning. This was allowed as long it was recognized that should they be required to get up early in the day for tests, etc. – then the rule would not apply. This was generally agreed!

Difficulties – managing change

When the Unit had been open for several weeks, staff became aware that parents seemed unhappy and at times appeared hostile towards the staff. Members of the POU multidisciplinary team seemed to disagree with certain practices on the unit and it appeared that these staff members were talking to the 'unhappy' parents about these issues without discussing it with the Unit staff. The 'caring–sharing' team was suffering a communication breakdown! This resulted in tension on all sides. However, the young people themselves seemed to be content with the Unit and the way in which it was running.

The Recreation Room was a major source of contention, particularly from the members of staff not working on the Unit on a day-to-day basis. The parents were angry that they were not allowed to use it as a sitting room, although there was a parents' room that they could use only 5 metres away! Some staff were unhappy that 8 year olds were not allowed in to play on the pool table! These particular issues were found to be difficult for those families who had 'moved' into the Unit with us. Although the newly imposed rules and guidelines had been developed by the Unit staff, along with the patients, professionals, more peripheral but still vital to the Unit, who had not been involved were feeling a lack of 'ownership'. It seemed that we were all reacting to change and lessons/strategies about change management were learned.

Our strategy

After discussion with our managers and members of the 'core team' it was decided to have a multidisciplinary meeting to discuss these issues openly and reach some sort of consensus.

The requirement to meet with the parents was also identified and it was decided to facilitate this meeting first. During this meeting with the parents it was identified that some of them felt that we were pushing them out and did not seem to want them involved. One of the issues, which we clearly had not thought about, was the fact that they had rules at home that we did not have on the ward, e.g. a 16-year-old young man had a girlfriend who we allowed into the day room and his single cubicle. At home, this would not have been allowed. We now ask the parents and the patient on admission if they would like to identify 'extra' rules that they would like us to instigate and have learned to work more with the parents in giving their son/daughter some 'control' over his or her situation.

We then held the multidisciplinary team meeting, to which everyone whose practice would involve work on the Unit was invited. The Unit psychologist was asked to chair the meeting, having been briefed on the difficulties.

The meeting identified those team members who were not ward based, who did not understand why the guidelines, some of which were thought to be too rigid, were in place. The Unit appeared to them to be run in a more autonomous way; they also felt that some of their 'boundaries' were being crossed, which in turn threatened their roles. This new way of working had been implemented, it seemed, almost overnight by a small team of professionals.

The rules of the day room and of the rationale for them, i.e. that the adolescents need their own space and autonomy, were explained. The fact that the adolescents had identified this in the questionnaire and had created their own guidelines for this room was a very powerful tool.

By the end of this very open discussion, it was clear that the core Teenage Unit team had unintentionally left the rest of the team behind when planning the way in which the Unit was run, and in the establishment of the guidelines. Other members of the wider team appeared to feel uninvolved and uninvited on the unit.

This was in some way corrected by the core team members giving presentations to the multidisciplinary team about the planning of the Unit and the rationale behind the decisions made, and also by inviting their involvement with the Unit.

Table 7.3 Recreation room

- It is strongly requested by everyone that you all clear up after yourselves. Various punishments have been suggested (by other patients) which we consider too harsh to implement!! However, we ask you to think of the other people who will be using this room. Keep it as you would wish to find it!
- No overnight sleepers are allowed in here!
- Parents and visitors are allowed in here by invitation only
- No medical procedures will be performed in this room at any time
- Patients or parents from the children's ward will not be able to use this room
- At all times you must be thoughtful towards the use and sharing of this room with the other patients

Assessing change

After the Unit had been running for 2 years it was decided that there should be an evaluation of the implemented rules and guidelines. As this was predominantly a different cohort of patients from when the original questionnaire had been issued, it was decided to send a similar questionnaire, with the addition of a few pertinent questions.

The results showed that no major changes were needed. They were generally happy with the amount of information they were being given and the way in which it was provided; they also felt that they had been fully involved in the decision-making process. Most of them liked the décor and there were adequate recreational facilities, although they felt that they would benefit from an Activity Coordinator. Many of the comments were of a 'personal-taste' nature, i.e. they did not like the colour of the curtains! The only major complaint was about the food!

They were asked if they had had any experience of staying on an adult oncology/paediatric oncology ward, and how they felt that it may have differed from the TCT Unit. Those patients who had answered stated that they much preferred the atmosphere and surroundings of the Teenage Unit.

Suggested changes included the installation of a coke machine, and the employment of an Activity Coordinator. There will be a further re-evaluation in the near future.

The psychosocial requirements of the teenager/young adult with cancer

Setting up a physical unit is only a part of the equation; there are many other issues to consider. Adolescence is a time of great conflict: dependence versus independence, maturity versus immaturity, and a time to develop new skills and emerge as an adult. It is also a time when adolescents are learning to take control of their lives and of their own behaviour. When the diagnosis of cancer is added to this scenario the adolescent can be cast adrift in a terrifying adult world. Helping these young people through this life-changing experience can, therefore, be the most challenging aspect of their care.

Family-centred care

Cancer in adolescence causes exceptional stress in the family. The development of a life-threatening illness has been identified as a parent's worse fear (Thompson, 1990). It is of paramount importance that the family and immediate carers, as in partner/best friend, are cared for as well as the patient.

A philosophy of 'family-centred care' (Langton, 2000) is integral to paediatric oncology nursing. This must carry through to the care of the adolescent, with the emphasis shifting slightly from the parents who lead the process in the care of a young child, to the young person who may now want to be in control of their treatment decisions.

Many parents struggle with this concept and will need support and reassurance throughout their son's/daughter's treatment, especially if there is a partner involved who may want to be the young person's chosen decision-maker. This partner may have only recently 'joined' this family unit and, in the parent's eyes, may not have yet proved his or her worth. The partner may also feel like an outsider in the family who has no voice or support.

It is a role of the nurse to help develop partnerships among the adolescent, his or her families and partners. In some cases this role includes being an advocate for all members of the group surrounding the patient in order to achieve support and appropriate control for all parties.

Control

Many of these young people are learning to leave their family nest and embark on independence and their own lives. Cancer can bring them back into the family fold, where parents take control again, and their personal independence is lost.

Nurses on adolescent units need to be their advocates throughout their cancer journey to re-establish the equilibrium and encourage independence and control. Part of receiving information about their disease and its treatment is about having control and choice over their lives throughout their disease trajectory.

Finding an effective way to provide information to these young people has been challenging. They are all individuals, covering a range of ages and different diseases, requiring different amounts and depth of information, tailor-made to suit them. With this in mind, it was soon identified that all information needed to be individualized and, although core information was possible, it was the facts pertinent to that person that were important.

Therefore, one of the early practices established was that of providing annotations of important discussions that took place between the doctor/nurse/patient and family. We had previously researched this change in practice, and found very little evidence/material. The idea of tape-recording important discussions was broached, but soon dismissed by the team. It was felt that it may be intrusive, that the main 'talker' may feel intimidated and that placing a copy in the notes would prove difficult.

However, the annotation of notes was time-consuming and involved the nurse present taking notes and then typing it up later. This was always a more senior nurse, and the annotations were checked and signed by the doctor who had led the discussion. A contact telephone number was always written on the paper for the patient to take away. Several copies were made, a copy given to the patient and their family, and a copy in each of the medical, nursing and social work notes. This innovation has several advantages:

- The patient and their family were able to relax a little, knowing that everything was written down, and that concentration, which is usually lost after they hear the word 'cancer', was not an issue.
- The patient is able to read the notes at home and ask for clarification on the phone, if needed.
- The professionals involved all know what has been said, and what the patient knows.

The only disadvantage to the professionals seemed to be that the process was time-consuming. Indeed, we have had very positive feedback about this practice, and we often see these pieces of paper pulled out for clarification. One 16-year-old girl was so tired of explaining to her friends about her Hodgkin's disease that she photocopied the annotation and gave them all a copy!

A difficulty of this process is also found when talking to patients whose first language is not English. In these cases a translator is always involved and they are asked to write some notes for the patient.

There are also textbooks for general loan to the patients and appropriate information leaflets. Access to the internet is a controversial area, but we feel that most families are likely to look there. We request that they let us see any information that they may have obtained, or look at it with the guidance of one of the members of staff. We also provide a list of the helpful sites to visit as with books.

'Patient-held records', which have also been recently developed, are given to all patients. This allows them to keep a diary and record of their care, treatment and feelings. It is also very useful when considering shared care with other hospitals.

Along with the cancer literature, there are also 'normal' adolescent health advice literature and leaflets available. These leaflets cover the areas of sex, sexuality, contraception, drugs, etc.

Consultations

A frequently asked question concerning consultations with medical staff relates to the provision of information to under 16 year olds. The Unit practice is always to give the information to the patient and the parents, but directing most of it to the patient. Some patients have expressed their concerns that their parents are being told one story and they are told another; we are able to reassure them that this is not the policy in this Unit. It is important to reassure them that the policy is always to talk honestly and openly and not to keep secrets. Absolute trust in the professional/patient/parent relationship is vital and communication channels should remain open at all times.

Parents often do not want their young charge to be told that they have 'cancer' – this is non-negotiable, and in this situation we talk to the parents explaining to them what their son/daughter will be told and why. An important aspect is that the young person will be admitted to a cancer unit with other young people with cancer. Any collusion makes professional relationships with the patient and the family untenable. Discussion with the parents almost always solves this dilemma.

Peer support

Peer support is pivotal to the care of these young people. Adolescence is a time when all-important peer groups are made, and these groups can be a very powerful resource in schools/colleges/employment. Even the short-est absence from such a group can create difficulties for the sick adolescent. It is not hard to imagine the difficulties that the teenager with cancer has in keeping up with 'peer pressure' when they spend the best part of a year in hospital.

Units need to be run in such a way that friends are able to visit regu-larly and when they come that they are made to feel important and welcome. Whenever possible, social activities for the teenagers should also include an invitation for their friends, so that they can see that life can still be normal in spite of the cancer. Contacts with schools/colleges or places of work should be maintained and visits, emails and telephone contact encouraged.

Peer support is also vital on the units; here they can interact with young people who are having similar experiences and a common bond is formed. Young adult and teenage support groups should be facilitated. The experience gained from the young adult support group is that, when they are together, they do not need to talk about cancer; just being in the same room as other cancer patients makes them feel comfortable.

A 'voice'

It is of great importance to listen to the patients and hear what they have to say. They often have a very clear view of what is happening to them and have a need to express it. One 23-year-old man, at the end of his treatment for a Ewing's sarcoma, was asked if he felt that he had been given enough control over his care and treatment. He replied that he had throughout the treatment, but that, at the very beginning, he had not been asked if it was something that he wanted; it had just been assumed that he would!

The TCT Multidisciplinary Forum recently held a conference for teenagers and young adults with cancer. One issue that was made very clear was that they have an opinion about what happens to them; they want to have a 'say' in what goes on and want to be a part of the nation-al agenda. The Director of the National Cancer Action Team had been invited and was asked to participate in a 'question and answer' session where the participants were given the opportunity to ask questions. Their questions were thought-provoking and appropriate, and gave insight into their global thoughts on the care of young people with cancer. One issue raised related to single sex wards/bays; 400 young people were unani-mous in their rejection of such an idea. This statement has been heard and practices altered in the light of it.

Disadvantages of teenage/young adult units

The teenager and his or her family can become dependent on the staff of a specialized unit (Allen et al., 1997). It would seem that they need to be managed in such a way that 'dependence' does not become an issue; however, this is a new field with little experience and evidence in this area.

Such issues need to be addressed with professionals working on these Units. Professionals are a small, but important, part of the patients' lives; however, they are not integral to them. As professionals, dependence on us should not be encouraged, but independence nurtured and great pride taken in allowing them to 'fly the nest'. Interestingly, when developing the TCT Unit in Leeds teenagers were asked whether nurses should wear uniforms or day-to-day clothes; one reply stated: 'Definitely uniforms, you are professionals, not our friends.'

Experiencing the relapse and death of teenagers can cause staff to become very demoralized. It is very important, therefore, to have a support network for all professionals working with these patients, because only then are they able to help support the other patients who are also struggling with this aspect.

Medical opinions about the use of teenage/adolescent units differ enormously throughout the specialities, and many doctors are reluctant to refer their young patients to such a unit. These young people are often viewed as being a welcome relief in the adult oncology practice because they respond better to treatment, have a better prognosis and can be a pleasure to have on the ward! Patterns of care can take years to alter, but the well-being of the patient is paramount.

Adult cancers can often cross the boundaries of age, e.g. a 19-year-old young man has recently been treated on the Unit for an oesophageal carcinoma. In these cases, i.e. an adolescent with an adult cancer, opinion must be sought from the adult oncologists about treatment, nurses educated about the different treatment protocols, and access to the adolescent multidisciplinary working is vital. Developing such a model of collaboration in care is the way forward when setting up adolescent services.

Palliative care has proved to be a difficult issue for the Unit. The patients now referred are older than the historical patient, and may have an adult-type cancer requiring differing aspects of palliation. Working with the adult Macmillan team has been an important link to share expertise and learn new skills. This, however, is being developed further with the aim of employing a liaison nurse to bridge this gap.

Another important issue to consider is caring for an adult-size patient on a Unit which has paediatric on-call cover. Again effective collaboration and communication with the adult oncology unit, informing them when such a patient is admitted to the teenage unit, has helped to overcome this difficulty.

However, professional jealousies do occur and diplomatic education, collaborative networking and liaison are pivotal to maintaining effective relationships.

Current practice

The TCT Unit has been open since June 1998. It is well established with referrals increasing from both the paediatric but, even more so from the adult service. Patients who are referred to the adult oncologists may be cared for on the TCT Unit, where their day-to-day care is delivered by the Unit's staff. However, their consultation and treatment are prescribed by the adult oncologist – a hotel-type arrangement. This also works in reverse, where older patients can be cared for on the Adult Oncology Unit, yet stay under the care of the paediatric oncologist. This is a new development, and this collaboration in care has helped to integrate further the paediatric and adult services. A specialist registrar from the Adult Medical Oncology Unit works on the Unit for a year as a part of his or her adult oncology training. This gives cross-pollination of skills and knowledge about therapies and treatment. It further develops the links across the services and may be producing the adolescent oncologists of the future.

The Unit frequently has more patients than beds and this often has had the effect of patients being cared for on other wards. However, in view of this growth of the Unit we have finally gained the support of the local commissioners, and from next year we will see funding to support the service that we have developed. Due to patient pressure, we also recruited an activity coordinator, following a successful bid to the Laura Crane Trust (a local charity). This has made a positive difference to the atmosphere and day-to-day activities on the unit.

The adolescent service

The TCT Unit primarily cares for those young people who are referred to the Unit; however, young people in other parts of the Leeds Cancer Centre are also cared for by this service. Over the last 5 years, the centre has developed a service to adolescent patients that encompasses a patient- and family-centred inpatient ward and a wider service to teenagers and young people outside the Unit. The MCNS now works alongside a Sargent

Social Worker and an Activity Coordinator. They work with young people who, for reasons of age, disease or place of referral/expertise or preference, are not admitted to the Unit, e.g. an 18 year old with malignant melanoma or a 19 year old with a testicular germ-cell tumour. These professionals see patients in other areas and offer them a level of support within the philosophy of that given on the Unit, working towards equal access to services. This includes patients who are cared for on the Adult Medical Oncology Unit at St James's, Cookridge Hospital and Leeds General Infirmary. Referrals are also received from areas outside Leeds.

The service has been able to provide support and practical help to patients. It has developed strong links with the Testicular Cancer Service and Lymphoma patients and, has received referrals from other disciplines. As a result of raising the awareness of this group of patients, monthly multidisciplinary meetings have been established where interesting cases are discussed and new patients are brought to the attention of the professionals attending. Professionals who attend these meetings are from both the Adult and Paediatric Oncology Units. This provides a forum for learning and greater understanding of the needs of this group of patients and promotes further integration of the service.

The Adolescent Service has also been instrumental in establishing, with patients and staff from the adult and paediatric sectors, a young adult support group. Charitable organisations and voluntary partners have been involved in this.

The aims of the Adolescent Service are:

- To establish communication with the patient/family within 2 working days of referral. They are contacted to arrange a meeting to discuss any issues with which they may need help. This may be in the form of psychosocial support and/or financial, educational, employment or relationship advice. They also have direct access to professionals who are able to answer any questions about their disease and its treatment.
- To offer a place of contact for any help, either practical or social, 5 days a week, with an answer phone to receive any messages.
- To offer visits from the team while the patient is hospitalized.
- To liaise with the professionals who are caring for the patient, in order to identify any developing issues and act appropriately.
- To attend outpatient appointments with them, in order to help explain any difficult issues or for moral support. The offer to annotate the discussions is also extended to this consultation.
- To provide access to a local network of young people with cancer, and their families. For those young patients aged 16 years and under a Teenage Social Support Group is available. This meets 3-monthly and is

funded by the local 'Candle lighters' charity. For the older patients a Young Adult Cancer Support Group is available which meets monthly at a local hotel.
- To provide access to a developing national network of young people who meet once a year in the form of a conference. This is funded by the TCT.
- To offer, in the event of the patient's death, bereavement follow-up to the families. This may include attending the funeral to represent the hospital, home visits and, if necessary, return visits to the hospital to discuss any unresolved issues with the medical staff.

Much of the development of this service has come from within the resources of paediatric oncology, with support from the charities identified above. The development of an Adolescent Service has led to improved working relationships across the service. It is important to recognize that the service was not in competition with other disciplines, but very much to complement existing teams and improve communications with the young patients. This has been its primary aim. The Adolescent Service has been instrumental in building bridges between the two disciplines and a vital link for the patients, their families and the professionals.

Traditional boundaries

The development of the Adolescent Service in Leeds has ensured that these young people and their families have access to a multidisciplinary team that is aware of these very individual and rapidly changing needs and allows access to all sectors of the service.

It is not unusual for patients and their carers to have very little say in their care and treatment. The TCT Unit and the Adolescent Service have been able to infiltrate these boundaries and can allow the young people to have a 'voice' in what happens to them. It is also building bridges across the disciplines, fusing adult and paediatric knowledge, in order to help the patient.

Literature has identified that coping and compliance with treatment improve when patients feel that they are in control of a situation. These young people have been encouraged, with much guidance from professionals, to lead in their cancer journey, and by giving them access to information and peer support they are able to feel in control.

Without walls

Currently, adolescents with cancer are treated in a variety of areas, areas where an adolescent unit may not be wanted, or where the financial resources for achieving one are not available. This means that there is no uniformity of care. Can virtual units exist until an adolescent unit can be developed? Can a service be developed that can provide these young patients with their very different needs? Is it the location or the philosophy of care that matters (Gibson and Edwards, 1997)? This philosophy of caring can be applied to other units by a motivated team of professionals. Peer groups should be developed so that all these young people and their carers can meet, should they wish, and not cope in isolation. If they are treated on other units, they can still have privacy, information, open visiting, and access to fertility treatment, cancer specialists, peer support, education, advice and committed professionals. They will also need a nest to return to when times are hard.

A service that meets these needs and empowers others to provide it, thus creating the previously discussed 'nest', is not expensive, but requires energy and commitment. It will almost certainly be contentious, causing healthcare professionals to question their own practice and philosophy.

A service, similar to that of the Leeds Adolescent Service, may be of some benefit in these instances. A small group of professionals, working peripatetically, may be able to fill the gaps, pull the available resources together and offer provision to a 'virtual unit.'

Provision of care

The question of for whom in this group of patients adult or paediatric oncologists should provide care is under debate. 'Ownership' of these patients can cloud professional judgement, create barriers and cause unnecessary friction among teams of professionals caring for them. Debates continue between adult and paediatric oncologists about the attributes and benefits of the service they offer. However, experts in both the adult and the child, experts in the spectrum of diseases that can affect these young people would provide the patient with the best of both worlds, when working alongside a multiprofessional team who would provide the bridge between the two. Until these two disciplines work together, the definitive service cannot be provided.

A business case to establish the service on a more robust basis in Leeds has now been accepted by the Commissioners, and we look forward to the continuing development of a high-quality service to meet the needs of teenagers and young people with cancer. This will involve the collaboration of adult and paediatric oncology services. However, discussion and debate need to remain on the agenda of all professionals involved in caring for these young people.

Conclusion

Many lessons have been learned during the process of setting up this Unit and, as it is evolving, learning is still taking place. Establishing a unit is very much about partnership and not about ownership; it is about team work and not about working in isolation. It demands constant involvement of other professionals and not making assumptions that they know what you are doing and the rationales for those decisions.

Change cannot happen overnight. It is a tedious and time-consuming process that does not always go right the first time. It happens slowly and in an orderly fashion, during which time it can be very difficult to take criticism on something about which one feels passionate. However, criticism can be used to advantage if handled well and not taken personally.

It is so important to listen and take the advice of the consumers, to keep the patient and his or her family at the heart of everything you do. Units such as these will become a second home to patients and their families for the duration of their treatment and it is vital that they have their 'say'. If change has occurred as a result of the consumer's point of view, this can become a very powerful tool to support change and instigate further development. Evaluation is also an important part of the change process.

Development of this 'nest' is pivotal to the care of adolescents with cancer; however, getting involved with these patients can be detrimental to relationships. It is a priority, therefore, to recognize professional boundaries and to have appropriate support networks for all healthcare professionals.

There is a dearth of research into adolescent cancers and their treatment and care, and very few groups of professionals are looking specifically into these issues. There is a need to establish patterns of care, and to develop national networks, policies and protocols. Looking specifically at the biology of adolescent cancers has not been on the national agenda, nor is there a national database for this particular age group.

Cancer in the adolescent is now being recognized as a specialty and, following the Calman–Hine Report (DoH, 1995), all cancer centres should have them on the agenda. As professionals caring for these young people, we need to ensure that they have the appropriate care, and give them a voice.

References

Allen R, Newman SP, Souhami RL (1997) Anxiety and depression in adolescent cancer: findings in patients and parents at the time of diagnosis. European Journal of Cancer – Part A 33: 1250-1255.

Barr RD (2001) The adolescent with cancer. European Journal of Cancer 37: 1523-1530.

Department of Health (1995) A Policy for Commissioning Cancer Services. A report by the Expert Advisor on Cancer of the Chief Medical Officers of England and Wales (Calman-Hine). London: HMSO.

Department of Health (2000) The Cancer Plan. London: DoH.

Eiser C (1996) The impact of treatment; adolescents' views. In: Selby P, Bailey C (eds), Cancer and the Adolescent. London: BMJ Publishing.

Gibson F, Edwards J (1997) Network of care for children and teenagers with cancer: an overview for adult cancer nurses. Journal of Cancer Nursing 1: 200-207.

Hollis R, Morgan S (2001) The adolescent with cancer - at the edge of no-man's land. The Lancet Oncology pp. 43-48.

Langton H (2000) The Child with Cancer. London: Baillière Tindall.

Lewis I (1996) Cancer in adolescence. British Medical Bulletin 52: 887-897.

Platt Report (1959) Welfare of Children in Hospital. London: HMSO.

Thompson J (1990) The Child with Cancer: Nursing care. London: Scutari Press.

World Health Organization (2000) Child and Adolescent Health Development. www.who.int/child-adolescent-health/site_map.htm

Whyte F, Smith L (1997) A literature review of adolescence and cancer. European Journal of Cancer Care 6: 137-146.

Chapter 8

Semen collection in adolescents with cancer

Neil Shaw, Howard Wilford and Beth Sepion

Adolescent cancer statistics demonstrate the dichotomy facing health professionals caring for this group of patients. Although advances in treatment and collaboration between cancer centres, both nationally and internationally, identify that 60% of adolescents are disease free after 5 years (Pinkerton et al., 1994) and that one in 1000 adults is a survivor of childhood cancer (Schwartz et al., 1994), it has also resulted in paediatric/adolescent cancer being acknowledged as a chronic disease with an unknown outcome for many youths (Blotcky, 1986). This has led to the recognition that, although survival is a major issue for children and adolescents diagnosed with cancer and their families (Kazak, 1993), over time issues change and the consequences of survival become paramount (Heiney et al., 1990) with late effects of treatment being well documented (Overbaugh and Sawin, 1992; Schwartz et al., 1994; Koeppel, 1995). Infertility in both male and female survivors is one of many documented side effects, with adult and adolescent male survivors of cancer being only 76% as fertile as the 'normal' population (Waring et al., 2000). The use of alkylating agents and/or radiotherapy, which both affect rapidly dividing cells such as sperm (spermatogenesis), results in an increased risk of azoospermia or oligospermia. Patients who are most at risk of being rendered infertile include:

- patients with:
  - Hodgkin's disease
  - genital malignancies
- patients receiving:
  - high-dose alkylating agents and/or
  - radiotherapy below the diaphragm.

Although these groups of individuals are at high risk it is suggested that all adolescents who are treated with cytotoxic agents are at some risk of infertility, however small. Spermatogenesis normally occurs in the testicles of healthy males at the onset of puberty, from 11 to 12 years of age (Waring et al., 2000). It is interesting, however, that there is evidence that, for some patients who have been treated for malignant disease, depending on the disease and type of treatment, spermatogenesis may return spontaneously up to 10–15 years after treatment (Kissen and Wallace, 1995).

Male infertility may create particular psychological complications in individuals (Connolly et al., 1992), which suggests that many survivors of adolescent cancer may have psychological difficulties in the future associated with the side effects of the treatment rather than because they have had cancer. However, improvements in technology mean that cryopreservation of sperm undertaken before the start of treatment offers young men with cancer the hope of fathering their own children in the future. The inability to be the biological father of a child, therefore, need not always be the automatic consequence of having received cancer treatment during adolescence.

A large proportion of adolescent males with a malignancy will be cared for in one of the 22 United Kingdom Childhood Cancer Study Group (UKCCSG) treatment centres where they can expect to receive similar considerations and uniformity of medical and nursing care through protocols and randomized trials (UKCCSG, 1997). Many practices of the UKCCSG centres follow either a local policy, i.e. the management of neutropenic fevers, or national protocols for the management of randomized trials. However, one area of healthcare where there is disparity in the approach to the management offered is sperm cryopreservation and the associated support and counselling services. Currently there are no national standards or guidelines.

Standardized guidelines such as *Long Term Follow Up Therapy Based Guidelines* have been developed to assist in the assessment of long-term effects of disease and/or treatment (Kissen and Wallace, 1995). However, even though the technology is widely available, guidelines for the preservation of a male adolescent patient's potential to reproduce in later life have not been developed. The recognition of the lack of service in this area prompted a review of the literature and current practices in UKCCSG centres to be undertaken in order to identify sperm cryopreservation services provided to adolescent patients receiving gonadal toxic drugs. The review also included exploration of the availability of appropriate counselling facilities by adequately trained and informed staff. The aim of the review was to identify recommendations for best practice.

Literature review

The issues identified through the review of the literature associated with adolescent patients experience with infertility are:

- physiological
- body image
- family
- communication
- patient information
- service provision.

It is acknowledged that religion, spirituality and sexuality are significant contributing factors that will influence the development and management of this service, but they are beyond the depth and scope of this chapter.

Physiological

There is a wealth of literature highlighting adverse effects of chemotherapy and radiotherapy on children and young people (Overbaugh and Sawin, 1992; Schwartz et al., 1994; Kissen and Wallace, 1995). In particular, long-term effects on gonadal function and infertility are well documented (Koeppel, 1995; Waring et al., 2000). Smith and Babaian (1992) suggest that cryopreservation is suitable for patients whose sperm count exceeds 20 million/ml with 60% motility. However, Ohl and Sonksen (1996) contend that thawed sperm maintain approximately 50% of their pre-thaw motility. Studies by Agarwal et al. (1995) and Sharma et al. (1997) proposed that all men with viable, motile sperm should be offered the opportunity for cryopreservation of their sperm whereas Levitt and Jenney (1998) recommended that this be offered to all peripubertal boys before the start of gonad-damaging treatment.

Research in this area has been available for over 25 years. Buchanan et al. (1975) identified that the return of spermatogenesis after cyclophosphamide could range from 15 to 49 months. This indicates that infertility/subfertility in male cancer patients can be temporary or permanent and may be influenced by the patient's physiological condition pre-treatment. The assessments of the risk of infertility post-treatment need, therefore, to be related to individual patients.

Family

The healthy adolescent has patterns of interaction, rules, organization principles and general belief systems, as well as those specifically regarding health and disease (Taylor and Muller, 1995). The healthy family projects a social image, which guides its function, adapting as influences change.

The reality for the adolescent with cancer is that from diagnosis through treatment they are thrust back into a dependent role, and parents return to a caring role (Kazak, 1993). Concerns of parents whose children have completed treatment, and those of adolescents, are mainly about the formation and sustenance of relationships with others, with the eventual hope of marriage and children, and ultimately how to deal with the uncertain future posed by the risk of relapse (Ellis, 1991; Overbaugh and Sawin, 1992). Parents' concerns could potentially bring further psychological and emotional pressure to bear on their children (Van Dongen-Melman and Sanders-Woodstra, 1986).

Fertility is considered by parents to be a critical concern for them. An infertile child restricts the potential for grandchildren, so limiting the continuation of the family's genetic legacy. In contrast, this fear is often not communicated by survivors themselves (Kazak et al., 1995).

Body image

The evolving body image of an adolescent is a delicate and complex subject, sensitive to influences that are both physical, with the onset of puberty, and psychological, with the potential reduction of dependency on parents (Drench, 1994). It is through the potential reduction in fertility of the adolescent that an insult occurs to their sexuality. This psychological burden of not knowing the outcome of their disease process can be very heavy to adolescents, particularly when attempting to be accepted within the peer group (Burt, 1995).

The limitation of healthcare professionals' abilities to communicate effectively with the young person with cancer who has a fragile body image is recognized. Healthcare professionals make an inadequate link between the issues of sexuality and body image (Price, 1992; Burt, 1995), not realizing that there may be a causal relationship between the two. It is suggested that nurses may find it difficult because of the nature of educational and professional development and their own sexuality. Williams and Wilson (1989) suggest a method of addressing issues of sexuality. They contend that cure is not only the absence of disease but also a return to health, both physically and psychologically. Sexuality and its development should be recognized as part of this process, acknowledging it is an area requiring effective communication skills. Nurses should, therefore, adopt a more positive and open attitude to their patients and employ an accepting and diverse approach, recognizing individual patients' needs; pivotal to this are effective communication skills.

Communication

Evidence suggests that nurses have communication difficulties, hindering patients from expressing their fears and anxieties (Wall-Haas, 1991). More specifically nurses need to develop communication skills to facilitate discussion of sexually related issues with adolescent patients (Hopkins, 1991; Bor and Watts, 1993). The need for open, effective communication has implications for multidisciplinary teams when forging initial relationships with adolescents with cancer (Hydzik, 1990). Discussing sexual issues is a vital area often neglected or avoided by nurses because of a lack of knowledge, embarrassment about the subject matter, personal abilities to discuss such issues and a misconceived idea that it is the domain of doctors (Koeppel, 1995). Healthcare professionals, once appropriately trained, are in a 'pivotal' role to assess and help the adolescent patient deal with his or her diagnosis of cancer (Koeppel, 1995).

Patient information

Hooker (1998) suggests that adolescents with cancer see truthful information about their illness as a right, a desire to be treated as adults. Attempts to exclude them from discussions or receiving information would generate fear and the feeling of inequity. Information offers some reassurance that the healthcare professional understands their position of uncertainty. Information-seeking by the adolescent is seen as a function of the coping process and source of threat elimination; through appraisal of the threat by obtaining knowledge, actions are informed by that knowledge and can be taken to reduce emotional stress.

Information provision for this group of patients must ensure confidentiality and be readily available even during the night or out of core working hours. With this in mind, Thompson (1990) held the view that the nursing assessment should be integrated with teaching and is dependent on a unique patient–nurse relationship. This could offer an ideal platform to address sexual issues, with the possibility of overcoming any normally preconceived misconceptions (Heiney, 1989).

The development of a relationship between health carer and adolescent would be enhanced by relevant literature, which is individualized and presented sensitively and unambiguously (Thompson, 2001). In identifying information to fulfil the adolescents' needs, a study by Chambas (1991) identified that adolescents with cancer did raise health and sexual issues not mentioned by the healthy adolescents, i.e. hair loss, feeling isolated, ability to have children, and having children with genetic or congenital effects. Therefore, adolescent patients need to be offered the opportunity to have access to support services in respect of these issues.

Policies and recommendations pertaining to sperm cryopreservation

Various policies and recommendations published in the last 10 years refer to consent of the adolescent and provision of cancer services.

In support of the cancer patient there are three formative reports on cancer services: *A Policy Framework for Commissioning Cancer Services* (DoH, 1995), *Standards of Care For Children With Leukaemia* (Royal College of Pathologists, 1996) and *Resources and Requirements of a UKCCSG Treatment Centre* (UKCCSG, 1997). These reports are about cancer patients having access to uniformly high standards of care and services, and also highlight some differences and similarities of services. However, what each of these reports overlooks is the provision of service that offers patients the ability to procreate or the provision of a facility to support and counsel the patients and families appropriately.

The current restricted use of cryopreservation facilities is highlighted by Foley (1996) and raises the issue of potential litigation. This could occur, if infertility results from treatment and sperm cryopreservation services were available and not accessed. Sweet et al. (1996) address the issues of infertility in men post-chemotherapy, suggesting that facilities readily available for such services as in vitro fertilization (IVF) could be accessed, at minimal cost, by these patients.

In summary, the Human Fertilisation and Embryology Authority (HFEA, 1992) recognizes the ability and need of the young person to be involved with and consent to procedures. The Joint Council for Clinical Oncology identified that all postpubertal male patients who are likely to be long-term survivors after treatment that could cause gonadal dysfunction should be offered sperm banking. They also recognize the importance of providing appropriate counselling and support facilities at all cancer centres. Each of the three formative reports on national cancer services proclaims the need for uniformity and equity of care service provision at each centre, but are not specific about preserving the individual patient's ability to procreate at an appropriate time. However, although sperm banking facilities are now widely available in the UK, the extent to which these services are uniformly offered to young men with cancer remains unknown.

The review of the literature on cryopreservation of sperm for adolescents was unable to identify research published in the UK identifying current services within the UKCCSG centres. Although the literature reviewed addresses the issue of gonadal toxicity and cryopreservation of sperm from a physiological perspective, identifying the problems and potentially how to overcome them, there is little evidence to illustrate how this particular patient group is assessed, counselled and supported through this difficult initial phase before treatment.

A survey of regional paediatric/adolescent oncology centres in the UK, together with an internal audit of current practice within one of those centres was carried out to identify issues of why the number of adolescent males offered these facilities is low. An internal audit of current practice, undertaken in 1995, collected information on the following issues:

- the way in which sperm banking is discussed with both the family and the patient
- the identification of the healthcare professional involved in the discussion
- the issues that are discussed
- identification of the adolescents who were offered the service
- identification of adolescents who were not offered the service
- the long-term outcome.

Before the presentation of the internal audit results, a description of past and current approaches is given.

The past

For many years sperm banking was offered on an ad hoc basis, with no specified person taking responsibility for this important aspect of adolescent care. The storage facility for donated semen was off-site, in a different town, and needed the cooperation of an already overstretched social work team to collect the fresh specimen and drive some 15 miles to the tissue bank. This meant that the donation had to be timed to coincide with an opportunity for the specimen to be transported, rather than at a time that would be convenient for the adolescent. The adolescent had to produce the specimen on the paediatric oncology ward, either in the patient's toilet or in the privacy of a single cubicle (if a cubicle was available), with the aid of appropriate reading material (soft pornographic magazines) provided by the social workers or nursing staff. The consultant paediatric oncologist initiated all discussions around the issue of sperm collection and storage; a male social worker was also present to facilitate further discussions. There is no information or records to indicate how the process was initiated or what was achieved.

The present

The current practice has evolved as the needs of adolescents have become more evident and the staff have become more proficient at the identification and management of these needs.

On referral to the ward or outpatient clinic, young men are assessed as to their physical and emotional maturity and, if appropriate, the issue of infertility is raised with the parents when side effects of chemotherapy are discussed. Once the issue has been raised with the parents, the teenager is then spoken to by one of the two male nurses who work on the teenage ward. The centre feels it appropriate to gain parental consent to discuss the subject with teenagers under the age of 16. Once the subject of potential infertility has been mentioned, it is explained to the adolescent that, through cryopreservation, it is possible to preserve semen specimens for future use if they so wish, providing that the collection and storage are successful. It is important at this stage to ascertain the adolescents' understanding of how the specimen is to be obtained. From experience, the auditor had found few teenagers able to discuss masturbation openly, especially in relation to admitting that they had masturbated. This is a very delicate subject matter for young men and appears to be one of the few remaining taboos.

Once it is established that the process of obtaining the sperm specimen is understood, contact is made with an embryologist within the assisted conception unit (ACU) situated within the hospital and arrangements are made to send the teenager to the unit at the earliest opportunity. Before the teenagers visit the ACU they are required to complete a consent form. The consent form includes a question about the use of their sperm in the event of their death. The adolescent is asked to make a decision about this within days or sometimes hours of being told that they have cancer. They are reassured that this question is asked of everybody who donates semen for storage, not just those who are about to undergo treatment for cancer. If a consultant from the unit is available, an urgent appointment is made for the adolescent and his parents if he is under 16, to sign a consent form. However, if the consultant is not available the collection will proceed in order to prevent delay in the commencement of treatment and an appointment is made for a later date. All discussions take place with the knowledge of the consultant paediatric oncologist, but rarely in his or her presence. A formal medical referral is also required by the ACU, but the absence of one does not prevent the adolescent from being seen. The embryologist meets with the adolescent to discuss the practicalities of collection and to confirm that the adolescent is aware of what is expected of him.

The facilities within the ACU consist of a small room with a couch and suitable reading material. The teenager is shown to the room and left with a specimen pot. The specimen is left in the room for the embryologist to collect; examination for storage viability is then assessed. Viable specimens are cryopreserved. Ideally, two or three specimens are required but this is not always possible because a 3-day gap between specimens is necessary and although chemotherapy may be delayed it is usually only for up to a week. If the adolescent is too ill to donate, currently there is no alternative but to commence treatment without obtaining a specimen.

If older teenagers with partners wish them to help with the collection, this is encouraged. There are no fees involved; the storage of the sperm is free of charge to the teenager.

Internal audit

The internal audit data identified 20 adolescent males admitted to the paediatric oncology unit, mainly as inpatients, who had been assessed as physically mature enough to discuss infertility and semen collection. The age range was 13–18 years. The development of secondary sex characteristics and achievement of puberty were used to assess maturity. On most occasions the subject of infertility was discussed with parents first and, depending on their reactions, subsequently with the teenagers. Of the 20 adolescent males identified only four produced viable specimens suitable for storage (Table 8.1).

Cryopreservation was not discussed with the parents of the patient who was assessed by the consultant as being too immature, both physically and emotionally, to consider semen collection.

Following discussion with parents, six adolescents were not offered the chance to donate sperm; reasons for these decisions again revolved around maturity, both physical and emotional, physical condition and prognosis.

Table 8.1 Internal audit results

No. of patients	Age range (years)	Reasons for not being offered the opportunity to donate semen
1	14	Physical and psychological immaturity
6	13-16	One prepubertal, two emotionally immature, two too unwell, one poor prognosis
		Reasons for non-production of viable sperm
4	13-16	Two too unwell, one refused to discuss masturbation, one angry and refused to proceed
5	14-18	Inability to masturbate as a result of previous experience, environment and disease symptoms such as pain

These six cases on their own raise serious questions as to whether it is correct to withhold information about long-term side effects and how they might be minimized. Only 13 teenagers, therefore, were offered, after discussion with their parents, the opportunity to have semen collection. At this stage four were unable to proceed, two as a result of their illness and the other two had difficulties discussing the practicalities of semen collection.

The five patients who produced non-viable specimens experienced problems such as lack of a conducive environment and appropriate reading material, having an appropriate person with whom they felt comfortable discussing masturbation, problems with symptom management such as adequate pain control and the ability to masturbate for the first time under such pressure. The following vignettes highlight the types of problems and pressures.

> An 18 year old was very keen to preserve semen for future use; however, he found that the experience of being left in the room with no reading material and in pain from his disease was too distressing. He was unable to produce a specimen on this visit; it was arranged for him to go to the more comfortable surroundings of the 'home from home', situated in the hospital grounds. He also asked his girlfriend to accompany him. Unfortunately, because of his ongoing pain/ discomfort, he was unable to produce a specimen.

> A 14 year old was approached via his parents and, on initial discussion, appeared very keen to preserve semen. He indicated that he knew what masturbation was and that this was how the specimen would be collected. It was arranged for him to visit the ACU on the

same day. Following his visit the ward received a telephone call from the embryologist to inform the staff that the specimen they had received was urine. The patient was approached and he knew that the specimen he had produced was urine. The subject of masturbation and ejaculation was discussed in more detail. He said that he did not masturbate but that he knew what an erection was. This was explored further and the male nurse, with the aid of a banana, demonstrated masturbation. Further discussions took place around the teenager's view of pornography because soft pornographic magazines are provided by the ACU for visual stimulation. He remained very keen to attempt a further donation and another appointment was made to visit the ACU. Unfortunately, he was still unable to produce a specimen; chemotherapy was commenced the following day.

The final four teenagers were able to provide viable specimens of sperm, which were successfully cryopreserved. Two 15 year olds visited the ACU on two separate occasions and were able to produce two viable specimens.

One teenager was seen as an outpatient and was spoken to by the consultant Oncologist and a nurse in the outpatient department. This 14 year old was able to produce one viable specimen; it was a small volume and a low sperm count but with good motility.

One teenager was unable to provide a specimen in the ACU, but when discharged home on weekend leave was able to provide two viable specimens.

There was evidence to suggest that an audit would highlight good and bad practice, which in turn would underpin plans for future provision. However, it was felt that a survey of the 22 regional paediatric oncology centres to establish current practice around the UK would add to the body of knowledge.

National questionnaire

A questionnaire was sent to each of the senior ward sisters at the 22 regional paediatric oncology centres within the UK. Fourteen of the 22 centres replied to the questionnaire, and Table 8.2 lists their replies.
The questionnaire addressed the following areas:

- Do you offer sperm banking to teenage boys before commencing chemotherapy?
- At what age do you consider sperm banking?
- What other factors do you take into account before offering the facility?

Table 8.2 National questionnaire

Type of service offered	Number
Sperm banking offered	8
Sperm banking offered to patients receiving specific chemotherapy protocols	3
Sperm banking offered sometimes, when staff who are aware of the service are on duty	1
No service offered on religious grounds	1
No service offered	1

- Who talks to the teenagers and/or their families about sperm banking?
- Is there anybody else involved in the discussion?
- Where is the donated sperm stored; is it on or off site?
- Is there a financial charge made for the storage? If so, who is liable for the charge?
- How successful is the process? i.e. over the past 2 years (for example) how many patients have been offered the facility and how many viable specimens have been collected?
- Under what circumstances would you not offer sperm banking?

The age range for the service was quite varied: from 11 years (one centre), 13 years (three centres) and 15 years (two centres). Puberty and the ability to produce a specimen were the criteria identified by two further centres.

Fourteen different factors were identified as being taken into consideration before the facility was offered; some of these were common to more than one centre. Nine centres identified the emotional maturity of the patient, whereas only four acknowledged the physical state of patient. The views of the parents were taken into consideration by six centres, the chemotherapy protocol by three and the physical state of patient by four. The remaining factors were:

- age of child
- prior success with patients
- storage facilities
- storage fees
- shyness of staff
- availability of male nurse to discuss subject
- stage of puberty
- previous treatment
- environment.

When questioned about who talks to the teenagers and their families, on the whole a multidisciplinary approach is taken (Table 8.3).

Table 8.3 Personnel involved

Person who talks to the patient	Number of centres
Nurse	2
Clinical nurse specialist	1
Consultant and male social worker	4
Parents	2
Male nurse	1
Adult medical staff	2

Other people identified as being included in the process were team members from the infertility team, e.g. the consultant or the embryologist. A member of the medical team gained consent for an HIV test.

Information about sperm storage facilities showed that six centres had on-site storage facilities; five were unable to offer the facility on site and one did not know. Only three centres responded to the questions about financial charges made for the storage. They stated that there was a fee: two were free for the first year, but incurred a charge to the family thereafter, and the other centre was charged directly by the infertility clinic involved.

The success of the process was questioned, i.e. over the past 2 years how many boys have been offered the service and how many have been able to provide viable specimens? The response was mixed but clearly very few centres kept accurate records and their responses are as follows:

- two sperm collections with only one viable specimen
- six to eight viable specimens
- one teenager offered, with one viable specimen
- one in last 12 months
- about 10 offered, with half donating viable specimens
- three offered with two viable specimens
- all viable specimens
- about 50% successful
- twenty teenage boys: twelve offered facility, with four viable specimens
- one centre had also taken a wedge testicular biopsy.

Finally the centres were asked to indicate the circumstances under which sperm banking would not be offered. The responses are shown in Table 8.4.

One centre said that they had no policy and one failed to respond to the question. It was reported by one centre that children under the age of 15 would not be offered the facility because the staff were unwilling to discuss delicate issues such as masturbation and the teenager's

Table 8.4 Reasons for not offering the service

Reason given by centre	Number of centres[1]
Physical: patient too unwell	2
Life-threatening disease at presentation	1
HIV positive	1
No previous experience of masturbation	1
Patient maturity	2
Designated chemotherapy	2
Previous chemotherapy	1
Prepubertal	1
Under the age of consent, without parents' consent	1
Ability to meet financial costs	1

1. some centres have provided more than one reason.

wishes for the sperm in the event of his death. They felt that they had not met any boy under the age of 15 who had been capable of discussing these issues.

Discussion

The data collection raises many questions for centres that treat adolescent males with cytotoxic drugs. It is well recognized that the main group of drugs that cause infertility is alkylating agents; however, there may be a small risk attached to the administration of any chemotherapy. The centre treating these individuals may need to identify to which teenagers it is prepared to offer sperm collection and storage. As part of this identification, guidelines may need to be outlined as to the necessary physical and emotional development required before sperm collection is discussed and/or offered.

Many centres appear already to take a multidisciplinary approach to the provision of this service. However, each centre may wish to examine their current practice and consider who are the most appropriate personnel to address the issues associated with sperm collection and storage with the adolescents. Methods of data recording and collection may also require a review in order to improve standards and service provision.

A recent survey of UKCCSG centres suggested an incidence of approximately 750 cases of teenage malignancies per annum (aged 13–19 years) (Waring et al., 2000). Given the simplicity of this survey and the fact that not all centres replied, it is difficult to draw conclusions. However, it does appear that as professionals we may be failing this client population in that, if there are 750 new cases per year, we are only able to demonstrate that sperm storage and collection has been offered to less than 10% of these individuals.

As previously mentioned guidelines have been produced in other areas to offer best evidence-based practice, and treatment protocols that suggest and prescribe the appropriate investigations to be performed before treatment starts. Currently there is no mention of sperm collection and storage. The reasons for this lack need to be investigated. Information from the literature on the concerns of long-term survivors indicates potential infertility as a real risk for male adolescents as a result of the treatment of a malignant disease. The literature suggests that nurses and healthcare professionals acquire communication skills and that communication is integral to nursing work; the reality appears to be, however, that healthcare professionals lack communication skills in issues of sexuality. The provision of an equitable service throughout the UKCCSG centres, in order to bring the facility of cryopreservation of sperm for the young person with cancer into line with the other standardized treatments and support services, is also required. The importance of this needs to be recognized and acknowledged as a priority for healthcare professionals caring for adolescents about to start chemotherapy.

The future

Currently sperm collection is established by masturbation and ejaculation. There does, however, appear to be a number of adolescents for whom masturbation is not possible as a result of ill-health, stress, physical discomfort or other cause.

Different methods of semen collection may need to be considered in order to give all adolescents a similar chance of naturally fathering their own children in the future. One possibility to be explored is that of transrectal electroejaculation. This method uses a rectal probe to stimulate ejaculation and may be performed under a general anaesthetic. Ohl et al. (1997) demonstrated, in spinal cord-injured men, that the semen produced via this method showed no difference in sperm count to that produced by vibratory stimulation. It did, however, show reduced motility, viability and motile sperm count. Given the choice between this and no specimens, this may be an option that professionals and teenagers wish to consider. Other options may include microsurgical aspiration of sperm from the epididymis. Marmar (1993) demonstrated that this method could be successfully used in IVF treatment for infertile couples. Testicular biopsy and subsequent re-implantation after chemotherapy may also be a viable option for all males who are receiving cytotoxic agents, both pre- and postpubertal.

All these innovative methods will necessitate the formulation of assessment criteria and appropriate guidelines by healthcare professionals who are skilled experts in the care of this group of patients.

It is intended that this piece of work should stimulate healthcare professionals involved in the care of adolescent cancer patients to consider the specific needs of this patient group in relation to their right to store semen for future use.

References

Agarwal A, Sidhu RK, Shekarriz M, Thomas AJ Jr (1995) Optimum abstinence time for cryopreservation of semen in cancer patients. Journal of Urology 154: 86-88.

Blotcky AD (1986) Helping adolescents with cancer cope with their disease. Seminars in Oncology Nursing 2: 117-122.

Bor R, Watts M (1993) Talking to patients about sexual matters. British Journal of Nursing 2: 657-661.

Buchanan JD, Farley KF, Barrie JU (1975) Return of spermatogenesis after stopping cyclophosphamide therapy. Lancet ii: 156-157.

Burt K (1995) The effects of cancer on body image and sexuality. Nursing Times 91: 36-37.

Chambas K (1991) Sexual concerns of adolescents with cancer. Journal of Pediatric Oncology Nursing 8: 165-172.

Connolly K, Eldetian RJ, Cooke ID, Robson J (1992) The impact of infertility on psychological functioning. Journal of Psychosomatic Research 36: 459-468.

Department of Health (1995) A Policy Framework for Commissioning Cancer Services. A report by the Expert Advisory Group on Cancer to the Chief Medical Officers of England and Wales (Calman-Hine). London: HMSO.

Drench ME (1994) Changes in body image secondary to disease and injury. Rehabilitation Nursing 19: 31-36.

Ellis J (1991) How adolescents cope with cancer and its treatment. MCN: American Journal of Maternal Child Nursing 16: 157-160.

Foley GV (1996) Family caregivers: the need for partnership. Cancer Practice: A Multidisciplinary Journal of Cancer Care 4: 174-176.

Heiney SP (1989) Adolescents with cancer: Sexual and reproductive issues. Cancer Nursing 12: 95-101.

Heiney SP, Wells LM, Coleman B, Swygert E, Ruffin J (1990) Lasting impressions: a psychological support programme for adolescents with cancer and their parents. Cancer Nursing 13(1): 13-20.

Hooker L (1998) The information needs of teenagers with cancer: developing a tool to explore the perceptions of patients and professionals. European Journal of Cancer Nursing 1: 160-168.

Hopkins M (1991) Sperm banking. Nursing Times 87: 38-40.

Hydzik CA (1990) Late effects of chemotherapy: implications for patient management and rehabilitation. Nursing Clinics of North America 25: 423-446.

Human Fertilisation and Embryology Authority (1992) Sperm and Egg Donors and the Law. London: HFEA.

Kazak AE (1993) Psychological research in pediatric oncology (Editorial). Journal of Psychology 18: 313-318.

Kazak AE, Boyer BA, Brophy P et al. (1995) Parental perceptions of procedure-related distress and family adaptation in childhood leukemia. Children's Health Care 24: 143-158.

Kissen GD, Wallace WH (1995) Long Term Follow Up Therapy Based Guidelines. London: UKCCSG.

Koeppel K (1995) Sperm banking and patients with cancer. Cancer Nursing 18: 306-312.

Levitt GA, Jenney M (1998) The reproductive system after childhood cancer. British Journal of Obstetrics and Gynaecology 105: 946-953.

Mackie EJ, Radford M, Shalet SM (1996) Gonadal function following chemotherapy for childhood Hodgkin's disease. Medical Pediatric Oncology 27: 74-78.

Marmar JL (1993) Microsurgical aspiration of sperm from the epididymis: a mobile programme. Journal of Urology 149(5 suppl): 1368-1373.

Ohl DA, Sonksen J (1996) What are the chances of infertility and should sperm be banked? Seminars in Urologic Oncology 14: 36-44.

Ohl DA, Sonksen J, Menge AC, McCabe M, Keller LM (1997) Electroejaculation versus vibratory stimulation in spinal cord injured men. Journal of Urology 157: 2147-2149.

Overbaugh KA, Sawin K (1992) Future life expectations and self esteem of the adolescent survivor of childhood cancer. Journal of Pediatric Oncology Nursing 9: 8-16.

Pinkerton CR, Cushing P, Sepion B (1994) Childhood Cancer Management: A practical handbook. London: Chapman & Hall.

Price B (1992) Living with altered body image: the cancer experience. British Journal of Nursing 1: 641-642.

Royal College of Pathologists, Clinical Standards Advisory Group (1996) Standards of Care for Children with Leukaemia. London: Royal College of Pathologists.

Schwartz CL, Hobbie WL, Constine LS (1994) The establishment of the follow up clinic. In: Schwartz CL, Ruccoine KS (eds), Survivors of Childhood Cancer, Assessment and Management. St Louis, MO: Mosby.

Sharma RK, Khon S, Padron OF, Agarwal A (1997) Effects of artificial stimulants on cryopreserved spermatozoa from cancer patients. Journal of Urology 157: 521-524.

Smith B, Babaian RJ (1992) The effects of treatment for cancer on male fertility and sexuality. Cancer Nursing 15: 271-275.

Sweet V, Servey EJ, Karrow AM (1996) Reproductive issues for men with cancer: technology and nursing management. Oncology Nursing Forum 23: 51-58.

Taylor J, Muller (1995) Nursing Adolescents: Research and psychological perspectives. London: Blackwell Science Ltd.

Thompson J (1990) The Child with Cancer. London: Scutari Press.

Thompson J (2001) In: Corner J, Bailey C (eds), Cancer Nursing Care in Context. Oxford: Blackwell Science, Chapter 32.

United Kingdom Childhood Cancer Study Group (1997) The Resources and Requirements of a UKCCSG Treatment Centre, unpublished.

Van Dongen-Melman J, Sanders-Woodstra J (1986) Psychological aspects of childhood cancer: a review of the literature. Journal of Child Psychology and Psychiatry 27: 145-180.

Wall-Haas C (1991) Nurses' attitudes toward sexuality in adolescents patients. Pediatric Nursing 17: 549-555.

Waring AB, Hamish W, Wallace B (2000) Subfertility following treatment for childhood cancer. Hospital Medicine 61: 550-557.

Williams H, Wilson M (1989) Sexuality in children and adolescents with cancer: pediatric oncology nurses attitudes and behaviours. Journal of Pediatric Oncology Nursing 6: 127-132.

Chapter 9
Teenagers' information needs
Louise Hooker

Each year in the United Kingdom about 600 people between the ages of 13 and, 20 are diagnosed with cancer, 60% of whom will be cured (Souhami et al., 1996). Treatment may take place in a variety of settings including paediatric oncology units or adult medical, surgical or oncology wards in cancer centres and units. Teenagers with cancer are increasingly being acknowledged as a distinct group with specific and complex needs and this has, in recent years, led to the development of adolescent oncology units. The provision of information has been identified as a fundamental component of care for all cancer patients, and has been enshrined in NHS policies for cancer services (Department of Health or DoH, 2000). Appropriate, timely information can offer teenagers with cancer the opportunity to develop coping strategies, and subsequently can give them the best chance of 'surviving' as psychologically intact adults. However, whether or not these needs are met is a consequence of the complex interrelationship of their priorities, the insight and skills of healthcare professionals, and the wishes of parents. This chapter describes work undertaken to explore the information priorities of teenagers with cancer and their perception of the role that information plays in their cancer experience.

Teenagers with cancer

Adolescence is a stage of physical, psychological, cognitive and social transition. Specific developmental tasks must be achieved if adaptation to adult roles is to be successful. These include establishing a gender-role identity and body image, achieving independence, preparing for self-sufficiency, and developing academic and social competencies. Teenagers have to challenge the boundaries imposed by parents, authority figures and society as they strive to adapt to adult roles (Coleman and Hendry, 1990). A cancer diagnosis during adolescence comprehensively challenges this developmental process. If young people with cancer are to be helped to achieve the transition to adulthood, it is necessary that professionals understand the particular problems that they face. Physical changes related to cancer and treatments challenge the teenager's ability to see him- or herself as normal. Teenagers with cancer are more troubled by the restrictions and changes demanded by treatment than younger children (Claflin and Barbarin, 1990), and this may precipitate diminished self-esteem and depression (Ritchie, 1992). Teenagers also understand their illness more fully than younger children, which can increase their sense of personal vulnerability (Eiser, 1993). In addition, the expectation is that parents will gradually 'let go' of their adolescent child, giving them the physical and emotional space in which to create an adult identity. Cancer threatens to disrupt this process and may reverse the emotional distancing from parents, which characterizes the move towards autonomy.

However, most teenagers with cancer do appear to have the resilience to survive the experience emotionally intact. There are reports of psychosocial dysfunction in teenagers during treatment, but, despite periods of anxiety and depression, most manage to maintain their self-image and social identity throughout therapy (Jamison et al., 1986). Lazarus and Folkman (1984) describe coping as a process that is activated in response to a perceived threat, with the purpose of managing emotional distress and eliminating the threat. They describe two main types of coping: problem-focused (behavioural) strategies, which entail taking action and emotion-focused (cognitive) strategies, which involve perceiving the threat differently. Coping is a dynamic and individual process, so variations in coping style between people and for each person over time are to be expected. This variation between and within individuals emphasizes that professionals should to be able to appraise needs and respond with interventions that are appropriate to each patient and the challenges as they perceive them at that point in time.

When compared with younger children, teenagers employ a greater repertoire of cognitive, as opposed to behavioural, methods and use them in a wider range of stressful situations (Claflin and Barbarin, 1990). They strive to retain their 'well' identity by developing strategies designed to reduce the differences that they perceive to exist between themselves and their healthy peers (Rechner, 1990). The process of psychological adaptation to cancer has been summarized in terms of gaining an understanding of their illness through knowledge and experience, and facing up to its challenges (Ellis, 1991). Lazarus and Folkman's (1984)

'Transactional Model of Stress and Coping' has been used as a framework for much research into cancer patient coping strategies (Degner and Sloan, 1992; Luker et al., 1995; van der Molen, 1999). Information seeking is seen as a key component of coping; knowledge supports a better understanding of the threat and this in turn can enable appropriate action to be taken. An important dimension of coping through information seeking is that the nature of information required is determined by the perceptions of each individual.

The information needs of people with cancer

In the field of cancer care, patient education has been the focus of much research. Not surprisingly, considering the demography of the cancer patient population, this has focused largely on the needs of adults. A smaller body of work exists about the information needs of children or teenagers. As adolescence is a period of transition between childhood and adulthood, it is important to consider findings from studies involving adults as well as those with teenagers and children.

Numerous studies with adults have established that the majority seek, rather than avoid, information, and that most want to be given both 'good' and 'bad' news, (Cassileth et al., 1980; Fallowfield et al., 1995; Jenkins et al., 2001). However, information needs change with time, and may vary with patients' age, gender, circumstances and experience of treatment (Butow et al., 1997; Boudioni et al., 1999). Patients rate disease concerns as having the highest priority, seeking information about their diagnosis, prognosis and treatment (Cassileth et al., 1980; Luker et al., 1995). Patients who receive the information that they desire are more hopeful, less depressed or anxious, and are more likely to express satisfaction with care (Cassileth et al., 1980; Derdiarian, 1989; Thomas et al., 2000).

The research about the information needs of teenagers suggests that, like adults, they seek information over a wide range of subject areas. (Pfefferbaum and Levenson, 1982; Ellis and Leventhal, 1993). However, Claflin and Barbarin (1991) found that only half of their teenage respondents were given specific information about their prognosis. These teenagers expressed concerns that information might be withheld, and fear about the nature of undisclosed details. The findings of studies with adult cancer patients demonstrated marked variation in the needs of individuals and in the same person over time. In child and adolescent cancer patients, it may be expected that the variations be exaggerated by developmental differences between individuals, and marked psychosocial changes during the illness experience. It may, therefore, be even more difficult to predict their needs, and the information offered to young patients might be particularly influenced by the preconceptions of professionals and family members.

In the past, it was considered acceptable to withhold information about a cancer diagnosis. In one study, 90% of doctors treating people with cancer exercised a policy of not disclosing the diagnosis (Oken, 1961). Since then, professionals' attitudes to patients, public attitudes to and knowledge of health matters, and the improvement in disease management have drastically altered the culture of cancer care and, by the, 1980s, most doctors told 'the truth' to their (adult) cancer patients (Novack et al., 1979). However, the issues surrounding information-giving to children and teenagers with cancer continue to create dilemmas for parents and professionals. Parents are naturally protective of their son or daughter, and may seek to conceal potentially distressing information from him or her. Historically, attitudes to informing children with cancer have changed with the improved chances of survival, and the growing awareness of the potentially damaging psychological effects of the sick child's enforced ignorance on the whole family. It is now widely accepted that information about diagnosis, prognosis and treatment should be honestly and openly discussed in language appropriate to their age and understanding. Disparities have been found to exist between adolescent cancer patients and their parents (Levenson et al., 1983), but Ellis and Leventhal (1993) found that for most issues these differences were not significant. Physicians' perspectives may, however, be less accurate than those of parents (Pfefferbaum and Levenson, 1982). The study described here was undertaken to gain a better understanding of the perspectives of teenagers with cancer about information related to their illness and treatment.

Methods

A number of approaches have been used in researching the information needs of children, teenagers and adults with cancer. Some studies have used quantitative tools to measure the relative importance of information needs, whereas a smaller number have employed qualitative methods. The use of both was indicated here, in order to gather data that were both specific in content and rich in meaning (Corner, 1991).

A research tool that offered a reasonably simple way for young people to prioritize their information needs was needed. Ranking items, here in order of perceived importance, is a complex cognitive procedure, requiring participants to compare items and make judgements about their relative value. Card-sorting techniques had been used both in research and as a clinical tool in a variety of health-related or counselling situations to assess clients' needs or emotional perspectives, or as a tool to stimulate discussion. Thurstone's law of comparative judgement (Thurstone, 1974) provided the theoretical framework for the collection of the quantitative data, and was selected because it had previously been used successfully in relation to cancer patients' information and decision-making preferences (Degner and Sloan, 1992; Luker et al., 1995). The development, application and analysis of the card-sort game is more fully described elsewhere (Hooker, 1998).

This small-scale study was undertaken with a convenience sample of seven teenagers with cancer at a regional paediatric oncology centre. Approval of the local research ethics committee was obtained and, after provision of written information and open discussion about the research with teenagers and their parents, written consent was gained from participants, and a parent if desired. Thirteen cancer-related information cards (Figure 9.1) were used, and participants undertook a structured sorting process to prioritize the information items. The raw card-sort data consisted of the rank order of information items according to each participant. To convert these data into interval scale values that could be plotted according to the relative importance of the items, a number of sequential procedures were performed, according to the paired comparison scaling model (Thurstone, 1974; Degner and Sloan, 1992). Following the card-sorting procedure, tape-recorded semi-structured interviews took place to explore the participants' perceptions of issues related to information-giving, according to an outline interview schedule. The interview tapes were transcribed, and the analysis was based on Burnard's (1991) approach, developed from grounded theory and content analysis.

Figure 9.1 Information items used in the teenager's card sort game.

Information about:

- Cancer
- How I can look after myself
- How my illness and treatment might affect the things I usually do
- How my illness and treatment might affect my appearance
- How my illness and treatment might affect my relationships
- How the treatments work
- How the treatment might affect my future
- My illness
- My treatment plan
- The chances that my illness can be cured
- The side effects of my treatment
- Whether the treatment is working
- Who I can talk to about what is happening

Findings and discussion

The age range of participating teenagers was 13–17 years; there were four boys and three girls, and a number of different diagnostic groups were represented. Two participants had completed therapy within the previous year, and the others were established on active treatment with curative intent. The small participant numbers, high intragroup variability, single-site setting and use of a new research tool all limit the generalizability of the results of this study. Therefore, in an attempt to appraise and put in context these findings within the body of evidence, results are discussed in the light of other published research.

The information profile (Figure 9.2) shows the perceived relative importance of each information item, a higher scale value denotes higher perceived importance.

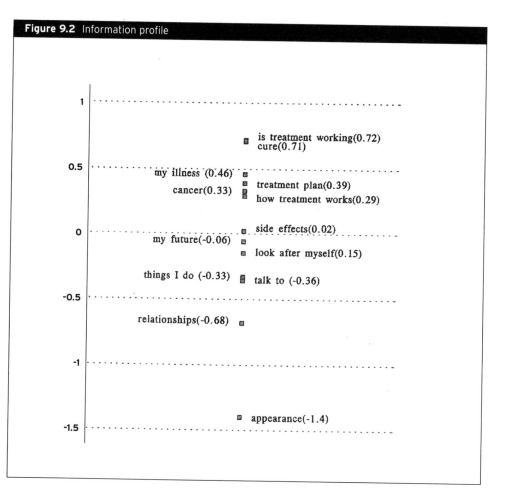

Figure 9.2 Information profile

Participant numbers were too small to conduct meaningful statistical analysis of variables within or between groups. The card-sort data indicate that those information issues most important to these teenagers with cancer were related directly to the life-threatening nature of their illness, their diagnosis and prognosis, and the plans for and the current effectiveness of their treatment. This reflects the results of studies with adults (Luker et al., 1995), and other work with children and teenagers (Pfefferbaum and Levenson, 1982; Ellis and Leventhal, 1993; Dunsmore and Quine, 1995). The fact that these issues are consistently reported across age groups and with different research tools substantiates the findings. Cassileth et al. (1980) found that most adult patients wanted information about their disease, cure and week-to-week progress. The teenagers in this study valued this information as highly as overall chance of survival, suggesting that timely communication of investigation results might help to reduce their anxiety. Information about the treatment plan was the teenagers' fourth priority item, highlighting their desire to know what to expect. The interview data seem to corroborate this finding, and are discussed further.

Information about the impact of treatment on the teenagers' everyday lives was given lower priority than these fundamental issues. Items concerning the potential effects of treatment on appearance, relationships and usual activities constituted three of the teenagers' lowest-ranked four information needs. This was also the case when adults were asked to consider the impact of treatment on their physical attractiveness, social life, and family and friends (Davison et al., 1995; Luker et al., 1995). The low priority given to these issues may seem surprising, but it is important to stress that the teenagers thought that all the information items were important, and that the priorities given to items were relative, not absolute.

During the analysis of the interview data, 16 themes emerged. These have been classified under four broad descriptive categories, and are depicted diagrammatically to show the relationship between categories and themes (Figure 9.3). Results are presented here as descriptions of the themes that comprise each category, with supporting evidence from interview transcripts. Minor alterations to verbatim text have been made where necessary to maintain the teenagers' anonymity.

Acknowledgement

Information sharing was perceived to be intrinsically valuable. Reassurance was gained from both the fact that information was disclosed and the content of discussions.

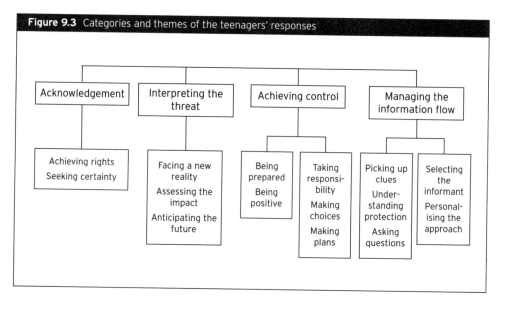

Figure 9.3 Categories and themes of the teenagers' responses

Achieving rights

The issue of the right to information was described. The teenagers expressed a sense of injustice when discussing the possibility that information might be withheld.

> It would be wrong not to tell, because people want to know. Because they could be sitting there thinking that they are going to get better, and then they find out later on, and they shouldn't do, if they can't or something.

Seeking certainty

It was deemed important to discuss the concrete facts around diagnosis and treatment even if the information was distressing, because this was preferable to the uncertainty of not knowing.

> I didn't think they wanted to tell me at one stage, 'cause Mum came in and she looked quite upset, and then when they took me here, I was thinking 'What is happening?', and everything. When they told me I thought 'Oh God'. It's a relief to know, but not very nice.

By discussing their diagnosis and planned treatment, the teenagers could allay some of their imagined fears, and seek reassurance. Teenagers expect to receive information (Ellis and Leventhal, 1993) and be involved in decision-making (Eiser, 1996), and if this is not offered they feel that their rights to have been denied. The teenagers in this study described positive results of receiving even distressing information. This is supported by Ellis and Leventhal (1993) and Claflin and Barbarin (1990), who found that withholding such information did not reduce, and can increase stress.

Interpreting the threat

Information enabled teenagers to interpret their illness in terms of how it potentially affected their present and future selves.

Facing a new reality

The need for information about how their circumstances had changed was described. The sense of disruption posed by diagnosis and treatment was evident, and information was considered the most immediately effective way of starting to manage the situation:

> . . . you would constantly be saying 'why am I having this done, and this done, why have I got to have this done?' You would get on everyone's nerves and also you would feel a bit strange doing all this stuff without actually knowing why.

Assessing the impact

The perceived threats to the teenager's body, emotions and social functioning were evident. The teenagers expressed this in terms of how their life was affected by treatment.

> I need to know the plans and stuff, what they are going to do to me, and will I be able to do all the things I used to?

Anticipating the future

The teenagers clearly expressed a desire to appraise what the future might hold, including the possibility of treatment failure.

> Because you need to know how you are going to be in the future, if the treatment's going to work, if you are going to survive the treatment, if you are going to need anything else in the future if the treatment isn't working, if you are going to need a bone marrow [transplant] or something.

The teenagers sought information that enabled them to understand and adapt to their changed circumstances and establish what aspects of their life might be altered. Lazarus and Folkman (1984) consider this process to be a fundamental aspect of the dynamic process of coping. Other studies with adults, children and teenagers support these findings (Bull and Drotar, 1991; Luker et al., 1995). By seeking information, the teenagers may assess the extent to which they can continue to perceive themselves as unchanged, and make plans to reduce the disruption to their lives. Teenagers are often assumed to focus on the present and the immediate future; however, it was clear that planning for the longer term was important to these young people. It is possible that teenagers with cancer have an increased awareness of their vulnerability and mortality, and consequently a greater degree of concern about the future.

Achieving control

The teenagers expressed the need to re-establish a degree of control and mastery. Five interrelated strategies were described, including both emotional adaptation and taking action. However, each strategy was seen as active and purposeful, rather than passive, because the teenagers sought out information that enabled them to decide what approach to take.

Being prepared

Information about what might happen to them enabled the teenagers to prepare themselves mentally for something that they could not actually change.

> I always ask questions. Y'know, when I'm having chemo, what the side effects are I'm going to have, so I can be prepared, and say 'I'm not going to have that side effect'.

Making plans

Rather different from psychological preparedness, this involved using information in active planning to assert themselves as individuals with a present and a future. By working towards goals, they sought to minimize the impact that their illness had on their lives.

> This is my main important year to decide what I'm doing, I've got to do work experience for what I want to do, so it's quite important, really important. Some people just don't bother planning, they can just take what comes to them, but people like me now have to plan and try to work something out.

Taking responsibility

The teenagers wanted specific information about how to look after themselves, and saw themselves as active agents in their own recovery.

> I don't want it to be my fault if I get a relapse or something. I want to get through this as quickly as possible and not do anything wrong, so I need to know what to do.

Making choices

The importance of selecting what information to believe and either accepting or rejecting advice was important in asserting their identity.

> Well I just had other things on my mind. Everyone was getting on to me, 'Oh [name] brush your teeth four times a day' and I was like 'No, my mouth will be fine' and it was fine, and I just felt it wasn't that important.

Being positive

This was seen as a priority:

> 'It was more important to keep positive, and, I dunno, just keep positive.'

For some this included acceptance of their limitations, and focusing on making their situation as bearable as possible.

> You just literally need to forget everything you used to do and get used to what you are doing now, because if you just keep thinking about what you could be doing and you would just not be having fun, when you could be doing something fun here [in hospital], but you would be moaning all the time and not doing it.

These teenagers felt that information enabled them to re-establish some control over their lives. In healthy adolescents, self-esteem is related to perceiving themselves as able to affect events and realizing their intentions (Coleman and Hendry, 1990). Loss of this sense of being in control is widely reported in relation to teenagers with cancer (Jamison et al., 1986; Ettinger and Heiney, 1993). Lazarus and Folkman's (1984) description of behaviour-focused and emotion-focused coping is reflected in these teenagers' efforts. By seeing themselves as able to make an active contribution to their survival, asserting their identity and maintaining some independence, teenagers perceive themselves as competent and are better able to cope (Evans, 1996). There seems to be a link between 'being positive' and the published work on 'hopefulness' among adolescent cancer patients (Hinds and Gattuso, 1991). Lazarus and Folkman (1984) also recognize the importance of hope as a psychological resource for coping.

Managing the information flow

These teenagers seemed to undertake thoughtful appraisal of their surroundings and the people they came into contact with, and used these insights to develop a range of strategies to meet their information needs.

Picking up clues

Knowledge was gained in a number of ways, and teenagers often based their assessment of any situation by gauging the reactions of those around them.

> I knew what I was expecting, like if they come in upset or something, I could see if it was bad, or just a general type of thing. When I saw they were upset, I could sort of prepare myself.

Understanding protection

The teenagers reported that some information was freely given, whereas some had to be actively sought, perceiving that the distinction between the two was related to the nature of the information.

> There are things they will tell you anyway, but some things you have to ask about. Like how likely you are to be OK, what your percentages are. No one told me, and I asked my mum and found out that they had been told, so I had to get them to tell me. And stuff about dying, they wouldn't want to worry you, looking on the bad side of things, so they wait to see if you want to ask about it.

Asking questions

The teenagers felt that they sometimes made direct enquiries about issues that worried them, but only after careful consideration:

> ... a couple of times, like I want to know, but I ain't got the guts to ask ... sometimes I want to know about it at that precise minute and then I think 'No', and when they say 'Do you want to ask any questions?', I just sit there and think about what it's going to be like to know.

Selecting a credible informant

The teenagers wanted information that was accurate and specific. For this reason they made careful decisions about whom to approach.

> The best person to ask is Dr [name], because he's qualified, he knows what he's talking about, really, it's not so good if they tell your Mum and your Mum tells you, if it's coming from your Mum and your Mum might not get it right.

The teenagers made judgements based on the adults' knowledge and expertise, and had little respect for, or trust in any professional who was found wanting.

> Some doctors didn't even know what I had, and stuff. Like this doctor came and he saw my scar, and he looked at it and said 'Oh that's a nice scar, what have you had?', and he was looking at my notes a couple of seconds ago, and he should have took that in and didn't.

Although parents were generally not seen the most useful sources of hard information, for some parents were the preferred informants because they gave information more sensitively.

> Doctors just sit there with their frowning faces and tell you, but parents break it to you slowly and stuff.

Selecting a 'teenager-friendly' informant

The teenagers valued certain personality characteristics: friendliness, positive attitude, a sense of humour, sensitivity and trustworthiness. It was also seen as important that professionals could communicate with teenagers and recognize their particular concerns. The people who met these criteria were regarded with great affection and respect. The teenagers appreciated the time and effort that was spent getting to know them.

> So they have to be nice, friendly, understanding, they can take it serious sometimes too, but mainly they have got to have an attitude to keep you up and going, not going to make you drop down 'cause you're not very happy, and they just come in and do their job and that's it, and get paid and that's all they want. But these want to be friends, and can still take it serious.

Personalising the approach

It became clear that individuals took steps to tailor the information-giving methods. They described how, initially, their diagnosis had been disclosed to their parents, in their absence. The teenagers had their own views about the acceptability of this strategy:

> The first time I came in, they took my Mum and Dad out first and told them, and they left me in the room. I said they should have told me right when they told Mum and Dad, because it's about me, and so I ought to know, so they just tell me stuff now.

Others felt differently:

> Like, yesterday he said, 'Is it alright if I speak to you here, or in the room?', and my Dad went, like, 'In the room'. I don't mind that, 'cause I know he wants to, like, check it out.

The teenagers were very perceptive, picking up information and inferences from the actions and reactions of people around them. This was used as a positive strategy for preparing themselves to receive distressing information. Teenagers noticed that sometimes adults sought to avoid giving them information, inferring that this was to avoid upsetting them, but were relieved when information was openly given once they had persuaded the adults that they really wanted to know. The issue of parental protection is widely reported. Previous studies have concluded that non-disclosure fails to mask the distressing nature of information, because children and teenagers are able to discern this from their experiences and others' behaviour (Pfefferbaum and Levenson, 1982; Claflin and Barbarin, 1991; Ellis and Leventhal, 1993).

The teenagers felt that they sometimes did ask direct questions to elicit information, but again described situations when they chose not to. They made thoughtful decisions about what information they sought from whom, about when to ask questions and what the impact of the answers might be. Asking a question was not always an easy, or a straightforward, issue. The teenagers expected professionals to give them accurate, knowledgeable information, and respected their honest, direct answers. This corroborates the work of Levenson et al. (1983), who found that teenagers valued information from 'straight-talking' physicians most highly. The teenagers in this study had acute awareness of professionals who 'knew what they were doing' and had little respect for those whom they perceived did not. The personality of professionals was also important; the teenagers cherished their relationships with those (nurses particularly) whom they perceived to be knowledgeable, friendly and trustworthy, and who respected them as individuals and maintained a positive outlook that reflected their own attempts to do so. Dunsmore and Quine (1995) also report this. At diagnosis, parents were initially given the 'bad news', with the teenagers being informed immediately afterwards, with their parents present. Individual teenagers in this study responded differently to this, highlighting the need to individualize approaches to disclosure of diagnosis. Ellis and Leventhal (1993) and Levenson et al. (1983) report that most teenagers want the opportunity to talk directly to the physician at diagnosis with their parents, but that a significant minority also want the opportunity to talk without their parents present.

Conclusions

The study attempted to describe the information needs of teenagers with cancer, and the role of information in their cancer experience. Further research is required, but these findings suggest that:

- Teenagers' priorities are for information about their illness, what treatment is available and how likely this is to be successful.
- Teenagers would benefit from accurate, timely 'progress reports' during treatment.
- There is likely to be much variation between and within individuals, requiring individualized assessment and discussion about preferred information-giving strategies.
- Teenagers perceive that they have a right to receive accurate truthful information about their illness. Attempts to exclude them precipitate anxiety and a sense of injustice.
- Teenagers rely on information to assess the impact of their illness and the threats that it poses.
- Teenagers use a range of active strategies to manage their information needs, and use information purposively to re-assert some control.
- Teenagers seek to construct positive attitudes to treatment and value the efforts of adults that mirror this. However, they sincerely wish their concerns, if voiced, to be taken seriously.
- Teenagers may not ask questions when given the opportunity. However, when they do they are likely to have considered the possible answers and to have chosen whom they ask, according to how credible and 'teenager friendly' they are perceived to be; these questions deserve our best attention and efforts.

These findings suggest the need for assessment of current practice, education and professional development. Nurses caring for teenagers with cancer and their families require specific abilities and competencies to facilitate the issues identified from this study. Effective communication skills are essential; establishing trusting relationships with adolescents takes time and yet many of the details raised by them need to be addressed at the time of diagnosis, the starting point of the relationship. Nurses, therefore, need to be able to establish a dialogue with the teenager in order to assess specific needs such as a preferred agenda for the delivery of information. Acting as the teenagers' advocate and meeting the needs of their family can sometimes create an additional challenge where skilful negotiation becomes essential.

Although a sound knowledge base about the disease and proposed treatment will underpin nurse credibility, other criteria must also be fulfilled. Involving them in decisions about their treatment (especially relevant when the adolescent is under 16 years of age), the provision of accurate, up-to-date information/results and the maintenance of hope through positive attitudes are significant issues. However, gaining and maintaining these skills is difficult as a result of the rarity of adolescent cancer. Theory relating to coping and adaptation strategies used by teenagers with chronic illness (Eiser, 1996) will also be valuable to underpin the development of ward/unit assessment and care planning documentation. Documentation generally should be reviewed to ensure that it facilitates the involvement of the teenager and assesses specific age-related issues. Involving teenagers in this part of their care may facilitate effective information and communication.

References

Boudioni M, McPherson K, Mossman J et al. (1999) An analysis of first-time enquirers to the Cancer BACUP information service: variations with cancer site, demographic status and geographical location. British Journal of Cancer 79: 138-145.

Bull B, Drotar D (1991) Coping with cancer in remission: stressors and strategies reported by children and adolescents. Journal of Pediatric Psychology 16: 76-82.

Burnard P (1991) A method of analysing interview transcripts in qualitative research. Nurse Education Today 11: 461-466.

Butow PN, Maclean M, Dunn SM, Tattersall MH, Boyer MJ (1997) The dynamics of change: cancer patients' preferences for information, involvement and support. Annals of Oncology 8: 857-863.

Cassileth BR, Zupkis RV, Sutton-Smith K, March V (1980) Information and participation preferences among cancer patients. Annals of Internal Medicine 92: 832-836.

Claflin CJ, Barbarin OA (1991) Does 'telling' less protect more? Relationships among age, information disclosure and what children with cancer see and feel. Journal of Pediatric Psychology 16: 169-191.

Coleman JC, Hendry L (1990) The Nature of Adolescence, 2nd edn. London: Routledge.

Corner J (1991) In search of more complete answers to research questions. Qualitative versus quantitative research methods: is there a way forwards? Journal of Advanced Nursing 16: 718-727.

Davison BJ, Degner LF, Morgan TR (1995) Information and decision-making preferences of men with prostate cancer. Oncology Nursing Forum 22: 1401-1408.

Degner LF, Sloan JA (1992) Decision making during serious illness: what role do patients really want to play? International Journal of Epidemiology 45: 941-950.

Department of Health (2000) The NHS Cancer Plan. London: DoH.

Derdiarian A (1989) Effects of information on recently diagnosed cancer patients and spouses' satisfaction with care. Cancer Nursing 12: 285-292.

Dunsmore J, Quine S (1995) Information, support and decision-making needs and preferences of adolescents with cancer: implications for health professionals. Journal of Psycho-oncology 13: 39-56.

Eiser C (1993) Growing up with a Chronic Disease: The impact on children and their families London: Jessica Kingsley.

Eiser C (1996) The impact of treatment: adolescents' views. In: Selby P, Bailey C (eds), Cancer and the Adolescent. London: BMJ Publishing, pp. 264-276.

Ellis JA (1991) Coping with adolescent cancer: it's a matter of adaptation. Journal of Pediatric Oncology Nursing 8: 10-17

Ellis R, Leventhal B (1993) Information needs and decision-making preferences of children with cancer. Psycho-oncology 2: 277-284.

Ettinger RS, Heiney SP (1993) Cancer in adolescents and young adults: psychosocial concerns, coping strategies and interventions. Cancer 71: 3276-3280.

Evans M (1996) Interacting with teenagers. In: Selby P, Bailey C (eds), Cancer and the Adolescent. London: BMJ Publishing, pp. 251-263.

Fallowfield L, Ford S, Lewis S (1995) No news is not good news: information preferences of patients with cancer. Psycho-oncology 4: 197-202.

Hooker L (1998) The information needs of teenagers with cancer: developing a tool to explore the perceptions of patients and professionals. Journal of Cancer Nursing 1: 160-168.

Hinds PS, Gattuso JS (1991) Measuring hopefulness in adolescents. Journal of Pediatric Oncology Nursing 8: 92-94.

Jamison RN, Lewis S, Burish TG (1986) Psychological impact of cancer on adolescents: self-image, locus of control, perception of illness and knowledge of cancer. Journal of Chronic Disease 39: 609-617.

Jenkins V, Fallowfield L, Saul J (2001) Information needs of patients with cancer: results from a large study in UK cancer centres. British Journal of Cancer 84: 48-51.

Lazarus RS, Folkman S (1984) Stress, Appraisal and Coping. New York: Springer.

Levenson PM, Copeland DR, Morrow JR, Pfefferbaum B (1983) Disparities in disease-related perceptions of adolescent cancer patients and their parents. Journal of Pediatric Psychology 8: 33-45.

Luker KA, Beaver K, Leinster SJ, Glynn Owens R, Degner LF, Sloan JA (1995) The information needs of women newly diagnosed with breast cancer. Journal of Advanced Nursing 22: 134-141.

Novack CH, Plumar P, Smith RL, Ochitill H, Morrow GR, Bennett JM (1979) Changes in physicians' attitudes towards telling the cancer patient. Journal of the American Medical Association 241: 897-900.

Oken D (1961) What to tell cancer patients. Journal of the American Medical Association 175: 86-94.

Pfefferbaum B, Levenson PM (1982) Adolescent cancer patient and physician responses to a questionnaire on patient concerns. American Journal of Psychiatry 139: 348-351.

Rechner M (1990) Adolescents with cancer: getting on with life. Journal of Pediatric Oncology Nursing 7: 139-144.

Ritchie MA (1992) Psychosocial functioning of adolescents with cancer. Oncology Nursing Forum 19: 1497-1501.

Souhami RL, Whelan J, McCarthy JF, Kilby A (1996) Benefits and problems of an adolescent oncology unit. In: Selby P, Bailey C (eds), Cancer and the Adolescent. London: BMJ Publishing, pp. 276-283.

Thomas R, Daly M, Perryman B, Stockton D (2000) Forewarned is forearmed: benefits of preparatory information on videocassette for patients receiving chemotherapy or radiotherapy - a randomised controlled trial. European Journal of Cancer 36: 1536-1543.

Thurstone LL (1974) A law of comparative judgement. In: Maranell GM (ed.), Scaling: A Sourcebook for Behavioural Scientists. Chicago: Aldine.

van der Molen (1999) Relating information needs to the cancer experience, part 1: information as a key coping strategy. European Journal of Cancer Care 8: 238-244.

Chapter 10

Shared care

Beth Sepion

Shared care was identified by Calman and Hine (Department of Health or DoH, 1995) as an important approach within cancer treatment. In paediatric oncology it was not a new concept and this was acknowledged in the NHS Cancer Plan (DoH, 2000a) with recognition for the success achieved by childhood cancer services in this area. Although it is more developed than in the adult sector, it has aspects that require adjustment and it is, therefore, still a significant issue for paediatric oncology nurses, paediatric nurses working in district general hospitals and the community, and children with cancer and their parents. Although there is a growing amount of literature describing the rationale for, and development of, this approach to care, there is little evidence of parents' experiences of participation. There is a paucity of knowledge and subsequently of understanding of the needs of parents who take part in this system, thus making us question the philosophies underpinning the fundamental principles of partnerships in care (Coyne, 1995) and family-centred care (Casey, 1988).

As part of an MSc in Child Health Nursing my thesis, in the form of a phenomenological study, set out to discover the experiences of parents whose child received cancer treatment that was shared between a regional centre and a designated shared care centre. The purpose of this chapter is to discuss some of the themes that emerged from the data, with a view to generating knowledge to encourage an holistic approach to care for children with cancer and their families. However, it must be recognized and acknowledged that qualitative research does not set out to provide data that can be generalized; the themes identified offer the opportunity to view care from different perspectives, thus providing a stimulus to examine current approaches to shared care. With reviews of the present services under way (DoH, 2000b), some of the experiences presented may no longer be issues for the new paediatric oncology shared care units

(POSCUs) in London. However, issues relating to another current Government initiative, that of involving patients and their carers (National Services Frameworks, Children's Taskforce – DoH, 2000b) may also emerge.

Incorporated within the chapter is a brief overview of the development of shared care, an outline of the study, the process of collecting and analysing the data, and a discussion of the identification of the themes. The remainder of the chapter explores the implications for current and future practice.

Shared care development

Shared care has developed within children's cancer services under the premise of improving treatment approaches for the child with cancer and his or her family (Muir et al., 1992). As documented in other chapters, the establishment of regional cancer centres for children began in the mid-1970s, when it was identified that they required the skills of an experienced multidisciplinary team (United Kingdom Children's Cancer Study Group or UKCCSG, 1997). This facilitated a coordinated physical and psychological approach for the child and his or her family, and resulted in the regional centres being deemed the 'experts' by local paediatricians and general practitioners (Pinkerton et al., 1994). The 'disappearance' of children with cancer from the district general hospitals (DGHs) resulted in healthcare professionals experiencing difficulties in keeping up to date with the treatment of children's cancer and the associated knowledge and skills (Patel et al., 1997), thus corroborating the notion of the experts elsewhere.

With this approach to care, although there was a significant improvement in mortality and morbidity rates (Stiller, 1988), long distance travel to regional centres had detrimental effects on the family and, therefore, not surprisingly financial (Bodkin et al., 1982) and psychological (Aitkin and Hathaway, 1993) problems were identified.

The development of shared care was to try to minimize these two issues while delivering safe treatment. Muir et al. (1992) demonstrated, through the measurement and comparison of survival rates, the feasibility for children with common acute lymphoblastic leukaemia (C-ALL) to receive part of their treatment in DGHs. The results claimed that it was of 'benefit for the child and family in that survival rates were comparable'. This was a quantitative study, based on comparisons of survival rates.

Shared care for paediatric oncology was introduced in the late 1980s. It was adapted from other shared cared models that have been in existence since the 1960s such as chronic diseases and obstetric care (Hickman et al., 1994; Chapple, 1995; Droongan and Bannigan, 1997). The significant difference between the models in practice was that care was primarily managed between the DGH and the GP and other community resources such as outreach clinics (Bennett et al., 1993; Orton, 1994), with little evidence of care being shared between a regional centre or tertiary centre and a DGH.

Although the UKCCSG recommended the implementation, the structure, management and organization were developed and implemented on an individual and local level. Each regional centre addressing specific elements depends on local services and geographical issues. The London region posed unique issues which, with hindsight, necessitated a multicentre collaborative approach. The current review of shared care has acknowledged this; however, the original review in the early 1990s was fragmented with individual regional centres in the London area developing their own system (Services for Children with Cancer in the South Thames Region, 1996). Unfortunately, as a result of the geographical location of regional centres and DGHs, and patterns of referral, this led to a system that posed challenges for all staff whether they were based in the regional centre, the DGH or the community, and for the patient and their family. The four regional centres within the London area share care with over 60 DGHs. Each DGH may participate in shared care with one, some or all of the London regional centres. Consequently, staff at DGHs may care for children with cancer who have received their initial treatment at different regional centres, where the approach to the management of common symptoms and procedures is dissimilar. This had the potential to cause confusion for the healthcare professionals and the child and family when comparisons were made.

It appeared, therefore, in the London area that, rather than improving care, shared care had created new challenges for the patient and his or her family and for childhood cancer healthcare professionals, in whichever area they were working.

The study

As previously mentioned Muir et al.'s (1992) study did not enquire into parents' experiences of participating in care that is shared between a regional cancer centre and a DGH, and yet they stated that such a practice would benefit the patient and the family. This was my stimulus. A central premise of family-centred care is negotiation (Coyne, 1995) and yet shared care is non-negotiable. It is the 'lottery' of paediatric cancer. Participation in shared care is determined by diagnosis and prognosis. Initially shared care was only for children who were diagnosed with C-ALL because it had been demonstrated that the side effects of the treatment, once remission was achieved, were manageable by DGHs (Muir et al., 1992). As knowledge about the management of side effects and prognostic features has increased and, in keeping with the drive to provide more outpatient care, the treatment or part treatment of other childhood cancers is now deemed manageable within the context of shared care.

There is a notion that there is pressure to increase shared care as a result of the increased demands for inpatient beds as intensive treatment regimens are developed for other childhood cancers. However, this approach is underpinned by the Calman and Hine Report (DoH, 1995), and the NHS Cancer Plan (DoH, 2000a) which both highlight the advantages of this approach towards achieving the 'seamless service'.

Participation in care

Following Government recommendations (the Platt Report – Central Health Services Council, 1959; the Children's Act [DoH, 1989]; the Welfare of Children and Young People in Hospital [DoH, 1991]; Audit Commission, 1993), parental participation in care is deemed normal practice for paediatric care. There is now an expectation that parents will become extensively involved in the care of their child (Callery and Smith, 1991). Parents are 'empowered' (Gibson, 1995; Valentine, 1997) to take on the role of caring for their sick child by nurses, through the provision of education about the illness and its treatment and new skills required to carry out 'nursing tasks'. Parent and staff negotiation is a key component of parent participation (Ahmann, 1994); however, Coyne (1995) suggests that this is an area where there are still problems attributed to the issues of knowledge and power. Parents of children with cancer need to have an understanding of several complex care issues relating to their child's disease and treatment strategy. They require information to care for central venous lines, recognize and manage infections and febrile episodes, and continue treatment and/or prophylactic medication regimens. For many parents, in order to do this they have to have some understanding of their child's illness and its treatment (Smith et al., 1983; Canam, 1986; Thompson, 1990; Eden et al., 1994; Pinkerton et al., 1994; Gibson and Evans, 1999); in short they have to become experts and develop their own expertise.

Although it is not well documented, there is evidence (Evans, 1994), and discussions at the Thames Paediatric Oncology Nurses Group (TPONG) and other paediatric oncology forums, that parents are extending their skills to access lines for taking blood samples and to administer intravenous drugs, in some cases chemotherapy. It appears, therefore, that participation in care is continuing to expand with some exploration of the perceptions of parents and nurses (Kawik, 1996), and encouragement by current Government initiatives such as National Service Frameworks (DoH, 2000b). The emphasis from these initiatives is, however, to involve the patients and their family in the negotiation – to listen to what they have to say.

My study, therefore, was to hear what parents wanted to tell me about what it is like to participate in care that is shared between a regional cancer centre and a DGH. The aim was to obtain in-depth accounts in order to gain a better understanding and, it is hoped, an increase in knowledge for nurses caring for families who participate in this approach to care.

Phenomenology is a naturalistic research methodology, a paradigm that is gaining recognition in nursing research because it offers the opportunity to explore issues that are different for every human being, and thus in keeping with the values and beliefs of the profession (Beck, 1994). It is criticized and has been referred to as a 'soft science' by some nurse researchers, with Salsberry (1989) arguing that it is not a scientific method because it does not generate new nursing knowledge. However, although it is acknowledged that studies of this type do not provide results that are applicable to the bigger picture, Munhall (1994) advocates their value by suggesting that a good study, rather than confirming truths or correctness, can liberate preconceptions, so enabling the original phenomenon to be viewed from a different perspective.

This different perception may then provide the opportunity to contemplate alternative strategies for the management or treatment of the phenomenon. Phenomenology is a philosophy, as well as a research approach (Pallikkathayil and Morgan, 1991), that has been applied to psychology, sociology and nursing (Taylor, 1993). It is complex, with confusing origins, but it provides a vehicle to explore the feelings of parents and legitimizes the use of narratives to expand/broaden nursing knowledge. Qualitative research is more frequently being used as a first step (Annells, 1999), in order to establish an understanding of an issue or area within nursing with a view to identifying appropriate methods to carry out quantitative studies.

Through discussion with supervisors I decided that interviews with six parents should provide sufficient data without making the task of analysing it too difficult. Having gained the appropriate ethical consent, a process that took a considerable amount of time and patience, data collection was undertaken. In-depth, semi-structured interviews (Rose, 1994) were used to facilitate the parents' description of their experiences.

The criteria for inviting parents to participate were: parents of a child with ALL who had experienced inpatient care in their designated shared care DGH. The criteria for participant selection were:

- parent of a child with cancer
- parent who had experienced care in their shared care hospital
- parent who understood the nature of the study
- parent who spoke and understood English.

The advantages and disadvantages of carrying out research in an area in which you are known and/or work had been explored with colleagues experienced in undertaking research in the 'field'. Ethical issues that I believed to be important in this study were those of confidentiality, informed consent, the absence of coercion, privacy, and accuracy of the presentation and interpretation of the data. I was concerned that parents may feel obliged to participate in case their child's care would be influenced in some way. The ward sister helped me to overcome this. She advised me when a family who fulfilled the criteria were admitted; she would then ask their permission for me to approach them to explain the study. If they agreed I would meet with them to explain the study further and make arrangements to return after a minimum of 24 hours to obtain written consent, at which point a mutually convenient time and venue for the interview would also be agreed.

Informed consent is not a static issue associated with the signing of a consent form (Beech, 1999). Therefore, when obtaining the witnessed signing of the consent form, I reiterated that the interview could be stopped at any time by them, they could refuse to answer any questions, all data would remain anonymous, names of the parents and their child would be changed, other family members, staff, names of hospitals would be recorded as sibling, husband, nurse, etc. and DGH or regional cancer centre. Finally, it was stressed that under no circumstances would their child's current or subsequent treatment be affected. I interviewed six parents – five mothers and one father – which is a realistic representation of the ward population.

The interviews were tape-recorded. Although a tape-recorder appears intimidating to both the researcher and the participant at the start, the positioning of the machine and nature of the interviews meant that it was usually soon forgotten and ignored. The advantages of using the tape-recorder include accurate collection of the data and the ability of the interviewer to concentrate on what is being said and to encourage the participant (Burns and Grove, 1987). It avoids the participant having to speak to the top of the interviewer's head, thus encouraging the maintenance of eye contact. Five of the interviews took place on the ward in rooms that maintained privacy but were easily accessible for the participants' child, and one took place in the participants' home. I had advised the parents that the interview would last for approximately an hour. One interview lasted longer than this – 75 minutes; the other five ranged between 40 and 55 minutes.

All the parents, although apprehensive of the tape-recorder at first, appeared to relax once the interview was under way and were able to describe their experiences clearly. It was an emotional experience for them because one of the questions asked them to tell me about when they first heard of shared care; this brought back memories of the time of their child's diagnosis.

The amount of data collected through six interviews of about an hour each was staggering. Transcribing the tapes took many hours but, when the transcriptions were printed, I could understand why it had taken so long.

Following data collection and transcription, the next stage in phenomenology is to describe the data in order to facilitate others understanding of the experience – not to analyse the experience but to provide a concept of the experience. There are methods available to assist the researcher; I chose the Giorgi method modified by Banonis (1988), which involves intensive reading of the transcriptions, looking for themes and identifying meaningful units.

Identification of the themes

As I had transcribed the tapes, I was already quite familiar with the data; however, initially the intensive reading identified 57 different themes. On re-reading I was able to assimilate these into 21 themes (Table 10.1).

The next stage is to re-read the themes to identify the focal meaning units. The initial 21 themes were re-examined to gain an understanding of the meaning of the experience. This process resulted in the identification of three focal meaning units: expectations, feelings and 'being more than a parent'.

Expectations

Parents described their expectations of both the regional cancer centre and the shared care hospital. The initial way that they were informed

Figure 10.1 Themes in the interview transcriptions

1   Child viewed as being different
2   Lack of skills
3   Experts
4   Parents placed in uncomfortable positions
5   Fighting for child
6   Feelings
7   Trust
8   Parent's knowledge and skills
9   Compromised care
10 Time
11 Facilities
12 Isolation
13 Information/communication
14 Care at diagnosis
15 Complaints
16 Risks
17 Pleasant staff
18 No choice
19 Safe
20 Advantages
21 What it is not

about transfer to the regional centre and then subsequently advised about participating in shared care influenced the parents' attitude to shared care.

Beverly was informed that:

> She was going to be transferred to the experts at the regional centre.

The staff at the DGH had been very efficient, professional and supportive at the time of pre-diagnosis, and she recognized that her son required specific care for his serious illness; however, she was concerned about the skills of nurses:

> Initially when they told us we would have shared care we were slightly nervous, this is such a specialized unit for a specific type of illness; you do worry whether the nurses at the local hospital are going to be trained well enough to look after your child, because obviously you want the best possible care for them.

Beverly said:

> I suppose the fact that the regional centre has approved them as a shared care centre you have some faith because I don't think you'd be able to go just anywhere.

The facilities was a common theme. The regional centre was purpose built with the help of funding by charities. The facilities are, as one parent described, 'like being in a posh hotel'. Parents have a kitchen to prepare food for themselves and their child. This practice is not feasible in all children's wards and it does cause additional stress for the parents if they are in hospital for a period of time. Food can become a focal point in the life of the child with cancer and their parents because the side effects of steroids and chemotherapy create a nutritional roller coaster.

Felicity explained that:

> There is no provision for you to eat, which doesn't sound much, but when you are in for long periods of time it is.

Beverly said:

> Our major worry when we went in was what are we going to do about food. With the drugs [patient] has become a fussy eater. If they don't like what comes round on the trolley and you can't cook it in a microwave, they don't eat.

The issue of time related to facilities/resources also created problems for the parents. Some of them had been advised by the regional centre that one of the reasons for shared care was to minimize the time spent travelling long distances for a 'quick blood test', when they could go to their local hospital (shared care centre). In theory this sounded logical; in practice it did not always work. For one family the regional centre was closer than the designated shared care centre. For another, there were a limited number of staff who could access a Port-A-Cath, and if they were attending on a day when only one was on duty they could wait longer than if they had travelled the extra distance to the regional centre.

Elizabeth described:

> We had the experience of going to shared care hospital when there wasn't anyone who could access his line. This proves very distressing because at the beginning he wasn't used to having people poking him around.

Chris was concerned:

> When you are going for bloods and you are waiting for 4 hours and there's no sort of awareness . . . children with a life-threatening illness who have a lot of hospitalization. They have a lot of normalization taken away from them.

Diana stated that:

> She was eventually accessed by a locum doctor in the end who bruised her; he was so rough and he'd obviously never done it before.

Feelings

The experiences described by the parents in this theme included isolation, having to cope with other people's reactions, including parents and healthcare professionals, being different, and having to relive the past.

Isolation was both physical and emotional. The physical isolation related to being isolated in order to prevent contraction of an infection by the child. Although parents could understand and appreciate the rationale and logic of this, it did mean that the child and parent were very alone. If they were allowed into the playroom, no other children were allowed in there at the same time. They felt isolated because often they were the only cancer family on the ward and parents of children with non-malignant illnesses did not always know how to react or to interact with them. This made them feel that they were different.

Elizabeth described:

> Its a bit like a gold fish bowl, when anyone's walking past and they see a bald headed little child.

Beverly explained:

> Isolation really does mean isolation; we understand why but it's very hard, he's very isolated, he's either in the play room on his own or in the room on his own with mummy and daddy.

Also:

> [doctors] relying on you to spout all the information all the time. You don't want to re-live the past 18 months.

Reliving the past was an experience that parents found distressing. Felicity also said:

> The other thing is the medical students coming up and asking to take a history because they find it fascinating. It doesn't help me much though having to talk about her illness.

Being more than a parent

Being more than a parent was a description given by one of the parents during the interview. Themes that contributed to this were: fighting for your child, being on your guard, monitoring your child's condition, being put into difficult conditions, and developing or extending your skills.

The difficulties occurred when parents had or felt that they had more knowledge and experience than the healthcare professionals caring for their child. They felt that they were placed in difficult situations when procedures were being carried out because the healthcare professional was unable to judge an individual situation.

Felicty said:

> We've been in the clinical room to have bloods taken and the doctor has got the guide book in front of them because they've never done it before. I don't blame her, but I just think no-one should be put in that position.

Extending their roles was a common issue. Teaching healthcare professionals to access and use central venous lines occurred frequently; occasionally parents administered antibiotics to meet a short-fall in the service provision. This again left the parents feeling isolated, different and vulnerable.

Diana described:

> I had to tell him how to do it. They couldn't take blood, so I had to write a protocol for them of how to do it.

Parental knowledge initially had been identified as a meaningful unit but it became apparent that it was the nucleus to the other three.

Diana explained:

> It was my child, how could I let anybody do anything to her without me knowing that was what should happen, it's your job to find out as much as possible . . . .

> She's the most important person in my life, how can I sit back and let someone do something to her that I don't know what they are doing.

Participating in shared care has a profound effect and invokes a range of intense emotions. The parents have to adapt to being cared for in environments where most of the healthcare professionals have received specific training and education or in environments where limited resources affect the standard of care. Assumptions are made by the parents that the standards will be the same because the regional centre has approved the shared care hospital.

There is now a range of literature exploring families' adaptation and coping mechanisms relating to chronic childhood illness. Canam (1986, 1993) identified that parents need information about their child's illness and treatment if they are to adapt successfully. There is a growing wealth of literature addressing the importance of parental knowledge relating to successful adaptation to cancer (Koocher and O'Malley, 1981; Blotcky et al., 1985; Brett and Davies, 1988; Clarke-Steffen, 1993, 1997; Thoma et al., 1993; Birenbaum, 1995). The pivotal component is information. Canam's (1993) study of parents' adaptation to the diagnosis of their child's cancer identified eight tasks (Table 10.2). The underlying assumption of each task is the acquisition of specific knowledge, skills and resources.

The complexity of the cancer treatments and the interrelationship between symptoms and side effects place tremendous pressure on parents in managing task 2. Understanding the disease, the treatment protocol,

Figure 10.2 Eight tasks identified by Canam (1993)

1   Accept the child's condition

2   Manage the child's condition on a day-to-day basis

3   Meet the child's normal developmental needs

4   Meet the developmental needs of other family members

5   Cope with ongoing stress

6   Assist family members to manage their feelings

7   Educate others about their child's condition

8   Establish a support system

Canam (1993, p. 46).

administering medications, caring for central venous devices, and monitoring and managing side effects require the skills of an experienced practitioner, and yet some parents may face going home within a week of the confirmation of the diagnosis and the start of treatment. It is hardly surprising that parents, by the time they visit the shared care hospital, are already becoming experts about their child's illness and treatment. However, it is stressed by Ahmann (1994) that the family is the constant in the child's life and their knowledge is crucial to the success of any healthcare plan. This has created a dichotomy. In some situations the parents have a greater understanding of their child's care needs related to the illness and its treatment/management than the healthcare professionals and this can create a problem for all concerned. The literature does not offer a solution because the issues of parental preparation for being cared for in different healthcare environments have not been researched.

The problem exists because to maintain expert practice and keep up to date with new knowledge there is a need to have regular practice. This is not always feasible for healthcare professionals working in DGHs. It is not realistic to train every member of staff and maintain their expertise/skills when the number of patients is small, and yet parents see this as a problem.

The problem has three components: the regional centre: the shared care centre, and the patient and their family. The Cancer Plan (DoH, 2000) talks about the 'seamless' approach to care. The description from some of the parents identified that the regional centre, once shared care was started, offered a 'seem less' to care approach. Felicity described that she felt like a:

> Second class citizen, that her daughter was not as important because of her diagnosis.

The term 'collaborative working' (Mercer and Richie, 1997) was introduced earlier and the development of the paediatric oncology shared care units in the London area is based more on a collaborative model, except for the inclusion of one of the key stake holders, the parents of children with cancer (Cardy, 2002).

One of the values of phenomenology identified earlier is that it offers the opportunity to review the approaches to current practice, to examine what is taken for granted. Shared care has, for many staff, become taken for granted. The way that parents are prepared for and supported through the illness may need to be reviewed, not only by the regional centre but also by the shared care centres, and strategies for parental preparation and support revised or developed. If parents are to be responsible for their child's care, effective negotiation, as identified by Callery and Smith (1991) is essential and effective assessment, preparation and teaching criteria need to be established. The opportunity to discuss the impact of this extended parental role on the whole family should be included, along with strategies to achieve Canam's (1993) tasks. In addition to this, parents also require advice and support to facilitate the establishment of relationships where they may be more knowledgeable than the healthcare professionals.

Of equal importance, if it is a given that parents are to become 'experts', the skills required by healthcare professionals to establish and maintain therapeutic relationships when working in areas where less childhood cancer experience is available need to be identified and appropriate development programmes devised.

Other areas that necessitate investigation include communication (Cooley, 2000). Parent-held records have been advocated as an effective method of communication by Hooker and Williams (1996), but these and other systems require evaluation. Communication facilities/networks should include advice for parents when they are unhappy about or unsure of issues related to the care of their child.

Another area for development is parental preparation for being cared for in different healthcare environments. Listening to the parents is an important part of developing appropriate family-centred care. Heller and McKlindon (1996) suggest making parents part of the 'faculty' in education establishments, in order that students hear first hand what it is like to have a child who is ill and cared for in hospital. It would, perhaps, help healthcare professionals to value the parents' journey of becoming more than a parent if they 'heard', from parents, about their experiences of participating in cancer treatment programmes.

References

Aitkin TJ, Hathaway G (1993) Long distance related stressors and coping behaviours in parents of children with cancer. Journal of Pediatric Oncology 10: 3-12.

Ahmann E (1994) Family centred care: shifting orientation. Pediatric Nursing 20: 113-117.

Annells M (1999) Evaluating phenomenology: usefulness, quality and philosophical foundations. Nurse Researcher 6(3): 5-19.

Audit Commission (1993) Children First: A study of hospital services. London: HMSO.

Banonis BC (1988) The lived experience of recovering from addiction: a phenomenological study. Nursing Science Quarterly 2: 37-42.

Beck CT (1994) Phenomenology: its use in nursing research. International Journal of Nursing Studies 31: 499-510.

Beech I (1999) Bracketing in phenomenological research. Nurse Researcher 6: 35-51.

Bennett L, May C, Wolfson D (1993) Sharing care between the hospital and the community: a critical review of developments in the UK. Health and Social Care 2: 105-112.

Birenbaum LK (1995) State of the science: Family research in pediatric oncology nursing. Journal of Pediatric Oncology Nursing 12: 25-38.

Blotcky AD, Raczynski JM, Gurwitch R, Smith K (1985) Family influences on hopelessness among children early in the cancer experience. Journal of Pediatric Psychology 10: 479-493.

Bodkin CM, Pigott TJ, Mann JR (1982) Financial burden of childhood cancer. British Medical Journal 284: 1542-1545.

Brett KM, Davies EMB (1988) 'What does it mean?' Sibling and parental appraisals of childhood leukemia. Cancer Nursing 11: 329-338.

Burns N, Grove S (1987) The Practice of Nursing Research, Conduct, Critique and Utilisation. Philadelphia: WB Saunders.

Cardy P (2002) NICE isn't listening. News, Cancer Nursing Practice 1: 4.

Callery P, Smith L (1991) A study of role negotiation between nurses and the parents of hospitalised children. Journal of Advanced Nursing 16: 772-782.

Canam C (1986) Talking about cystic fibrosis within the family: what parents need to know. Issues in Comprehensive Nursing 9: 167-178.

Canam C (1993) Common adaptive tasks facing the parents of children with a chronic conditions. Journal of Advanced Nursing 18: 46-53.

Casey A (1988) A partnership with child and family. Senior Nurse 8: 60-61.

Central Health Services Council, Ministry of Health (1959) Platt Report: The Welfare of Children in Hospital. London: HMSO.

Chapple CR (1995) Prostate shared care in practice. Geriatric Medicine July: 34-36.

Clarke-Steffen L (1993) A model of the family transition to living with cancer. Cancer Practice 1: 285-292.

Clarke-Steffen L (1997) Reconstructing reality: family strategies for managing childhood cancer. Journal of Pediatric Nursing 12: 278-287.

Cooley C (2000) Communication services in palliative care. Professional Nurse 9: 103-105

Coyne IT (1995) Parental participation in care: a critical review of the literature. Journal of Advanced Nursing 21: 716-722.

Department of Health (1989) The Children Act. London: HMSO.

Department of Health (1991) Welfare of Children and Young People in Hospital. London: HMSO.

Department of Health (1995) A Policy Framework for Commissioning Cancer Services. (Calman-Hine Report). London: HMSO.

Department of Health (2000a) The NHS Cancer Plan. A plan for investment. A plan for reform. London: DoH - www.doh.org.uk/cancer

Department of Health (2000b) The NHS Plan. A plan for investment. A plan for reform. National Service Frameworks, The Children's Taskforce. London: DoH www.doh.gov/nsf/children

Droongan J, Bannigan K (1997) Organisation of asthma care: what difference does it make? Nursing Times 93(34): 45-46.

Eden OB, Black I, MacKinlay GA, Emery AEH (1994) Communication with parents of children with cancer. Palliative Medicine 8: 105-114.

Evans M (1994) An investigation into the feasibility of parental participation in the nursing care of their children. Journal of Advanced Nursing 20: 477-482.

Gibson CH (1995) The process of empowerment in mothers of chronically ill children. Journal of Advanced Nursing 21: 1201-1210.

Gibson F, Evans M (1999) Paediatric Oncology: Acute nursing care. London: Whurr Publishers.

Heller R, McKlindon D (1996) Families as 'faculty': parents educating caregivers about family centred care. Pediatric Nursing 22: 428-431.

Hickman M, Drummond N, Grimshaw J (1994) The operation of shared care for chronic disease. Health Bulletin 52: 118-126.

Hooker L, Williams J (1996) Parent held shared care records: bridging the communication gaps. British Journal of Nursing 5: 738-741.

Kawik L (1996) Nurses and parents perception and partnership in caring for hospitalised child. British Journal of Nursing 5: 430-434.

Koocher GP, O'Malley JE (1981) The Damocles Syndrome. New York: McGraw Hill.

Mercer M, Ritchie JA (1997) Tag team parenting of children with cancer. Journal of Pediatric Nursing 12: 331-341.

Muir KR, Parkes SE, Boon R, Stevens MCG, Mann JR (1992) Shared care in paediatric oncology. Journal of Cancer Care 1: 15-17.

Munhall P (1994) Revisioning Phenomenology: nursing and health science research. New York: National League for Nursing Press.

Orton P (1994) Shared care. The Lancet 344: 1413-1415.

Pallikkathayil L, Morgan SA (1991) Phenomenology as a method for conducting clinical research. Applied Nursing Research 4: 195-200.

Patel N, Sepion B, Williams J (1997) Development of a shared care programme for children with cancer. Journal of Cancer Nursing 1: 1-4.

Pinkerton CR, Cushing P, Sepion B (1994) Childhood Cancer Management. London: Chapman & Hall.

Rose K (1994) Unstructured and semi-structured interviewing. Nurse Researcher 1: 23-32.

Salsberry PJ (1989) Phenomenological research in nursing: commentary and responses. Nursing Science Quarterly 2: 9-13.

Services for Children with Cancer in the South Thames Region (1996) Report of the South Thames Paediatric Oncology Working Party. London: UKCCSG.

Smith CE, Garvis MS, Martinson IM (1983) Content analysis of interviews using a nursing model: A look at parents adapting to the impact of childhood cancer. Cancer Nursing 6: 269-275.

Stiller CA (1988) Centralisation of treatment and survival rates for cancer. Archives of Diseases in Childhood 63: 32-40.

Taylor B (1993) Phenomenology: one way to understand nursing practice. International Journal of Nursing Studies 30: 171-179.

Thoma ME, Hockenberry-Eaton M, Kemp V (1993) Life change events and coping behaviors in families of children with cancer. Journal of Pediatric Oncology Nursing 10: 105-111.

Thompson J (1990) The Child with Cancer, Nursing Care. London: Scutari Press.

United Kingdom Children's Cancer Study Group (1997) The Resources and Requirements of a UKCCSG Treatment Centre. University of Leicester.

Valentine F (1997) Empowerment: family centred care. Paediatric Nursing 10: 24-27.

Chapter 11

A survey of staffing levels

Rachel Hollis, Alison Arnfield and Guy Makin

Services for children and young people with cancer in the United Kingdom and Ireland are provided in the 22 regional centres of the United Kingdom Childhood Cancer Study Group (UKCCSG) and the district general hospitals with which they share care. Significant improvements in outcomes for paediatric cancers have been associated with the development of specialist treatment centres for children and young people (Stiller, 1994). Centralization of treatment has occurred partly as a result of the move towards increased specialization in paediatrics, and partly as a response to the need to see sufficient patients to generate a critical mass for involvement in innovative new treatments and clinical trials. Experience and evidence over the last 25 years in paediatric oncology have shown that developing expert multidisciplinary teams in the regional treatment centres of the UKCCSG, and the subsequent development of clinical expertise in the management of critically ill children, have been important factors in improved overall survival (Mott et al., 1997). Expert nursing care, from highly qualified nurses educated in both paediatrics and oncology, is recognized as an essential element of that specialist support required by children, young people and their families.

The UKCCSG acts as a coordinating body for clinical trials, so that children and young people treated in any of the regional centres, which stretch from Aberdeen and Belfast to London and Bristol, should all receive the same treatment. It also provides peer support to team members, and develops and critically evaluates programmes of care. This is in line with the recommendations of the Expert Advisory Group on Cancer (Department of Health, 1995), commonly known as the 'Calman–Hine Report', which gave guidance on the provision of services to cancer patients. The Report set out, as its first principle, that 'all patients should have access to a uniformly high standard of care'. Within the specialty of paediatric oncology, there has been a growing recognition of the need for equity and accountability in the quality of service provision. In the actual treatment of disease, there is generally a greater equity in the provision of care to children than in the adult population (Department of Health, 2000a), although the care of adolescents and young people remains fragmented and subject to local referral patterns (Hollis and Morgan, 2001).

Although regional centres generally give the same medical treatments, using the same protocols, they do so in very different clinical environments and with different resources. Paediatric oncology is a relatively new specialty and has had to compete for resources at a time of stringent budgetary control and an increasingly cost-conscious culture. There have been attempts to address this variation in service provision with the development of standards and guidance for the care of certain patient groups, notably children with leukaemia (Royal College of Pathologists, 1996), and children with brain and spinal tumours (Royal College of Paediatrics and Child Health – UKCCSG, 1997a). An attempt has also been made to define more broadly the requirements and resources needed in a treatment centre for childhood cancer (UKCCSG, 1997b). These documents go some way towards identifying national standards for service provision in the care of children and young people with cancer. This brings the specialty into line with the most recent developments of the Government's policy on health and the need to develop national standards, as set out in both the 'NHS Plan' and the subsequent 'Cancer Plan' (DoH, 2000a, 2000b). The Cancer Plan, however, makes little reference to services for children, and none at all to services for adolescents and young people. Within paediatric oncology, it is recognized that the current guidance documents are not sufficiently comprehensive in their recommendations to form a robust framework for the development of national standards for services for children and young people with cancer and their families. Although a National Service Framework for children is being developed it is unlikely that this will offer specific guidance for standards of care in any particular specialty.

Nurse staffing levels

One of the key elements of a high-quality service is the workforce that delivers the care and support to children and their families. The Cancer Plan (DoH, 2000b) recognizes that nurses are the largest single group within the cancer workforce, and their contribution to care is crucial to the delivery of safe, efficient, timely and empathetic treatment. Paediatric oncology patients place considerable demand on the nursing team, much greater than an 'average' paediatric patient. These are very sick children who require intensive nursing input, alongside considerable non-clinical support for the whole family, who are devastated by the diagnosis of cancer and the impact of the treatment. Although the overall numbers of children with cancer in the UK have remained much the same over the last few years, many more are now surviving treatment and/or embarking on more intensive treatments, which has greatly increased the requirement of the nursing workforce. No clear and comprehensive national guidance or recommendations for nurse staffing levels within paediatric oncology are available.

The Cancer Nursing Society of the Royal College of Nursing (RCN, 1996) addressed the needs of cancer patients for appropriate nursing care and support in the light of the recommendations of the 'Policy Framework for Commissioning Cancer Services'. They referred to the need for 'specialist nursing services' to be available to children, but stated only that there should be a 'minimum of two Registered Sick Children's Nurses, who are also trained in paediatric oncology, available on each shift to supervise in-patient care and treatment for children and families'. This document makes use of long-standing national guidance on the staffing of any children's wards which recommends *at least* two qualified children's nurses at any one time (DoH, 1993), although this is recognized as a minimum requirement on a general children's ward. It is certainly not a total number for any specialist unit with highly dependent and complex patients.

These recommendations made no reference to the numbers of nurses needed in relation to the number of patients on a ward or unit or the dependency of those patients. A key earlier report on service needs from the UKCCSG (1987) recommends that, in paediatric oncology, 'of the beds provided, one third should be staffed to high dependency nursing standards and the remainder to medium dependency levels'. This was reiterated in the guidance for the care of children with leukaemia (Royal College of Pathologists, 1996). This reflects the complexity of the clinical workload on these specialist wards, and the dependency of patients. There has been no comprehensive attempt to translate this into more concrete terms. The Calman–Hine Report (DoH, 1995) states that 'the provision of specialist nursing in paediatric oncology must remain a high priority for purchasers'. The nature of that 'specialist nursing' and the level of nursing support remain ill defined.

Background to the work

The issues of workload and staffing levels within units have long been a matter of concern to both the UKCCSG and the Paediatric Oncology Nurses Forum (PONF) of the RCN. PONF brings together nurses working with children and young people with cancer, and works closely with the UKCCSG. The 1987 UKCCSG report was written with input from the PONF and addressed many of the key concerns relating to staffing levels. In certain areas little seems to have changed, and some of the same problems persist in many units today. In 1999 these concerns became more critical for a number of reasons. A number of regional treatment centres were undergoing external staffing reviews, which in some cases benchmarked paediatric oncology wards against general paediatric medical wards, without any recognition of the complexity of the workload and the dependency of patients in the specialty. The complexity of this particular specialty is well understood within paediatrics, but is not well described or documented. No tools, benchmarks or best practice guidance are available on staffing, although the nursing role is highly technical, and the skills and knowledge that it requires are in many ways akin to paediatric intensive care.

All specialist centres expect nurses to work well beyond traditional nursing boundaries, e.g. in the delivery and management of cytotoxic drug treatment regimens and complex intravenous therapy. Their assessment skills are highly developed in managing vulnerable, often very sick and haemodynamically unstable children. The supportive role of nurses, which demands strong interpersonal skills in a difficult area of practice, is well recognized. All the regional centres have a consistently heavy caseload and many of them face unremitting pressure on beds, yet few have effective tools for measuring and quantifying either activity or patient dependency. A number of centres have major and in some cases chronic problems of recruitment and retention, and this obviously contributes to pressure on beds and on the nursing workforce.

Methodology

After discussion at a meeting of the Link Members of PONF, where all centres are represented, the forum steering group decided on a national study to map out staffing provision within the specialty. The aim was to establish current staffing levels, and identify patterns, differences and issues in the 22 centres. A project group was formed and met with an independent children's nursing consultant with a particular interest in both paediatric oncology and staffing in an initial 'brainstorming' exercise. An attempt was made in this group towards representation of the clinical and geographical diversity of the UKCCSG centres. Representatives were sought from centres that share the care of their patients with their local district general hospitals (DGHs) and those that undertake all the treatment themselves, units with integrated bone marrow transplantation (BMT) units, those with separate units, and those that send their patients elsewhere for transplantation.

A literature search carried out before the meeting yielded little in the way of useful published work in relation to the staffing of children's' wards, and nothing at all in relation to the staffing of children's cancer wards and units. Some work on guidance for staffing of paediatric wards was available (RCN, 1999a, 1999b) but revealed no categorical numbers or formulae for numbers of staff. All members of this group were asked to look for any useful local methods of workload or dependency measurement that might be useful in the work.

The aim of the initial 'brainstorming' exercise was to try to identify the most critical factors when looking at nursing staffing levels specifically in paediatric oncology. It was recognized that the regional centres all worked in very different ways and that, with so many variables, comparison of like with like, to establish a benchmark, would be complex and difficult. Local issues were important, as was the ability to identify common factors that would enable the development of meaningful ways of establishing comparisons across the centres. At the end of the meeting a list of critical elements that affected staffing levels were established, which included:

- the availability of dedicated oncology inpatient provision, or the mix of inpatients on the ward.
- the dependency of children cared for on the ward, the availability of, and access to, high dependency unit (HDU)/intensive care unit (ICU) beds and criteria for transfer of patients.
- the use of complex, high-dose chemotherapy regimens and facilities for BMT on the ward.
- availability of separate, dedicated, oncology day care and associated resources.
- the impact of 'shared care' on the centre.
- medical staffing numbers and the experience of medical personnel.
- pharmacy support, including personnel, and the service provided, in particular, centralized intravenous additive (CIVA) or aseptic services.
- play provision.

- the role of support workers, including administrative support, housekeeper and similar roles, and phlebotomy.
- development of specialist, educational and other nursing roles to support the work of the unit.

The factors identified during this exercise emphasized once again the complex nature of the specialty, and the difficulty of trying to develop a tool that would capture that complexity. The next task was to try to fashion a tool to do this, initially through the development of a self-completed questionnaire.

A copy of the first draft of a questionnaire was circulated to all members of the working group. While responses were awaited, the Chair of the PONF was approached by a representative of the UKCCSG with the draft of a questionnaire that had been designed to address some of these same issues of staffing levels in the regional centres. The audit project, under the broad auspices of the UKCCSG, intended to look not only at medical staffing levels, but also at nursing and pharmacy numbers and configurations. It was clear that this was an opportunity to look at this as a multidisciplinary project, with the backing of both the PONF and the UKCCSG.

There was some work to be done in merging the two draft questionnaires. The 'PONF' version was too complex, trying to identify as many as possible of the factors raised by the working group. The UKCCSG version was too brief, and would not provide the detail needed for meaningful conclusions to be made. So began a time-consuming process of amalgamation and refinement. The outcome of this was a questionnaire that, it was felt, would yield the information needed, and prove reasonably 'user-friendly' to complete.

It was decided to pilot it in three organizationally different centres, where link nurses were asked to complete the questionnaire, and comment on its ease and applicability. It was also important to establish whether it was possible to obtain all the information requested and to ascertain whether there were other questions that should be asked. This pilot was sent out and completed in May 2000 and some small changes were made in response to the results. The questionnaires were then sent to all 22 regional centres of the UKCCSG in August 2000. One copy went to the (medical) UKCCSG Centre Co-ordinator and another to the (nursing) PONF Link Member. A covering letter from both the Chair of the PONF and the UKCCSG representative emphasized the importance of the project, and the expectation that the questionnaire would be completed with input from pharmacists and other members of the multidisciplinary team.

The eventual response rate was 100%, although the initial analysis of the questionnaires showed a considerable amount of missing data, and also revealed the difficulty that had been anticipated in 'fitting' the very different centres into one framework of analysis. It quickly became clear that the particular circumstances of local centres had a considerable impact on the way that they worked, and that it was going to be difficult to make meaningful comparisons. However, it was equally clear that all centres shared common challenges of a complex clinical workload, which the data would reflect.

It was necessary to go back to some centres on a number of occasions to obtain missing fundamental information on patient numbers and bed numbers. Frequently occurring problems included difficulty in establishing actual staffing levels, and the difference between funded nursing establishments and actual nurses in post. This was most marked in those centres where facilities for oncology patients were 'shared' with other patients. In one centre with multiple sites, the data were particularly complex, and in much of the analysis it was not possible to include this centre. Finally, when all the missing data were available, it was possible to begin to draw together some conclusions. The findings presented here describe the service provided in the regional treatment centres, and look in particular at the nursing establishments providing that core service.

Findings and discussion

Inpatient wards

The first question asked whether centres had dedicated inpatient wards. Of the 22 centres, only 5 did not have a ward dedicated to oncology, although a number of other centres used their beds for an additional small number of non-malignant haematology patients. This is a marked improvement on the earlier work carried out by the UKCCSG (1987) when only 4 of the 20 centres in existence at that time had wards specifically designated for paediatric oncology. That report highlighted concerns about the difficulties of shared wards, whether they were shared with other paediatric subspecialities or general paediatrics. These comments were echoed in this study through the questionnaires returned by those centres that still shared their wards (Table 11.1).

Of the five wards identified above, two shared their ward with cardiology, which is clearly a mix of two subspecialities with highly dependent patient groups, who share complex but quite discrete needs. Both are demanding and highly technical specialities which require expert nurses with different sets of skills. Putting them together can create an unacceptable workload and high levels of stress. The other three centres

Table 11.1 Shared wards

Centre	Total beds	Oncology beds	Shared with
1	23	4.5 (but variable)	Acute medical
2	14	Not known	Acute medical
3	17	13	Acute medical
4	14	8	Cardiology
5	16	8	Cardiology

share with general paediatrics but, for two of those centres, the emphasis of the ward activity is very much dominated by oncology, which may lead to some difficulties in providing an equitable standard of care and commitment to general patients. It was noted that, with the exception of one centre, all had between 40 and 60 new patients a year, and so certainly had the number of patients to warrant separate provision.

In shared wards the sister or charge nurse may not be an oncology specialist, which raised the issue of expert nursing leadership and whether or not an oncology nurse led the service. In the survey it was noted that specialist oncology nurses at G grade or above are clinical leaders on three of the five centres that have shared wards. This is in line with existing guidance (Royal College of Pathologists, 1996).

Inpatient activity

To determine activity and then make comparisons between centres, it was necessary to look first at the number of patients seen in that centre, the number of beds and the number of patients in those beds, i.e. actual bed occupancy. It soon became evident that most centres did not appear to have robust information systems for provision of accurate figures of activity data or, if they did, that the respondents did not have access to those data.

Once it was established that most centres do now have separate inpatient provision, the next question asked how many inpatient beds there were for oncology patients, an apparently simple question, which actually caused a number of difficulties, both for respondents and for the team interpreting the data. In a number of centres, beds were closed, as a result of staff shortages (primarily nursing). In other centres, the service had access to beds other than on the designated oncology ward, e.g. on a surgical ward or an adolescent unit.

To assess workload, it is necessary to gain a clearer picture of bed occupancy because previous work had established that dependency scoring was not widely used to assess workload. Centres were asked to give their average bed occupancy, in order to give a clearer measure of activity than simply the number of beds. It became clear that this too was information to which most respondents did not have access. Most respondents could say only that occupancy was 'full', '100+%', '> 90%'. This was also complicated by the fact, discussed below, that in a number of centres day-case work is still carried out on the inpatient ward. In the absence of robust occupancy data, it was felt that there was no alternative but to work on overall bed numbers when looking at activity. It is certainly the case that paediatric oncology wards are known for high occupancy rates and frequent 'overspill' or 'outlie' to other clinical areas; 100% occupancy rates are, however, unlikely to be statistically accurate.

Nursing establishments

One of the most frequently asked questions in relation to staffing is: How many nurses do you need on a paediatric oncology ward? The next section of the questionnaire addressed the current nursing establishments on the inpatient wards. Information requested included both funded establishments (i.e. the numbers and grades of nurse agreed and financed by the trust), and the actual nurses in post (usually a lower number than the funded establishment, although occasionally in this work higher!). It was necessary to return to some respondents a number of times to clarify the figures given. To establish a useful benchmark, funded establishments were compared. In the course of the analysis, it was reported that a number of centres had major recruitment and retention problems, and did not reach their funded establishment. This has clear implications for both the service and the nursing staff providing that service, in terms of both workload and morale, because working below that establishment must be to the detriment of patient care.

As noted above, bed occupancy data were not consistent or robust enough to allow for meaningful comparison between centres. In looking at the number of nurses on the inpatient wards, therefore, this was related simply to the number of inpatient beds, not to the activity in those beds. For that reason only those wards dedicated to oncology/haematology are shown in Table 11.2.

Table 11.2 shows all nurses on the establishment (as at August 2000), from H to D; it does not include play or support staff and, therefore, is only the number of qualified nurses. It will be noted that there is a marked difference between the ratios of D to E to F grades on the units, with some

Table 11.2 Number of nurses on inpatient wards

Hospital	H	G	F	E	D	Total no. of nurses G–D	Total no. of beds	No. of nurses/beds
1		1	1	4.09	9	15.09	8	1.9
2		1	4	10.16	1.27	16.43	9	1.8
3	1	1	3	10	5	19	10	1.9
4	0.5	1	4.7	9.2	5.4	20.3	10	2
5	1	1	3.07	11.27	7.07	22.41	14	1.6
6	1	2	5.1	10.87	5.98	23.95	14	1.7
7	1		3.4	11.76	9.62	24.78	14	1.8
8	1	2	6	20	3.5	31.5	15	2.1
9	1	1	6	19.32	2	28.32	15	1.9
10	1	1	2	30		33	18	1.8
11	2.8	1	4	16	2	23	19	1.2
12		1	3	21.96	7.61	33.57	22	1.5
13	1	2	5	28	4	39	23	1.7
14	1	4	14.54	26.92	11.31	56.77	26	2.1
15	2	3	15.7	37	10	65.7	29	2.3

centres enjoying a notably richer grade mix than others. This is an area that needs greater exploration. The survey also showed marked differences in the number and roles of support staff, whether this was in posts providing administrative and clerical support, 'housekeeper' roles or phlebotomy. These posts clearly have a great impact on the workload of qualified nurses, and again this warrants further exploration.

When looking at the ratio of nurses to beds, a decision was taken to exclude the H grades. This was based on the assumption that, in many cases, their role would keep them away from regular direct patient care. This assumption was recognized as contentious, because the research team were aware that a number of H grades are in fact very much part of the nursing establishment, and play a very direct clinical role. Table 11.2 does not include nurses in specialist roles such as nurse practitioners and lecturer/practitioner; these were addressed separately in the study. The nature of specialist role development and clinical leadership in paediatric oncology will be the subject of further work.

The survey identified a significant variation in the number of nurses to each inpatient bed. This is particularly notable bearing in mind the recommendation cited above, in a succession of reports in relation to paediatric oncology, that 'one third [the beds] should be staffed to high dependency . . . and the rest to medium dependency levels' (UKCCSG, 1987; Royal College of Pathologists, 1996). It should also be noted, however, that a number of the key factors that impact on activity, which are identified below, need to be taken into account when looking at this local variation.

Shared care

When looking at these local variations, one of the most important factors to recognize in looking at the ways in which particular centres manage both their patients, and their resources, is the practice of 'shared care' in individual units. Most UKCCSG centres share care to some extent with their surrounding DGHs. The aim of 'shared care' is to maintain access to specialist services, alongside the convenience of local provision for some of the less intensive aspects of cancer treatment and supportive care. The practice of 'shared care' is variable, with some centres doing very little and some (principally in and around London) doing a great deal. For some centres, it is the only way that they can manage their patients with the beds available to them. Some of these centres share care with a large number of different DGHs. Table 11.3 illustrates the variability that there is in the practice of shared care in the UK. Only two centres declared that they did no shared care.

Shared care impacts on the service in the regional centre in a number of ways:

- It may reduce the number of beds needed for inpatient episodes.
- It can increase the dependency of patients in the regional centre, especially in centres where the DGH manages the neutropenic inpatient episodes.
- It impacts on day-care activity for those who do all their own outpatient chemotherapy, in comparison to those who devolve work through their DGH shared care hospitals.

Some centres are heavily reliant on DGHs to provide supportive care whereas others keep all aspects of care within the regional centres. The 'shared care' role also varies between different hospitals, which may take on different levels of care. There are a number of larger shared care centres in both the south and south-west of the country where there are specialist paediatric oncology nurses in post to support the service. These nurses were not included in this survey. Shared care creates new pressures on both the DGH and the regional centre, with an enormous requirement for good communication, and a responsibility to meet training and

Table 11.3 Shared care

Centre	Number of shared care centres	Comments from centre
1	1	Induction treatment for ALL in one centre; OP chemotherapy in one centre; management of febrile neutropenia one centre
2	1	
3	2	OP chemo x 2; neutropenia x 1
4	2	Limited – no inpatient work
5	2	OP chemo x 2; neutropenia x 2
6	2	OP chemo x 1; neutropenia x 1; developing shared care with three further centres, currently will do blood tests
7	2	OP chemo x 2; neutropenia x 2
8	2	DGHs will take bloods only
9	4	Occasional neutropenia; limited OP chemo
10	7	ALL induction x 2; IP chemo x 4; OP chemo x 2; neutropenia x 7
11	8	Rely heavily on shared care as a result of staffing difficulties and bed closures
12	9	
13	9	Induction x 10/year; OP chemo and neutropenia
14	10	Induction x 1; OP chemo; IP chemo x 2; neutropenia – ALL but not AML
15	12	Well-developed systems in place
16	15	ALL induction and treatment x 2; OP chemo x 1; neutropenia 70% in shared care
17	36	
18	35-40	OP chemo and management of neutropenia
19	51	
20	58-60	Shared care administrator in post

ALL, acute lymphoblastic leukaemia; AML, acute myeloid leukaemia;
DGH, district general hospital; IP, inpatient; OP, outpatient.

education needs. The driving force for the development of 'shared care' is varied, pressure on beds and resources being perhaps the most common. In some centres where a number of local hospitals and clinicians have historically cared for children with cancer, or leukaemia, 'shared care' has always been part of the referral pattern. In others it is driven by the geography of a region, primarily where the centre is a long way from some of its patient population; alternatively it may develop as a response to patient or family demand. Rationalization of 'shared care' to a few well-chosen sites is likely in some parts of the country in the future, along the lines described for adult patients in 'The Cancer Plan' (DoH, 2000b). This is an area that warrants further research and clarification, to help to establish models of good practice and effective clinical governance.

Patient dependency

Shared care is just one of a range of factors that affects the dependency of patients seen on the inpatient wards at the regional centres. There was no attempt in this study to quantify the amount of nursing care given by each unit, as there were not the data to do so. To indicate the complexity of the clinical environment on the wards however respondents were asked what the criteria were for the transfer of patients to HDU and paediatric ICU. It became apparent that, in most centres, most children requiring high dependency care remained on the oncology ward. A few centres used HDU for postoperative care, or on occasion when staffing was poor, but most centres would retain children who fitted accepted criteria for high dependency care (DoH, 1997; National Health Service Executive, 2000). Transfer to paediatric ICU was primarily for ventilation, increased circulatory support or multiorgan failure.

Many of the patients cared for on paediatric oncology wards fitted accepted criteria and definitions of high dependency care (sometimes described as level 1), including:

- close observation and monitoring of respiratory/circulatory/renal and neurological systems.
- complex multidrug therapy – both cytotoxic chemotherapy and the requirements of intensive supportive care.
- patients with complex fluid management requirements – again in relation to both complex chemotherapy regimens and the need for supportive care.
- circulatory support and fluid resuscitation – particularly in relation to the management of sepsis. Most oncology wards keep patients on single, low-dose inotrope and only transfer them if they require greater circulatory support.
- renal dysfunction – either related to disease processes, e.g. tumour lysis syndrome or a common acute side effect of both cytotoxic and supportive care therapies.
- electrolyte instability – with the need for supplementation and monitoring, again a common side effect of chemotherapy and related to renal dysfunction.
- intensive blood product support.

As well as the need for expert clinical nursing assessment and intervention in the management of these patients, they and their families also require intensive psychosocial care and support. This further enhances the argument for greater staffing provision than was found in place for such high-dependency patients at ward level, despite consistent recommendations in reports and guidance documents within the specialty (UKCCSG, 1987; Royal College of Pathologists, 1996).

Bone marrow transplantation activity

Bone marrow transplantation is an integral part of treatment in some childhood cancers. Access to BMT facilities is required in all the regional treatment centres. In some centres, this means sending patients off-site, sometimes to another centre. Other centres will treat all patients in a BMT unit, which may take children only, or may be shared with adult patients. In most centres transplantations are done on the wards (Table 11.4) either in side rooms or in a dedicated area of the ward. The provision of BMT within the ward adds to the probable complexity of nursing workload. All BMT patients are nursed in isolation, thus impacting on staffing levels. Even where no BMTs as such are done, or there is a separate transplant unit, peripheral blood stem cell transplantations are carried out on most wards. This modality of treatment also uses complex conditioning regimens, and these patients may well require intensive supportive care and high levels of nursing.

Table 11.4 Variations in bone marrow transplantation practice

No bone marrow transplantation facilities	2 centres	Patients sent elsewhere for transplantation
Separate bone marrow transplantation unit	4 centres	Two paediatric-only units Two mixed: adults and children
Bone marrow transplantations on the ward	13 centres	May be a separate part of ward for HDU/transplantation only
Autograft and peripheral blood stem cell transplantation only	3 centres	

HDU, high dependency unit.

Day care

In line with national guidance and good practice recommendations, which recommend that children should be admitted as inpatients only if absolutely necessary, increasingly complex care is being given on a day-case basis (Hooker and Palmer, 1999). The survey looked at paediatric oncology day care, and found that only half of the UKCCSG centres (11 of the 22) had a separate, dedicated day-care unit. Of the rest, five shared a unit with other paediatric specialities, or general paediatrics, and six had no day care and used the inpatient ward, often with no extra, identified resource. A degree of special provision was made for oncology patients in some of the shared care centres, but all centres reported a growing workload and stretched facilities. In the earlier report to the UKCCSG, only five centres (of twenty) had dedicated day care. It was one of the recommendations of that report that 'each centre be provided with day-care beds and out-patient services sufficient to meet its needs' (UKCCSG, 1987).

It is disappointing that 14 years later only half of the centres now have day care, despite a huge swing towards day-care treatment, and changing protocols in line with this preference, which makes many existing services inadequate and under-resourced. A number of centres still carry out day care on the inpatient wards, with little or no additional resources in terms of staffing or service provision. The scope of practice in day care varies considerably, as do staffing resources and opening hours. Most provide day-case chemotherapy and therapeutic interventions, whereas others deliver anaesthetic procedures in the department. Hours of opening vary (with best practice identified in a unit that was open from 8am to 8pm) and it is reported that, where hours are not extended beyond 5pm, there is frequent overflow in the evenings to the inpatient wards, which are not staffed for this extra workload. Indeed, in areas where there is dedicated day care, a considerable amount of activity still spills over onto the inpatient wards even within day-care hours.

In the rapidly expanding and increasingly complex clinical setting of day care, staffing levels have not appeared to keep up with complexity of services, with an even greater variation than was apparent on the inpatient wards. Looking at the number of nurses in relation to actual 'beds' would be misleading, because much of the activity in day care goes on outside of physical beds! In many units the number of beds is now recognized as inadequate in relation to activity. Senior leadership roles were also less consistently well provided in the day-care setting. Of the eleven centres with dedicated day care, two were led by an H grade, six by G grades, two by an F and one by an E grade. It is clear that there is some important further work to be done on looking at day-care provision in more depth.

Conclusion

The work outlined here is an initial exploration of the data provided by the survey of regional centres, and begins to describe the service provided within those centres, with the emphasis on the nursing establishments providing that core service. It aims to demonstrate the complexity of the service provided, and has identified some of the key variables in looking at service provision, which is critical when looking at any benchmarking between different centres. The results of the questionnaire support previous recommendations for the provision of dedicated oncology provision. They also demonstrate areas where more work is needed to look at certain key variables that have a particular impact on service provision, notably the prevalence of 'shared care', and how it is accessed and used, and the availability and resourcing of day-care provision. This survey did not look at the service provided by outreach and community nursing teams.

This is the first exploration of data; it needs more work and will form the basis of a report to the PONF and the UKCCSG. The results demonstrate the need for better activity data than are currently available – in particular in relation to bed occupancy and patient dependency. By using crude indicators of activity, it has been possible to map out current levels of nurse staffing in the regional centres. As a result of the complexity of individual units some of the data may be misleading; it is not intended to be so, nor is this a 'league table' of who has what availability of resources. This is information that those individual centres will be able to access when addressing the needs of their own particular service in relation to staffing levels. There is further work to be done by looking in more depth at grade mix and the role of support staff. Nurses cannot be seen in isolation from other members of the multidisciplinary team, and detailed work looking at medical staffing levels remains to be done. The data collected in relation to both pharmacist support and the provision of services such as aseptic preparation show considerable variation between centres, and areas of best practice will be identified.

This work set out to address some of the variations in service provision in the 22 regional treatment centres of the UKCCSG, and to offer guidance on staffing levels within paediatric oncology. It was an ambitious piece of work, which is still in the process of being developed and which has in many ways raised more questions than it has answered. The information gathered maps out current levels of staffing nationally within the specialty. It is expected that subsequent work will further clarify the picture, identifying areas of best practice, and allowing the development of clearer recommendations in relation to the staffing levels required to provide the high-quality service towards which all units aspire. This is work that will feed into the development of more robust national standards of care and service guidance for children and young people with cancer.

References

Department of Health (1993) The Welfare of Children and Young People in Hospital. London: DoH.

Department of Health (1995) A Policy Framework for Commissioning Cancer Services. A report by the Expert Advisory Group on Cancer to the Chief Medical Officers of England and Wales (Calman-Hine). London: HMSO.

Department of Health (1997) Paediatric Intensive Care 'A Framework for the Future'. London: HMSO.

Department of Health (2000a) The NHS Plan. London: HMSO.

Department of Health (2000b) The Cancer Plan London: HMSO.

Clinical Standards Advisory Group (1996) Standards of Care for Children with Leukaemia. London: Royal College of Pathologists.

Hollis R, Morgan S (2001) The adolescent with cancer – at the edge of no-man's land. The Lancet Oncology 2: 43–48.

Hooker L, Palmer S (1999) Administration of chemotherapy. In: Gibson F, Evans M (eds), Paediatric Oncology Acute Nursing Care. London: Whurr Publishers, pp. 48–58.

Mott MG, Mann JR, Stiller CA (1997) The United Kingdom children's cancer study group – the first 20 years of growth and development. European Journal of Cancer 33: 1448-1452.

National Health Service Executive (2000) Paediatric High Dependency Care. NHSE North West.

Royal College of Nursing, Cancer Nursing Society (1996) A Structure for Cancer Nursing Services. London: RCN.

Royal College of Nursing (1999a) Skill-Mix and Staffing in Children's Wards and Departments. London: RCN.

Royal College of Nursing, Paediatric Nurse Managers' Forum (1999b) Children's Services: Acute Health Care Provision. London: RCN.

Royal College of Pathologists (1996) Standards of Care for Children with Leukaemia. London: Royal College of Pathologists.

Stiller CA (1994) Centralised treatment, entry to trials and survival. British Journal of Cancer 70: 352-362.

United Kingdom Childhood Cancer Study Group (1987) Report on cancer services for children, unpublished. London: UKCCSG.

United Kingdom Childhood Cancer Study Group (1997a) The resources and requirements of a UKCCSG treatment centre, unpublished. London: UKCCSG.

United Kingdom Children's Cancer Study Group and Society of British Neurological Surgeons (1997b) Guidance for Services for Children and Young People with Brain and Spinal Tumours. London: Royal College of Paediatrics and Child Health.

Part 3

Perspectives on care

Tom Devine

Outside calls for clinical nursing practice to be based on best available evidence are growing increasingly louder (Department of Health, 1993, 1998, 2000). The following contributions provide the reader with a platform from which not only to explore current perspectives in paediatric oncology nursing practice, but also to provide the interested practitioner with an insight into the sometimes torturous, yet rewarding, process of generating research evidence in clinical settings. Laudably many of the contributors are paediatric nurses primarily engaged in clinical practice. Reduction in the gap between good clinical nursing research and clinical practice is one of the major ways of ensuring that clinical practitioners can best appreciate the contribution that sound evidence can make to their practice. Opportunities for paediatric oncology nurses to gain the necessary skills to carry out good quality clinical research are vital if paediatric oncology nursing is to take the lead in generating its own best evidence. At the same time, nurses need to be equipped with the necessary critical appraisal skills with which to evaluate clinical research findings (Richardson et al., 2002). An excellent introduction and clear guide to the process of evaluating healthcare research can be found in Trisha Greenhalgh's book, *How to Read a Paper* (2001).

The contributions in Part 3 highlight how paediatric oncology nurses have started to go about identifying clinically focused nursing research questions and their efforts to answer them. Addressing the clinical nursing priorities of nurses in practice is one means of forging strong collaborative relationships between nurse researchers and clinical nursing staff. In Chapter 12, Soanes et al. describe the process of involving stakeholders in deciding on nursing research questions and prioritizing the order in which they would be addressed. The authors' self-critical style in describing the challenges of using a Delphi survey technique to access nursing opinion is to be applauded, serving as it does as an object lesson in what problems can be encountered using the approach and, importantly, how such problems might be avoided or their consequences minimized. The survey's findings overwhelmingly indicated that clinical nurses wish for nursing research to address nursing care issues. Three of the four emerging categories were care based, with symptom assessment and management seen as a top priority. Soanes et al. rightly highlight the need for a strategic research framework relevant to patient care if those in the best position to implement research findings are to appreciate fully the need for their clinical practice to be based on best available evidence.

In Chapter 13, Gibson and Hayden critically examine the practice behind what they describe as 'one of the most basic of all nursing activities', the oral care offered to children with cancer. The authors, rightly, point out that 'children undergoing treatment for cancer experience many invasive procedures, therefore each and every procedure must be justified'. Once again the clear step-by-step approach taken by the authors is presented. From an initial recognition of oral care practices, lack of consistency to the development and introduction of patient-centred oral assessment guidelines (OAG), the reader is systematically guided through the process of carrying out action research, a commonly used collaborative approach to enquiry. The approach relies very heavily on the researcher's skill in facilitating and mediating the process of practice change (Meyer, 1993). One of its powerful attributes is that clinical practitioners bring about the process of change themselves. The OAG and associated recommendations were based on what the authors term 'expert' opinion, arguably the weakest form of evidence, given the subjective and biased nature of what is fundamentally personal opinion. It is to be hoped that the authors will have the opportunity to develop this work and look at the evidence underpinning their recommendations for practice.

It is now recognized that cancer-related fatigue (CRF) is a common and disturbing symptom for adults with cancer (Richardson, 1995; Richardson and Ream, 1996; Stone et al., 1998; Curt, 2001). Hockenberry-Eaton et al. (1998, 1999) have recently investigated the phenomenon, as experienced by children and teenagers with cancer, and clearly demonstrated the existence of CRF in this age range. In Chapter 14, Edwards et al. describe the process of designing two comparative studies currently being undertaken in the UK, designed to investigate the dimensions of CRF as experienced by three groups of adolescents: those receiving cancer treatment, those having completed cancer treatment and a non-cancer group. The authors use the middle-range theory of unpleasant symptoms, as put forward by Lenz et al. (1997), to provide the framework for their studies.

The theory suggests a cyclical relationship between symptoms and the interrelated influences – physiological, psychological and situational factors – affecting an individual's response. Such an approach is sound given the multidimensional nature of the symptom. The authors share their 'journey of discovery' from the formulation of the research question to decisions about the most reliable method of answering the question, given the population under study. It is written in such a lucid way that the reader is able to follow the research route taken, the obstacles encountered and the steps taken to overcome them. When the authors start out on their journey, they genuinely question whether research with a population of adolescents receiving treatment for cancer is feasible. At the heart of their research is the desire to establish an effective evidence-based response to a symptom that has been rated as the most highly distressing by adolescents with cancer (Hinds et al., 1990, 2000).

The routine placement of a central venous catheter (CVC), to facilitate the treatment and associated supportive care required for most children with cancer, is currently standard practice. In Chapter 15, Sanderson examines, from the child's perspective, the experience of living with a CVC. Phenomenological research, with its emphasis on the subjective experience, is an extremely useful approach to theory generation when exploring the personal meaning of a common experience. Researchers should always go for the words children use, because it is out of these that they are making meaning. As the author points out, it is no easy option; would-be users of the approach should be aware of the rigorous nature such enquiry demands if theoretical saturation is to be achieved without being undermined by researcher bias or a lack of insight in interpreting and ascribing meaning to data. The main value of this section is its clear demonstration of young children's ability to self-report clinically relevant information about their lived experience of having and being treated for cancer, a finding supported by Collins et al. (2002) in their study of the ability of 7- to 12-year-old children with cancer to report accurate and relevant information concerning their symptom experience.

Information about the illness experience of pre-school children relies heavily on observation or proxy reporting, usually using parental or healthcare professional perspectives. The usual reason sited for adopting these approaches is the cognitive limitations such young informants pose. In Chapter 16, Hedström and Von Essen describe a proxy report approach used to investigate disease and treatment-related distress among children, aged 4–7 years, on and off treatment for cancer. For each child, the researchers carried out semi-structured interviews with the child's parent and a member of the nursing staff who had cared for the child on at least three previous occasions. Clinical nursing staff need to be careful when interpreting second-hand accounts of personal experience. The reader needs to keep this in mind when assessing the validity of what is being reported on and interpreted by the researcher, e.g. in a population who had all received chemotherapy, the authors found that nearly all parents of children with leukaemia reported that their child had found it positive to receive chemotherapy whereas none of the parents of children with solid tumours did so. The authors suggest that this might be the result of children with leukaemia having a greater understanding of the need for chemotherapy. Alternatively, it may more accurately reflect the different levels of toxicity experienced by the two groups. Overall analysis of the data identified several sound categories of children's responses to cancer and its treatment. Paediatric oncology nurses would do well to account for these when planning interventions, especially in relation to combating feelings of alienation and isolation.

In Chapter 17, Chesterfield explores the lived experience of parents administrating intravenous chemotherapy, via a central venous catheter, in the home. The analysis of 9 semi-structured interviews uncovered 14 themes relating to parental experience. When presented to parents in a follow-up interview, all parents concurred with the themes that had been generated. The major overarching concern for these parents, it would appear, relates to their mastery of the situation, e.g. 'a way of regaining care of their child' and 'managing the many other aspects of life'. This is unsurprising in the sense that these parents were sufficiently self-motivated, in the first instance, to want to undertake this extended parental role.

This part of the book provides clinical nursing staff with sound practical advice, based on parental experience, with which to inform guidelines for the education and supervision required to give the best support to those parents wishing to carry out this role safely and with confidence.

Together, the parts of the book provide the reader with a broad introduction to the kinds of theory and models that underpin the nursing research approach to generating evidence for practice. For all of the research questions posed, the authors have had to be inventive and in some cases extremely flexible in the approach taken to gaining access to the information required to illuminate the question. Examples include the Delphi technique, an action research approach, self-reporting, proxy reporting semi-structured interviews and personal diaries, none of which, the reader will be left with no doubt, is a soft option when it comes to generating evidence – all have their strengths and weaknesses (Parahoo, 1997). What I hope will come through is that all the informants, young and old, involved in the various studies were treated not merely as informants but as co-researchers in the quest for new knowledge. The direct involvement of children in research designed to uncover optimum nursing practice is essential. No longer is it permissible to use a proxy report design with all children, when it is abundantly clear that children, down to the age of 7, can report clinically relevant and consistent information when given the opportunity to do so (Collins et al., 2002).

A common feature of the studies described and many other nurse-led clinical research initiatives is the availability of sufficient patients who are suitable for inclusion within the time constraint imposed when the research is, as is often the case, carried out as a part requirement for a postgraduate qualification. As a result, many important questions contained within otherwise well-designed studies remain unanswered. The UK urgently needs to develop a competent core of paediatric oncology nurse researchers and establish a collaborative research programme designed both to extend theory and, together with clinical colleagues, to drive practice. As Glanville et al. (1998) point out, 'a national dissemination strategy . . . combined with local support mechanisms may increase the uptake of changes in practice'. Although many questions remain to be answered, the growing agreement that nursing practice can benefit from a more systematic approach to the problems that it encounters in everyday practice is an encouraging sign for the future nursing management of children and adolescents with cancer.

References

Collins JJ, Devine TD, Dicks GS et al. (2002) The measurement of symptoms in young children with cancer: the validation of the memorial symptom assessment scale in children aged 7-12. Journal of Pain and Symptom Management 23: 10-16.

Curt GA (2001) Fatigue in cancer. British Medical Journal 322: 1560.

Department of Health (1993) Report on the Task Force on a Strategy for Research in Nursing, Midwifery and Health Visiting. London: HMSO.

Department of Health (1998) First Class Service: Quality in the new NHS. London: HMSO.

Department of Health (2000) The NHS Plan. London: HMSO.

Glanville J, Haines M, Auston I (1998) Finding information on clinical effectiveness. British Medical Journal 317: 200-203.

Greenhalgh T (2001) How to Read a Paper: The basics of evidenced based medicine. London: BMJ Books.

Hinds P, Scholes S, Gattuso J, Riggins M, Heffner B (1990) Adaption to illness in adolescents with cancer. Journal of Pediatric Oncology Nursing 7: 64-65.

Hinds P, Quargnenti A, Bush A et al. (2000) An evaluation of the impact of a self-care coping intervention on psychological and clinical outcomes in adolescents with a new diagnosed cancer. European Journal of Oncology Nursing 4: 6-17.

Hockenberry-Eaton M, Hinds PS, Alcoser P et al. (1998) Fatigue in children and adolescents with cancer. Journal of Pediatric Oncology Nursing 15: 172-182

Hockenberry-Eaton M, Hinds P, Brace O'Neill JB et al. (1999) Developing a conceptual model for fatigue in children. European Journal of Oncology Nursing 3: 5-11.

Lenz ER, Pugh LC, Milligan RA, Gift A, Suppe F (1997) The middle-range theory of unpleasant symptoms: an update. Advances in Nursing Science 19: 14-27.

Meyer JE (1993) New paradigm research in practice: the trials and tribulations of action research. Journal of Advanced Nursing 18: 1066-1072.

Parahoo K (1997) Nursing Research: Principles, process and issues. Basingstoke: Macmillan.

Richardson A (1995) Fatigue in cancer patients: a review of the literature. European Journal of Cancer Nursing 4: 20-37.

Richardson A, Ream E (1996) Fatigue in cancer patients receiving chemotherapy for advanced cancer. International Journal of Palliative Care 2: 199-204.

Richardson J, Boath E, Metcalfe A (2002) Helping nurses to interpret and evaluate research. Nursing Times 98: 38-39.

Stone P, Richards M, Hardy J (1998) Fatigue in patients with cancer. European Journal of Cancer 34: 1670-1678.

Chapter 12

A Delphi survey: establishing nursing research priorities

Louise Soanes, Faith Gibson,
Julie Bayliss and Julia Hannan

Many people reading this chapter will acknowledge that developing practice can be challenging to say the least. A lack of consensus, the fear of
leaving secure positions and inadequate planning are three of the most
common reasons for this situation (McPhail, 1997). To overcome these
difficulties and to increase the chance of successful implementation of
new initiatives, it is recommended that staff of all levels are involved in
the decision-making and implementation processes, the so-called 'bottom-
up' approach (Cutcliffe and Bassett, 1997). Although an honourable sen-
timent and in line with current Government thinking (Department of
Health or DoH, 1997, 1998), this is not as easy as it seems; when applying it to the implementation of evidence-based nursing the practical
challenges are rather more complex than those suggested by McPhail
(1997).

The current drive within nursing to develop evidence-based practice
continues to gain momentum (DoH, 1993, 2000; Sackett et al., 1996;
Callery, 1997; Cullum, 1997; Kitson, 1997). Although at the macro-level
evidence continues to be produced, at the micro-level, despite long-
standing encouragement, nurses still appear reluctant to use research evidence to support their practice. Hunt (1987) suggests that this is because
nurses do not understand research, do not believe in research findings and
do not know how to apply research to practice. Ten years later, Walsh
(1997) confirmed these findings and, in addition, found that nurses identified pressures of work and lack of research training as barriers to
implementing research.

Paediatric oncology is not immune from these problems (Hinds et al.,
1990), and it has been suggested that, in order to improve participation
in nursing research, a strategic research framework relevant to patient
care must be advocated (Hinds et al., 1990; Stevens, 1997). Returning to
the opening statement, it is now accepted by many that, for research to be

successfully integrated and applied to practice, ownership and identification must come from those who are most likely to implement research (Baessler et al., 1994; Walczak et al., 1994; Cavanagh and Tross, 1996). This chapter outlines one approach to ensure that key stakeholders – nurses, doctors and parents in a haematology, oncology and immunology unit – were involved in the decision-making process in developing a research strategy for the unit. As nursing research was the focus of this work, the Delphi survey will form the main part of this chapter; later, the methods used to seek the opinions of parents and medical staff are explored (for a detailed description see Soanes et al., 2003) with the results of all three approaches brought together in the discussion.

A Delphi survey was undertaken with nurses working in the unit to identify and rank their clinical research priorities (for a detailed description, see Soanes et al., 2000). These priorities would then form the focus of a future research programme within a strategy of evidence-based nursing on the unit. As a means of structuring the study the working party decided to use the published work of Hinds et al. (1990) as a framework. This was chosen because their enquiry closely reflected the client group of the unit being studied. In addition the steps of the Delphi survey were clearly documented by Hinds et al. (1990) and offered a guide to researchers who were novices to this method of data collection.

Within Hinds et al.'s (1990) study, two groups of nurses were asked to identify their research priorities. One group included nurses at a children's hospital, and the second group included participants at a paediatric oncology nursing conference. All participants provided direct care to children with cancer. Using the classic Delphi technique, three rounds of questionnaires were completed. Participation level was high (91% and 81% respectively). The two groups identified similar types of research priorities but rated them differently. The predominant focus of the 10 research priorities identified was professional issues (1–9); only the tenth related to patient care. The low priority given to patient care research may result partly from the hospital in which the survey was undertaken. St Jude Children's Research Hospital has a strong history of nursing research focused on patient care; for this reason nurses may have chosen areas not adequately addressed in current research, but nevertheless important to their role as paediatric oncology nurses. The consensus reached by the Delphi survey has, according to Hinds et al. (1990), some degree of generalizability to other paediatric oncology units. It is considered that British paediatric oncology nursing is experiencing similar professional issues to those identified by Hinds et al. (1990), e.g. changes in the care delivery system and the stress of nursing children with cancer.

The Delphi method

The Delphi technique is a survey method of research that aims to structure group opinion and discussion using a multi-stage process. First developed by the Rand Corporation 50 years ago, it was introduced in an attempt to eliminate interpersonal interactions in decision-making (Dalkey and Helmer, 1963). In healthcare the Delphi technique has a much shorter history, but it has been used to determine the priorities and future alternatives by a number of nurses (Lindeman, 1975; Bond and Bond, 1982; Hitch and Murgatroyd, 1983; Hinds et al., 1990; Broome et al., 1996). Lindeman (1975) was one of the first nurse researchers to determine the research priorities of clinical nurses, using the Delphi survey. Since then the Delphi survey has been used in a variety of nursing specialities: clinical nursing (Bond and Bond, 1982; Fitzpatrick et al., 1991; Daly and Chang, 1996), cancer nursing (Western Consortium for Cancer Nursing Research, 1987), paediatrics (Broome et al., 1996; Schmidt et al., 1997) and paediatric oncology (Hinds et al., 1990, 1994).

The Delphi technique is now used primarily to reach a consensus in the absence of an acceptable body of knowledge or where there is a desire to gather opinion and initiate debate (Goodman, 1987). Reid (1988, p. 232) defines the Delphi approach as 'a method for the systematic collection and aggregation of informed judgement from a group of experts on specific questions and issues'. The results of a Delphi exercise are perceived by Sackman (1975) as a structured brainstorming session, and by Pill (1971) as 'picking the brains of a group', as opposed to a rigid, positivist and scientific exercise (McKenna, 1994).

The Delphi technique is essentially a series of questionnaires used to structure group communication (Duffield, 1989); three to five questionnaires are normally required before consensus is reached (Beretta, 1996). It consists of questioning a known group of experts about a specific issue. The term expert may imply an élitist approach but Pill (1971) defines an expert as anyone with relevant input in to the purpose of the Delphi. In the first round participants are asked to make judgements or comment on the items presented. Individual responses are then collated for re-submission to the group. In the second and subsequent rounds, participants receive statistical feedback on the group's responses and are asked to reconsider their judgement. Repeat rounds are carried out until consensus of opinion, or a point of diminishing returns, is reached (Williams and Webb, 1994). Strauss and Zeigler (1975) have identified six key characteristics that are common to the Delphi process:

1. They use panels of experts for obtaining information or data
2. They are conducted in writing, using sequential questionnaires interspersed with summarized information.
3. They systematically attempt to produce a consensus of opinion and to identify opinion divergence.
4. They guarantee anonymity of both the panel members and their statements.
5. They use iteration and controlled feedback.
6. They are conducted in a series of rounds, between which a summary of the results of the previous round is communicated to the panel members.

The advantages of the Delphi technique are that responses are anonymous to other participants and that it allows consensus to be reached without the overt influences of peer pressure. These last two issues were thought to be important in encouraging junior members of staff to respond, who otherwise might be reluctant to offer their opinion if it is in conflict with that of senior colleagues.

Further advantages to the Delphi survey are its adoption of both quantitative (more appealing to policy developers) and qualitative (more appealing to nurses) approaches (Reid, 1988). Disadvantages, as identified by Beretta (1996), are the reliability and validity of results, the influence of the researcher and ethical issues of consensus methods of research. Furthermore, results may be affected by panel attrition and fatigue, reducing the response rates of each round (Berretta, 1996).

Purpose of the study

The purpose of this study was to provide an opportunity for all nursing staff on the unit to identify and rate their priorities for nursing research, and so hopefully disseminate the message that everyone's views were important and valued. The Delphi survey was part of a wider (and ongoing) project to develop a clinical research strategy within the unit. According to Street (1995), in such a culture ownership and importance of setting research priorities are key factors in its success. However, recognition that nursing research does not take place in a vacuum, the opinions of two other parties were sought, namely doctors and parents. Although these two parties were not involved in the initial stages of this work, they informed the final outcome and the methods used to seek their opinions, and the outcomes of these are discussed later.

Methods

Sample and demographic data

The nurse sample included all qualified nurses ($n = 98$) working within the unit, comprising four inpatient wards and an outpatient area (Table 12.1). This included, clinical nurse specialists (CNSs) working in palliative care, haematology, oncology, immunology, hepatitis C, haemophilia, bone marrow transplantations, HIV and intravenous therapy, and the senior nurse of the unit.

Table 12.1 Area of specialty, number of beds and total numbers of nursing staff at the time of the final round

Specialty	No. of beds	Total no. of nurses	No. who responded
Bone marrow transplantation	8	20	5 senior 1 junior 30% of total
Haematology/oncology (area 1)	8	19	5 senior 5 junior 52% of total
Haematology/oncology (area 2)	16	20	3 senior 15% of total
Immunology	7	14	3 senior 1 junior 28% of total
Unit day care and outpatients	N/A	7	3 senior 42% of total
CNSs and others	N/A	11	11 (100% of total)

CNSs, clinical nurse specialists; N/A, not applicable

Methodology

Procedure

Data collection, for the nurses' Delphi survey, was undertaken in four rounds from May 1998 to June 1999. Data collection for doctors and parents took place between October 1999 and December 2000. The time scale for this work may raise questions, but it does illustrate the complexities of research in the clinical area, the difficulties of undertaking part-time research in addition to a full-time job and studying for a higher degree, as many of the working parties were. An overview of the procedure and response rates for each round is shown in Figure 12.1.

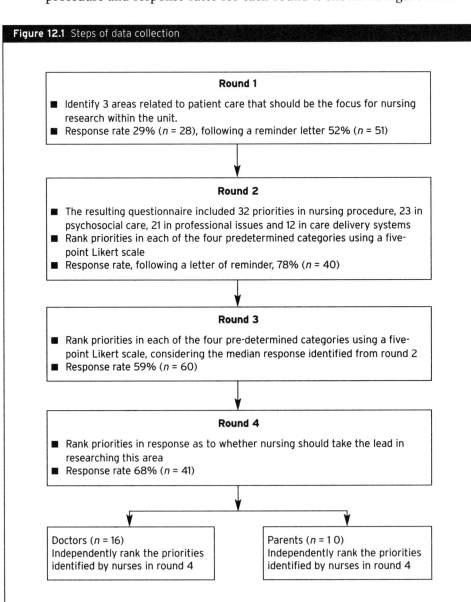

Figure 12.1 Steps of data collection

Round 1
- Identify 3 areas related to patient care that should be the focus for nursing research within the unit.
- Response rate 29% (*n* = 28), following a reminder letter 52% (*n* = 51)

Round 2
- The resulting questionnaire included 32 priorities in nursing procedure, 23 in psychosocial care, 21 in professional issues and 12 in care delivery systems
- Rank priorities in each of the four predetermined categories using a five-point Likert scale
- Response rate, following a letter of reminder, 78% (*n* = 40)

Round 3
- Rank priorities in each of the four pre-determined categories using a five-point Likert scale, considering the median response identified from round 2
- Response rate 59% (*n* = 60)

Round 4
- Rank priorities in response as to whether nursing should take the lead in researching this area
- Response rate 68% (*n* = 41)

Doctors (*n* = 16)
Independently rank the priorities identified by nurses in round 4

Parents (*n* = 1 0)
Independently rank the priorities identified by nurses in round 4

First round

For the first round every nurse on the unit (n = 98) was asked to identify up to three key areas related to patient care that they felt should be the subject of nursing research within the unit. This initial process identified 151 priorities. Following the steps identified by Hinds et al. (1990) areas of overlap were addressed. Three of the researchers independently reviewed the list of priorities, clarifying areas of overlap, reducing the list to 89. The fourth researcher collated the work from this refining process, noting any lack of consensus. This combined list was confirmed as the final list of priorities by one of the researchers, ensuring that any merged priority still accurately reflected the initial priority described.

The next step was to group the list of priorities using the three category headings identified by Hinds et al. (1990) (Table 12.2) in order to provide structure and a user-friendly format to the second round questionnaire. Clarification of care delivery systems (category 4) was felt to be necessary for a UK audience (clarification provided in brackets) in Table 12.2. The priorities were then categorized under these headings, as discussed and agreed by the researchers.

Table 12.2 Research categories identified by Hinds et al. (1990), adapted for use in this work

Categories	Category definition
Nursing procedures	Responses in this category relate to areas of care concerning direct care actions by a nurse to respond to immediate child/family needs, potential child/family problems or altered child/family status
Psychosocial care needs	Issues related to needs, values, perceptions, coping and quality of life of children and their family members, and the role of nurses in those issues
Professional issues	Concerns about the continued existence of the specialty, definition of scope of practice and unique knowledge base, and aspects of the nursing role such as patient advocacy
Care delivery systems	Issues related to the management of healthcare resources (are the appropriate people caring for the appropriate patient group?)

Second round

The second round questionnaire was sent to the 51 (of 98) nurses who had responded to the first round. They were then asked to rate priorities in each category (see Table 12.2) using a 5-point Likert scale with a rating of 1 meaning 'strongly disagree' and 5 meaning 'strongly agree'. The questionnaires were analysed using Excel 97 to determine the median score.

At this point concerns about the sample size for the third round were raised. Following the Delphi procedure the third round questionnaire should have been sent to the 40 nurses (of 98) who had responded in round 3. However, 40 nurses, when considered in terms of the total population of nurses working on the unit, was thought to be a small and unrepresentative sample. To address this issue the third round questionnaire was once again sent to all the nursing team (n = 101). The increase from 98 in the first round was as a result of recruitment to the unit. This approach to a poor response rate had been used, with success, by Broome et al. (1996).

Third round

The third round questionnaire was a repeat of the second round with the addition of the median scores. Using the same 5-point Likert scale, respondents were asked to rate the priorities once again considering the median and their own score; where their response varied from the median they were asked to comment.

The median and mean scores were calculated from the data. The mean score was used to rank the priorities identified by respondents. Respondents were then asked to rank the top 25% statements from each category (highest score the most important and lowest the least important). A percentage rather than number was used to ensure equity within the categories. Each statement was considered on its own merit and in response to the question: Whether nursing should take the lead in researching this area?

Fourth round

Of the 41 questionnaires returned for round 4 only 37 were completed correctly. Some respondents had clearly not understood the instructions and principles of ranking, awarding the same ranking to a number of listed priorities. The final rated priorities for each category can be found in Table 12.3, 1 being the most important research priority for that category.

Table 12.3 Rank order of priorities on completion of the study

Nursing procedures	Rank order	Psychosocial care needs	Rank order
If nurses have knowledge to implement effective symptom management to their patients on a day-to-day basis	1	Quality of life from the children's perspective	1
How well nausea and vomiting is controlled for patients having chemotherapy, after discharge	2	Preparation for procedures (is there adequate use of play specialists?)	2
If we are appropriately assessing and treating children's nutritional needs	3	Whether families are being given adequate information to give informed consent	3
The most appropriate way to assess antibiotic levels	4	What are the options for children regarding their future fertility? Are children/teenagers offered opportunities to bank sperm/ovaries and are these opportunities equal?	4
Ward-based isolation procedures using a multidisciplinary approach involving infection control, nurses, play specialists	5	If sibling donors are getting adequate support and preparation before, during and after bone marrow transplantation	5
Methods available to pre-medicate children	6		
The necessity of 4-hourly observations on all patients and their significance	7		
The evidence on chlorhexidine/alcohol-based hand-washing products: are they more effective than 'ordinary dispensed soap'?	8		

Professional issues	Rank order	Care delivery systems	Rank order
Retaining staff: what incentives do staff need, e.g. study time, time owing?	1	Whether effective and appropriate negotiation takes place between nursing staff and families	1
The incidence of stress/burnout on the unit and support available	2	Information giving to families at diagnosis – who tells the child about the cancer	2
The most effective form of documenting care	3	If parent-held records assist in communication between the regional centre and district general hospital	3
What support/information do shared care hospitals want from the regional centre	4		
Whether parents who have English as their second language really understand their child's illness and protocols	5		

Findings

Category 1 nursing procedures resulted in the highest number of research priorities, 32 in total. The top priorities reflected concerns such as symptom management, assessment of children, preparation for procedures and effectiveness of care (Table 12.3). In category 2 psychosocial care needs, the priority was on helping children and families deal with their disease and treatment throughout their cancer experience, 23 priorities in total. Support, information and the impact on quality of life were the top priorities (Table 12.3), in the psychosocial care category. Professional issues (category 3) resulted in 21 priorities, with the top priorities reflecting concerns about the role of the nurse in terms of scope of practice, advocacy and stress/burnout (see Table 12.3). The final category (4), care delivery systems, encompassed the least number of priorities, but still reflected a focus of family care in terms of who gives information to families, and negotiates and communicates with the different service providers. Overall, the findings highlight patient/family-centred priorities, with the top ranking of each category being management of the child's symptoms, negotiation of care with the child and family, quality-of-life issues and the effects of high staff turnover within the unit.

Although there was also a section for comment within each round of the Delphi survey, very few comments were made. Of the 60 respondents in round 3, only 16 (of 101) took the opportunity to offer further comment. Most of these offered clarification of why they were voting in a certain way, reinforcing the importance of their score, or commenting that some areas were already a focus of research on the unit and elsewhere. Also highlighted in the comments was the view that some of the priorities had more of a 'medical focus' than nursing. The fact that some of the priorities would be difficult to 'research' was also addressed and the use of 'expert' opinion was identified as a way forward in some of these areas, e.g. methods available to pre-medicate children.

Concern was expressed in some of the comments about the 'cancer' focus. The overwhelming number of responses came from the haematology/oncology areas within the Host Defence Unit. This is the largest specialty on the unit. The working party was concerned that this factor may bias the priorities towards this specialty, and this seemed to be the case in the first round. However, as the later rounds progressed generic issues, applicable to all specialities, were given higher priority (see Table 12.3).

Seeking the opinions of doctors and parents

Doctors

The working party acknowledged that, whatever the outcome of the Delphi survey, the chosen research priorities would impact on doctors as the second largest group of healthcare professionals working in the clinical area. Involvement of doctors in this process was thought to be important for three reasons. First, as the overriding aim of this work was to improve the quality of care offered by the unit to children and their families, multiprofessional debate on this issue could be stimulated by sharing the outcome of the nurses' opinions. Second, by researching shared priorities the encouragement from Government for multiprofessional working (DoH, 1997) could also be met. Furthermore, a recent concern of health-related research is that small populations of patients and their families, such as those that form the population on the unit, are at risk of becoming 'over-researched', and collaboration in research could lessen this risk. Thus, potential overlap in research priorities between the two main professional groups working in the high defence unit (HDU) could possibly be identified.

Sample

The working party wished to involve all levels of medical staff. Pragmatic reasons, specifically the time it takes to complete all the rounds of a Delphi survey and the short time many of the junior doctors spend on the unit, ruled out a full Delphi survey. Therefore, another method was needed to access as many and as varied a group of doctors as possible. A solution to these challenges was found using the Directorate Breakfast Meeting. This takes place every 6 weeks and is a multiprofessional forum to discuss and share issues common to the unit; it is well attended by doctors of all grades, offering a convenient sample of the medical team. At the chosen meeting the working party were able to approach junior and senior medical staff for their opinions on the priorities for research on the unit; 16 questionnaires were returned.

Method

After explaining the rationale and process of the original Delphi survey and why their involvement was being sought, it was clarified that participation was optional and anonymous. After this each doctor was given a copy of the priorities identified by the nurses in each of the four categories shown in Table 12.3, although not in rank order. The doctors were then asked to rank them according to their perceived priority. An invitation to comment on the content and process of the Delphi was also given. The mean score was calculated and used to rank the priorities.

Findings

The results from the doctors' survey are shown in Table 12.4. Consensus with nursing priorities is shown in the top priority for nursing procedures, i.e. nurses' knowledge and effectiveness in symptom management. Results from the other three sections, unsurprisingly, reflect issues pertinent to the day-to-day working lives of medical staff, e.g. whether families receive adequate information to give informed consent, the needs of shared care hospitals and who tells the child about the cancer.

Parents

Consultation with stakeholders is seen as crucial in the current climate of healthcare (DoH, 2000), and the working party wanted to be sure that the priorities of healthcare professionals reflected the needs and wishes of children and families using the unit. However, seeking the opinion of children proved impossible. At the time of data collection no school-aged children were available to take part in the questionnaires; although unusual in comparable units, the unit in question cares predominately for babies and very young children, and the situation described is not unusual.

Sample

The sample for this stage of the work came from the population of parents of children being treated as inpatients, outpatients or at home on a randomly chosen day, a day convenient for the nursing staff collecting the data. Two members of the working party approached parents resident with their children in the four inpatient and outpatient areas. A third member of the group, working as a paediatric oncology outreach nurse (POON), approached parents of those families whom she was visiting that day. Exclusion from this sample included parents whose child was acutely ill, receiving a major investigation or procedure that day, had recently received news of relapse or was in the palliative phase, or newly diagnosed families, families for whom English was not their first language and no appropriate interpreter could be found. Some parents chose not to take part; others agreed but did not return the completed questionnaire; in all 10 completed forms were obtained

Table 12.4 Rank order of priorities of doctors

Nursing procedures	Rank order	Psychosocial care needs	Rank order
If nurses have knowledge to implement effective symptom management to their patients on a day-to-day basis	1	Whether families are being given adequate information to give informed consent	1
How well nausea and vomiting is controlled for patients having chemotherapy, after discharge	2	Quality of life from the children's perspective	2
If we are appropriately assessing and treating children's nutritional needs	3	Preparation for procedures (is there adequate use of play specialists?)	3
Ward-based isolation procedures using a multidisciplinary approach involving infection control, nurses, play specialists	4	If sibling donors are getting adequate support and preparation before, during and after bone marrow transplantation	4
The necessity of 4-hourly observations on all patients and their significance	5	What are the options for children regarding their future fertility? Are children/teenagers offered opportunities to bank sperm/ovaries and are these opportunities equal?	5
Methods available to pre-medicate children	6		
The most appropriate way to assess antibiotic levels	7		
The evidence on chlorhexidine/alcohol-based hand-washing products: are they more effective than 'ordinary dispensed soap'?	8		

Professional issues	Rank order	Care delivery systems	Rank order
What support/information do shared care hospitals want from the regional centre?	1	Information giving to families at diagnosis – who tells the child about the cancer	1
Whether parents who have English as their second language really understand their child's illness and protocols	2	If parent-held records assist in communication between the regional centre and district general hospital	2
Retaining staff: what incentives do staff need, e.g. study time, time owing?	3	Whether effective and appropriate negotiation takes place between nursing staff and families	3
The incidence of stress/burnout on the unit and support available	4		
The most effective form of documenting care	5		

Method

Parents were approached the day before data collection to explain the rationale and process of the original Delphi survey, to clarify parental participation, and to obtain verbal and written consent in accordance with national and local guidelines. On the day of data collection parents were given a copy of the priorities identified by the nurses in each of the four categories shown in Table 12.3, although not in rank order. They were then asked to consider these and rank them according to their perceived priority; parents could do this alone or the nurse collecting the data could complete the form with them. Most parents were happy to complete the form alone, although some of the terminology and context used in the priorities occasionally needed clarification. Parents were asked the additional question: What three things could be done to improve your child's experience of hospital?

Findings

Data were analysed using the same approach as for the doctors' data. Once again the priorities chosen by parents (Table 12.5) reflect their needs as a group, although the priorities match those chosen by nurses in three of the four categories: nursing procedures, psychosocial care needs and professional issues. Doctors and parents agreed on the category of care delivery systems (Tables 12.5 and see Table 12.4), a major issue for these parties who form the receivers and givers of this information, and for whom the impact of their role in this situation is reported (Lowden, 1998; Strachan, 2000).

Discussion

The use of the Delphi technique has enabled the unit to identify the top research priorities around which to structure a research strategy for the next 3 years. Alongside other activities introduced on the unit, the research priorities will contribute to an evidence-based approach to nursing care, by initiating further research into the areas identified or by identifying areas where further dissemination of current research findings is needed.

In terms of the participants who took part in the Delphi survey, a large number of nurses had over 2 years' experience on the unit or in paediatric oncology, indicating that they were confident to identify areas that would benefit from nursing research. There was a wide range of experience

Table 12.5 Rank order of priorities of parents

Nursing procedures	Rank order	Psychosocial care needs	Rank order
If nurses have knowledge to implement effective symptom management to their patients on a day-to-day basis	1	Quality of life from the children's perspective	1
Ward-based isolation procedures using a multidisciplinary approach involving infection control, nurses, play specialists	2	Whether families are being given adequate information to give informed consent	2
The necessity of 4-hourly observations on all patients and their significance	3	Preparation for procedures (is there adequate use of play specialists?)	3
How well nausea and vomiting is controlled for patients having chemotherapy, after discharge	4	What are the options for children regarding their future fertility? Are children/teenagers offered opportunities to bank sperm/ovaries and are these opportunities equal?	4
If we are appropriately assessing and treating children's nutritional needs	5	If sibling donors are getting adequate support and preparation before, during and after bone marrow transplantation	5
Methods available to pre-medicate children	6		
The most appropriate way to assess antibiotic levels	7		
The evidence on chlorhexidine/alcohol-based hand-washing products: are they more effective than 'ordinary dispensed soap'?	8		

Professional issues	Rank order	Care delivery systems	Rank order
Retaining staff: what incentives do staff need, e.g. study time, time owing?	1	Information giving to families at diagnosis – who tells the child about the cancer	1
What support/information do shared care hospitals want from the regional centre?	2	Whether effective and appropriate negotiation takes place between nursing staff and families	2
The most effective form of documenting care	3	If parent-held records assist in communication between the regional centre and district general hospital	3
The incidence of stress/burnout on the unit and support available	4		
Whether parents who have English as their second language really understand their child's illness and protocols	5		

among nurses who responded to the first round; however, in subsequent rounds the number of nurses with less than 2 years' experience who responded dropped significantly. This may indicate that these nurses felt less able to prioritize issues in a new specialty. On reflection, the 100% response rate from CNSs may be because they know the researchers and feel obliged to complete the Delphi questionnaires, thus reflecting the influence of familiarity between researchers and respondents (Beretta, 1996).

A concern of the researchers at the beginning of the project was that the views of nurses working in immunology would not be represented, because fewer nurses work in this area of the unit. However, there is a rotational system in operation between the oncology and immunology settings for junior members of staff, resulting in nurses currently working in one specialty having an insight into the needs of other client groups. This was reflected in the final top priorities. Still, the problems of reaching a consensus in a unit that encompasses a number of clinical specialities should not be underestimated. Nor are there any easy solutions to this problem. Likewise, in involving other groups in this work, the priorities identified were those that affected them; although consensus was achieved in some priorities between parties, the only priority in which all three agreed was when nurses have the knowledge to implement effective symptom management (Table 12.6). Effectiveness in symptom management undoubtedly has an impact on all those involved who have a vested interest in the well-being of the child and the quality of care that the child receives.

Several of the top research priorities from the study were similar to those identified by Hinds et al. (1990). Similarities included retention of staff, staff burnout, nurses' knowledge about symptom control, sedation/pre-medication for painful procedures, and communication between tertiary centres and shared care centres. The existence of these similarities indicates that these issues continue to be important to many paediatric oncology nurses, indicating that research is required in these areas.

Respondents commented on the 'medical focus' of some of the priorities initially identified, e.g. measuring the efficacy of drug regimens and methods to pre-medicate children, responses may have been influenced by issues that were clinically important to nurses, but not nursing research questions. When considering what was important to nursing research, the overlap highlights that the multidisciplinary approach to care on the unit was evident. Some nurses required clear guidance to focus on nursing research in the final fourth round, and some doctors commented that some of the priorities identified by nurses were in the field of other healthcare professionals. This also reflects the nature of the specialty

Table 12.6 Top priority from each group

Nursing procedures	Rank order	Psychosocial care needs	Rank order
If nurses have knowledge to implement effective symptom management to their patients on a day-to-day basis	N, D, P[a]	Quality of life from the children's perspective	N, P
		Whether families are being given adequate information to give informed consent	D
Professional issues	**Rank order**	**Care delivery systems**	**Rank order**
Retaining staff: what incentives do staff need, e.g. study time, time owing?	N, P	Whether effective and appropriate negotiation takes place between nursing staff and families	N
What support/information do shared care hospitals want from the regional centre	D	Information giving to families at diagnosis – who tells the child about the cancer	D, P

[a] P, parents; D, doctors; N, nurses.

where nurses undertake medical work within the context of nursing. Parents, on the other hand, focused on their child and their experience, and did not seem to mind who 'owned' the priority although for them it mattered more how further research would affect families following a similar path to their own.

The fact that some nurses and doctors identified priorities that were currently part of the unit's research programme, e.g. use of pain assessment tools and symptom management, was worrying. This could be a problem in trying to communicate research activities to a large team of nurses and failing to ensure that other healthcare professionals are aware of current nursing practices. Added to which, some nurses were clearly not aware of published research that had already impacted on care. Clearly, if evidence-based nursing is to become a reality, the importance of a culture that facilitates such awareness and encourages the use of research findings in practice must be the focus of the research implementation strategy for the unit, in addition to undertaking more research.

One reason for choosing to use the Delphi technique was its ability to facilitate 'grassroots' involvement while also reducing the effect of dominant individuals. As a result nursing staff of all grades were encouraged to participate, ensuring that powerful individuals alone did not influence the focus of research, and avoiding the potential for unrepresentative individual agendas to dominate. Although the total sample of nurses who participated in the study remained small ($n = 41$) in relation to the population ($n = 101$), the aim of 'grassroots' involvement was still realized because the sample reflected all levels of nurses involved in direct clinical care. Doctors working in haematology, oncology, immunology and infectious diseases were included in the sample, and representation from all rungs of the medical career ladder was thus achieved. The creative approach to capturing their involvement appears to have worked well. Involving parents in the study was a challenge and is reflected in the small number of respondents ($n = 10$); again parents with children being treated across the illness trajectory for conditions from the four main specialities treated on the unit were involved.

Limitations

The limitations of this Delphi survey fall into the three main categories previously identified in the literature: reliability, validity and researcher influence (Goodman, 1987; McKenna, 1994; Williams and Webb, 1994; Beretta, 1996).

The reliability of the nurses' Delphi survey is at risk of being reliant on the time it was undertaken. However, the final identified priorities appear to be consistent with those identified by Hinds et al. (1990), and consensus with doctors and parents in one area suggests a level of replication that is said to be rare in Delphi surveys (Beretta, 1996). In the early rounds, areas of current concern and interest to the unit were reflected in the responses from nurses. Although this is to be expected, and potentially unavoidable, the reliability of the consensus may be limited to the length of time that these issues remain areas of concern over time. A further threat to the reliability of the findings is a changing workforce in the unit. In common with other teaching hospitals turnover of staff, particularly junior nursing and medical staff, is high. Hence the research undertaken in response to the priorities identified from the Delphi survey may not be perceived as a priority by the subsequent staff, a problem identified by Reid (1988).

Although it has been suggested that the content, and face and concurrent validity of the Delphi may be high (Beretta, 1996), the validity of results will be affected by response rates. A high level of participant motivation is important to maintain the momentum of the Delphi survey. The response rate to all stages of the survey was low and waned despite the use of reminder letters. Reasons for this may vary. First, the questionnaires were sent to participants and addressed to work rather than home; during a busy shift they were not a priority and once at home other concerns took priority. In both cases, the respondents may have rushed the completion of the questionnaire, resulting in answers that are not a true reflection of their research needs. Second, in sending the questionnaires to the workplace, this may have encouraged discussion and collaboration in responses, again a potential risk to the reliability of the final outcome. Finally, some nursing staff felt that it was almost impossible to decide which areas were a priority for future research and therefore felt unable to respond. This seemed especially true for nurses with less than 2 years' experience in the unit, leading to potential bias (Duffield, 1989), in this case, towards meeting the needs of senior staff and the ongoing reliability of the consensus. Response fatigue was also evident. The survey was time-consuming and took place over some months, resulting in a loss of motivation that was reflected in the poor response rates.

A further limitation of the study is the fact that the researchers all worked within the unit. Although this may have raised the profile of the Delphi survey and encouraged staff to respond, it may also influence nurses' responses and threaten the anonymity of the respondents. The presence of the researchers on the HDU may have been discerned as silent coercion to complete the questionnaire. Contact with the researchers (and knowing other panellists) had the potential to sway respondents' opinions, leading to a less objective final outcome (Bond and Bond, 1982; Goodman, 1987).

Finally, the use of category headings identified by Hinds et al. (1990), although providing structure to the questionnaires, may have biased responses, forcing respondents towards a judgement because of the category heading.

Conclusion

The purpose of this study was to provide an opportunity for all nursing staff within the unit to identify their priorities for clinical nursing research and to seek the opinions of parents and doctors. Although a long and time-consuming process, it nevertheless proved to be a valuable experience for all involved. The final step of the dissemination of findings to the nursing and medical staff through the unit will, it is hoped, result in feedback to the working party on the process, as well as the outcome, which will influence the future project work of the 'Nurses Research Group'.

Overall, the findings highlight the continuing patient/child focus of nurses and doctors working in increasingly technical/interventionist areas of care. Quality of life and care remain central to the concerns of nurses in these areas, but so too does the impact of working in such areas on their own and their colleagues' lives. The consensus of these areas as a priority for additional research was also reported by Hinds et al.'s (1990) work.

The four priorities identified in this survey are directly linked to practice and are well documented in the literature (Hinds et al., 1990, 1994; Broome et al., 1996) as concerns of specialist and general children's nurses. It would be of interest to explore the outcomes of replicating this study with nurses working in a non-specialized children's unit in the UK, to see whether participants identified similar influences on the healthcare of children. In combining research priorities drawn from three categories of informants, an integrative approach to future nursing research and the research culture on the unit will be undertaken.

References

Baessler CA, Blumberg M, Cunnigham JS (1994) Medical-surgical nurses utilization of research methods and products. Medsurg Nursing 3: 113–117, 120–121, 141.

Beretta R (1996) A critical review of the Delphi technique. Nurse Researcher 3: 79–89.

Bond S, Bond J (1982) A Delphi survey of clinical nursing research priorities. Journal of Advanced Nursing 7: 565–575.

Broome ME, Woodring B, O'Connor-Von S (1996) Research priorities for the nursing of children and their families; a Delphi survey. Journal of Pediatric Nursing 11: 281–287.

Callery P (1997) Using evidence in children's nursing. Paediatric Nursing 9: 13–17.

Cavanagh S, Tross G (1996) Utilizing research findings in nursing: policy and practice considerations. Journal of Advanced Nursing 24: 1083–1088.

Cullum N (1997) Evidence-based nursing: an introduction. Evidence-Based Nursing Pilot issue 4–5.

Cutcliffe JR, Bassett C (1997) Introducing change in nursing: the case of research. Journal of Nursing Management 5: 241–247.

Dalkey N, Helmer O (1963) An experimental application of the Delphi method to the use of experts. Management Science 9: 458–467.

Daly JP, Chang EML (1996) A study of clinical nursing research priorities of renal specialist nurses caring for critically ill people. Intensive and Critical Care Nursing 12: 45–49.

Department of Health (1993) Report on the Task Force on a Strategy for Research in Nursing, Midwifery and Health Visiting. London: HMSO.

Department of Health (1997) The New NHS: Modern and dependable. London: HMSO.

Department of Health (1998) First Class Service: Quality in the new NHS. London: HMSO.

Department of Health (2000) The NHS Plan. London: HMSO.

Duffield C (1989) The Delphi technique. Australian Journal of Advanced Nursing 6: 41–45.

Fitzpatrick E, Sullivan J, Smith A et al. (1991) Clinical nursing research priorities: a Delphi study. Clinical Nurse Specialist 5(2): 94–99.

Goodman C M (1987) The Delphi technique: a critique. Journal of Advanced Nursing 12: 729–734.

Hinds P, Norville R, Anthony LK et al. (1990) Establishing pediatric cancer nursing research priorities: a Delphi study. Journal of Pediatric Oncology Nursing 7: 101–108.

Hinds P, Quargneti A, Olson MS et al. (1994) The 1992 APON Delphi study to establish research priorities for pediatric oncology nursing. Journal of Pediatric Oncology Nursing 11(1): 20–27.

Hitch PJ, Murgatroyd JD (1983) Professional communications in cancer care: a Delphi survey of hospital nurses. Journal of Advanced Nursing 8: 413–422.

Hubbard S, Doneower M (1980) The nurse in a cancer research setting. Seminars in Oncology 7: 9–17.

Hunt M (1987) The process of translating research into nursing practice. Journal of Advanced Nursing 12: 101–110.

Kitson A (1997) Using evidence to demonstrate the place of nursing. Nursing Standard 11: 34–39.

Lindeman C (1975) Delphi priorities in clinical nursing research. Nurse Researcher 24: 434–441.

Linstone HA, Turoff M (eds) (1985) The Delphi Method: Method, technique and applications. Reading, MA: Addison.

Lowden B (1998) The health consequences of disclosing bad news. European Journal of Oncology Nursing 2: 225–230.

McKenna HP (1994) The Delphi technique: a worthwhile research approach for nursing? Journal of Advanced Nursing 19: 1221–1225.

McPhail G (1997) Management of change: an essential skill for nursing in the 1990s. Journal of Nursing Management 5: 199–205.

Pill J (1971) The Delphi Method: substance, context, a critique and annotated bibliography. Socio-economic Plan Science 5: 57–71.

Polit DF, Hungler BP (1995) Nursing Research: Methods, appraisal and utilisation, 5th edn. Philadelphia: Lippincott.

Reid N (1988) The Delphi technique: its contribution to the evaluation of professional practice. In: Ellis R (ed.), Professional Competence and Quality Assurance in the Caring Professions. London: Chapman & Hall.

Sackett DL, Rosenberg WMC, Gray JAM, Haynes RD, Richardson WS (1996) Evidence medicine what it is and what it isn't. British Medical Journal 312: 71–72.

Sackman H (1975) Delphi Critique. USA: The Rand Corporation.

Schmidt K, Montgomery LA, Bruene D, Kenny M (1997) Determining research priorities in Pediatric nursing: a Delphi study. Journal of Pediatric Nursing 12: 201–207.

Soanes L, Gibson F, Bayliss J, Hannan J (2000) Establishing nursing research priorities on a paediatric haematology, oncology, immunology and infectious diseases unit: a Delphi survey. European Journal of Oncology Nursing 4: 108–117.

Soanes L, Gibson F, Bayliss J, Hannan J (2003) Establishing nursing research priorities on a paediatric haematology, oncology, immunology and infectious diseases unit: involving doctors and parents. European Journal of Oncology Nursing 7: 110–119.

Stevens J (1997) Improving integration between research and practice as a means of developing evidence-based health care. NTresearch 2: 7–15.

Strachan H (2000) Handling bad news: an innovative training approach. European Journal of Oncology Nursing 4: 118–121.

Strauss JH, Ziegler LH (1975) The Delphi technique and its uses in social science research. Journal of Creative Behaviour 9: 253–259.

Street A (1995) Nursing Replay, Researching Nursing Culture Together. Melbourne: Churchill Livingstone.

Walczak JR, McGuire DB, Haisfield ME, Breezley A (1994) A survey of research-related activities and perceived barriers to research utilization among professional oncology nurses. Oncology Nurses Forum 21: 710-715.

Walsh M (1997) How nurses perceive barriers to research implementation. Nursing Standard 11: 34-39.

Western Consortium for Cancer Nursing Research (1987) Priorities for cancer nursing research: a Canadian replication. Cancer Nursing 10: 319-326.

Williams PL, Webb C (1994) The Delphi technique: a methodological discussion. Journal of Advanced Nursing 19: 180-186.

Chapter 13

Development of an oral care protocol

Faith Gibson and Sharon Hayden

The effect of cancer therapies on the oral mucosa is a major concern for paediatric oncology nurses. Within cancer care oral complications are associated with certain modalities of treatment. In addition, some types of malignancies themselves may also predispose to various oral complications. Many of these complications, however, can be avoided, or at least minimized, when symptom management follows a validated oral care protocol. This includes ongoing assessment, prevention and treatment, coupled with specific nursing measures instigated to prevent, minimize or reverse changes in the oral cavity. There is certainly no dispute that regular oral care is essential in reducing the detrimental effects of a compromised oral cavity. A number of authors, however, suggest that oral care regimens are often based on tradition, anecdote and subjective evaluation (Maurer, 1977; Daeffler, 1980; Holmes, 1991; Peate, 1993; Campbell et al., 1995). This is not surprising considering the vast array of conflicting information about the appropriateness of oral care regimens: the choice of implement, the use of cleansing agents and frequency of oral care (Beck, 1992; Moore, 1995). This has resulted in nurses being uncertain of which oral care regimens they should follow. Nevertheless, nurses must be accountable for the care that they give and whenever possible scientific-based evidence should inform their decision-making and underpin the rationale for the care given, resulting in clinically effective nursing interventions (Kitson, 1997).

Children undergoing treatment for cancer experience many invasive procedures so each and every procedure must be justified. In the absence of national clinical guidelines for oral care clinical guidance was required in order to (Royal College of Nursing, 1995):

- reduce unacceptable or undesirable variations in clinical practice
- offer a way of implementing research findings

- provide a focus for discussion among both healthcare professionals and their patients/families
- help professionals from different disciplines to come to an agreement about treatment
- provide a quality framework against which to measure practice
- give managers useful data for assessing treatment costs.

As part of an ongoing programme of research and audit undertaken by a 'mouth care working party' on a paediatric haematology/oncology unit, clinical guidance was developed in the form of an oral care protocol to guide healthcare professionals in providing individualized oral care to children receiving chemotherapy. This protocol encompasses an oral assessment guide and a pictorial algorithm. Both aim to facilitate decision-making and inform the nursing care delivered. The protocol is based on a synthesis of the available literature, and the knowledge and clinical experience of the experts who contributed to the working party. The following discussion reflects on the development and evaluation of the oral care protocol and algorithm which have been used systematically to guide nurses, doctors and pharmacists in the decision-making process pertaining to oral care. This chapter offers a summary of the activities of the working party; more detail can be found in Gibson et al. (1997) and Nelson et al. (2001).

Background to the development of an oral care protocol

Care of the mouth is one of the most basic of all nursing activities, and maintenance of oral health is essential to ensure comfort, protect against infection, and maintain nutritional status and patient well-being (Perry and Potter, 1986). In relation to chemotherapy treatment, oral stomatitis occurs as a result of damage and destruction of epithelial cells, usually 5–7 days after administration of therapy. Stomatoxic therapy affects the oral epithelial cells both directly and indirectly: directly by interfering with actual cell production, maturation and replacement; indirectly as a result of bone marrow depression, where subsequent neutropenia and thrombocytopenia increase risks from bleeding and infection. The agents that are most often stomatotoxic are the anti-miotic antibiotics and the antimetabolites; however, some alkylating agents may also cause problems (Beck, 1992). The degree of stomatitis appears to be influenced by the dose, frequency and rate of administration, coupled with the combination of drugs used (Macko, 1983; Sonis, 1983; Lawson, 1989; Beck, 1992).

It is a known fact that oral care cannot prevent the chemotherapeutic inhibition of cell replication in the basal oral mucosa; systematic oral care may, however, prevent or minimize infections, thus limiting further damage to the oral tissue (Daeffler, 1980; Allbright, 1984; Holmes, 1991). Beck (1992) suggests that a realistic objective of oral care is to decrease the intensity and duration of stomatitis and to minimize the complications of pain, oral and systemic infection, bleeding and malnutrition. Oral care is therefore the responsibility of the multidisciplinary team, as well as the patient and the family care-giver (Beck, 1992). This is a negotiated role in which the nurse may often be in a supportive role. The nurse's role is to facilitate family-centred care and therefore, whenever possible, oral care is performed by the child or family. However, where there are specific concerns, the nurse may be required to assist/support, educate/advise or refer the child or family (Casey, 1993) for more specialized oral/dental assessment or treatment. Two issues were highlighted as separate concerns for nurses on the unit in relation to oral care: assessment and management of symptoms.

Assessment

Picture the following scene, which took place on the unit in 1988:

> In a nurse-to-nurse handover the oral status of a 10-year-old boy who was receiving chemotherapy for a B-cell lymphoma was being described. The nurse described the oral mucosa as red, sore and looking like a cheese grater has been used on its surface. Two experienced children's cancer nurses on hearing this description asked of each other a number of questions:
>
> - What does this information communicate to other nurses?
> - How far did this description reflect a shared understanding of the symptom?
> - How would a nurse receiving this handover prioritize this boy's oral care?
> - How far could this type of terminology be used to provide baseline data, predict or minimize oral complications, and evaluate nursing interventions?
>
> These questions led the two nurses to reflect on the current assessment of oral stomatitis, as well as the methods used to communicate this symptom. This reflection led to the formulation of two final questions: how did nurses assess the oral status of children and what methods were used to communicate their assessment to all members of the multi-professional team?

Management of symptoms

Picture the following scene:

> A paediatric oncology ward where a mother is resident with her child who has been receiving chemotherapy for leukaemia. For the fourth time that day the mother is struggling to cleanse her child's mouth with an antibacterial mouthwash. And for the fourth time that day, her attempt subsides into a distressing struggle, which ends up with both participants in tears. This scenario, unfortunately all too familiar on many paediatric oncology wards, highlights some important issues: what justification was there for the implementation of the oral care regimen currently practised on the unit? Had those children who actually experienced oral complications been identified so that specific oral care regimens could be implemented to suit their individual needs? Or was this just another aspect of nursing practice that had been taken for granted and become a ritualized routine (Walsh and Ford, 1989)? These questions highlighted fundamental issues about this nursing intervention: was the current oral care procedure based on research, and how did nurses make decisions about the care delivered?

To facilitate answers to all these questions, thus ensuring that all children undergoing chemotherapy received appropriate oral care, a working party was established in 1988. The working party included expert practitioners, one of whom was an educationalist. The working party chose action research as their change strategy because this had been suggested as the most appropriate method for the investigation of nursing problems (Greenwood, 1984).

Change strategy

Greenwood (1984) proposed action research as the method most suitable for research in nursing because of its situational, collaborative, participatory and self-evaluative nature. It has been described as a 'new paradigm' research, i.e. research with and for people rather than on people (Meyer, 1993), which rejects both empiricist and interpretational models of science (Badger, 2000). Action research is not easily defined because it is an approach to research, rather than a specific method (Meyer and Batehup, 1997). However, it has been described as a type of applied social research differing from other varieties in the immediacy of the researchers' involvement in the action process (Lathlean, 1996). Many writers have discussed different types of action research and debated which types can be justified as 'real' (Webb et al., 1998).

The value of action research to bridge the gap among theory, research and practice, using a process similar to developing evidence-based practice (Wallis, 1998), was the rationale behind selecting the approach in the first instance. The recognition that generation of research data was not enough to influence practice meant that the approach appealed for documented reports to motivate practitioners to use their findings within the methodology (Wallis, 1998). In selecting the approach, the problems of ensuring reliability and validity were acknowledged (Greenwood, 1994; Badger, 2000). Some key characteristics of action research do emerge from the literature and highlight clearly the author's reasons for selecting the approach:

• There is collaboration between researcher and practitioners.
• The aim of the research is the solution of practical problems.
• The research results in change in practice.
• Theory is developed from the results.
• It is a cyclical process.
• The process includes reflection on practice.

Development of the oral care protocol

The process of moving through several action research cycles, which allow for refinement of ideas and practice, is well documented (Lauri, 1982), and features in many of the action research studies reported (e.g. Owen, 1993; Rolfe and Philips, 1995; Manley, 1997). It was, therefore, an expectation of the working party that ongoing evaluation and reflection would reveal developments within practice that contribute to the ongoing action research cycles. Although the direction of the study was clear at the start (to introduce a validated oral care protocol and thus improve care), the actual journey and route could not be predetermined and therefore the research remains open-ended, with information gained from one cycle informing the next (Hope, 1998–99). By keeping the research open-ended, issues that arose from practice could be dealt with through subsequent cycles of diagnosis, action planning, action taking, evaluation and learning specification (Susman and Evered, 1978) see Figure 13.1. The period of development reported below spans over 12 years and began with the introduction of an oral assessment tool, followed by the development and implementation of a clinical algorithm.

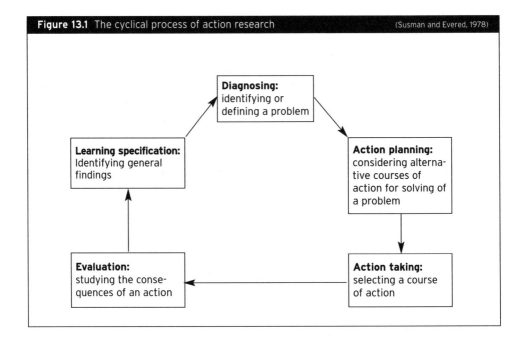

Figure 13.1 The cyclical process of action research   (Susman and Evered, 1978)

Oral assessment

Theory

As previously stated, it is known that oral care cannot prevent the chemotherapeutic inhibition of cell replication in the basal oral mucosa; systematic oral care may, however, prevent or minimize infections, thus limiting further damage to the oral tissue (Daeffler, 1980; Holmes, 1991). As discussed earlier, the objective of oral care is to decrease the intensity and duration of mucositis and to minimize the complications of pain, oral and systemic infection, bleeding and malnutrition. To achieve these goals, paediatric nurses must be able to identify those children with the potential to develop oral complications as early as possible. Knowledge and understanding of the chemotherapy agents children receive, supported by a nursing assessment, will be the first steps in realizing these goals. Based on this assessment, an individualized care plan can then be developed which identifies either prophylactic or treatment-specific measures.

Oral assessment is considered to be central to planning effective care and begins with a history of previous dental care, which includes the child's usual brushing regimen, as well as recording any previous oral problems. Assessment begins before the first dose of chemotherapy is given and should include a dental check-up, planned intervention, and education of the child and family. Ongoing assessment is then dependent on the child's baseline oral status, intensity of the chemotherapy regimen and expected mucosal toxicity.

The use of an oral assessment tool can facilitate this process because historically the measurement of stomatitis has been far from standardized, with care often being underpinned by subjective evaluation alone (Dodd et al., 1996). Therefore, in order to help clarify terminology and provide accurate descriptions of a child's oral status, effective objective measurement is recommended whenever possible. Assessment has the potential to provide baseline data: to predict, prevent or minimize oral complications, and to evaluate nursing interventions (Richardson, 1987). In addition, Beck (1992) suggests that a numerical assessment tool would ensure consistency of assessment between assessors. The literature reveals a number of oral assessment tools (Beck, 1979; Eilers et al., 1988; Crosby, 1989; Dibble et al., 1996); however, the oral assessment guide by Eilers et al. (1988) appeared to be the most appropriate and with minor adaptations has been in use on the unit since 1988 (Table 13.1). The oral assessment guide (OAG) was chosen for several reasons: its validity and reliability have been verified, albeit in an adult population; it is concise, yet comprehensive; and it appeared suitable for adaptation for use in the paediatric setting.

Practice

As mentioned previously nurses on the unit had no common language in which to communicate symptoms of oral problems. This was compounded by the fact that there was an absence of a structured oral assessment tool in use on the unit. Using action research members of the working party identified and implemented an OAG on the unit. The steps taken are highlighted within the cyclical process of action research in Table 13.2.

The OAG has proved to be a successful tool for assessing deterioration and resolution of oral complications. In addition, the general perception of nursing staff is that the OAG has:

- improved nurse-to-nurse communication
- improved communication among the multiprofessional team
- ensured that all aspects of the mouth are assessed at least daily
- enabled the care delivered to be evaluated
- provided a record of a child's response to chemotherapy
- introduced a valuable 'tool' used to teach children, parents and nursing staff about oral care.

Table 13.1 Oral assessment guide

Category	Method of administration	1	2	3
Voice	Converse with patient; listen to crying	Normal	Deeper or raspy	Difficulty talking, crying or painful
Swallow	Ask patient to swallow	Normal swallow	Some pain on swallowing	Unable to swallow
Lips and angle of the mouth	Observe and feel tissue	Smooth and pink and moist	Dry or cracked	Ulcerated or bleeding
Tongue	Observe appearance of tissue	Pink and moist and papillae present	Coated or loss of papillae with a shiny appearance with or without redness Fungal infection	Blistered or cracked
Saliva	Insert depressor into mouth, touching centre of the tongue and the floor of the mouth.	Watery Excess salivation as a result of teething	Thick or ropy	Absent
Mucous membranes	Observe the appearance of the tissue	Pink and moist	Reddened or coated without ulceration Fungal infection	Ulceration with or without bleeding
Gingival	Gently press tissue Visual	Pink and firm	Oedematous with or without redness, smooth Oedema caused by teething	Spontaneous bleeding or bleeding with pressure
Teeth (if no teeth score as 1)	Observe appearance of teeth	Clean and no debris	Plaque or debris in localized areas (between teeth if present)	Plaque or debris generalized along gum line

Oral assessment guide adapted and reprinted from Eilers et al. (1988)

Prevention and management of symptoms

Theory

There are no 'best practice' guidelines available advising nurses of the most appropriate way to provide oral care. The frequency of oral care

Table 13.2 Steps taken to implement an oral assessment tool

Diagnosis	Action planning	Action taking	Evaluation
Absence of a structured assessment tool	Undertook a review of published literature on assessment tools	Three oral assessment tools selected	Informal feedback was positive
No common language to report oral problems		Tools circulated between working party and nurses on the unit	Diagnosed problems with treatment and management of symptoms
Problems in reporting accurate descriptions of the oral status		Tool by Eilers et al. (1988) chosen	Returned to the start of the action research cycle
		Tool circulated and teaching sessions arranged	
		Following preparation of staff, tool implemented	

and the materials used to perform safe and effective care are often debated in the literature. There is a vast array of proprietary products and materials available to provide prophylactic oral care, and this has resulted in nurses being unsure which are the most appropriate to use (Adams, 1996; Holmes, 1996). Added to this there is much conflict over the efficacy and safety of various oral care regimens (Holmes, 1991, 1996), with some regimens having the potential to do more harm than good (Daeffler, 1980; Miller and Rubinstein, 1987; Peate, 1993).

Regular brushing is imperative in plaque removal and, although some studies have shown that nurses prefer using foam sponges (Pearson, 1996), there is a general agreement that a small-headed, soft, multi-tufted, nylon-bristled toothbrush is the best tool for cleaning the teeth (Madeya, 1996; Pearson, 1996; Kennedy and Diamond, 1997) and massaging the gingiva. Teeth should be cleaned effectively twice a day, as soon as possible after meals if eating, and before bedtime. Young children will need to have their teeth brushed for them, up to an age when the parent or carer feels that they have the dexterity to do it properly for themselves. The easiest and most effective way is for the adult to sit down and have the child stand in front with the child's head against the adult's chest and brush the teeth (Lloyd, 1994). For babies and very young children they may lie in the adult's lap. Even when the child is not eating, regular and thorough mouth care is just as vital.

The use of very soft toothbrushes enables children to continue brushing even when their platelet count is low; however, where the child is experiencing pain or spontaneous bleeding, a foam sponge may be more acceptable during that period (Kennedy and Diamond, 1997). In addition, if required, a foam sponge soaked in water or chlorhexidine is more appropriate for babies who have no teeth.

Rinsing the oral cavity after brushing is also important. This activity removes loose debris and further irrigates the tissues. Tap water, or for some children sterile water (unit dependent), is the most common mouth rinse. Only those patients at high risk of mucosal deterioration are advised to use an antibacterial mouth rinse such as chlorhexidine 0.2% (Coleman, 1995a, 1995b). The rationale for using an antibacterial mouth rinse in this small group of children is that many of the micro-organisms responsible for causing systemic infections can be isolated from the oral cavity.

In addition to tooth brushing and rinsing with water/chlorhexidine, children who are profoundly neutropenic and at risk of developing fungal infections should use a prophylactic oral fungal agent. The most commonly cited oral antifungal agent is nystatin; however, its prophylactic use has been questioned (De Gregorio et al., 1982). The use of oral fluconazole has several advantages over nystatin. It is required to be taken only once a day, compared with oral nystatin which is taken every 4–6 hours. Once a day is particularly attractive to children who often dislike taking oral medications. In addition, the use of fluconazole allows the concurrent use of a chlorhexidine-based mouthwash. Previously, where oral nystatin had been used, a gap of 1 hour had to be observed between chlorhexidine and oral nystatin (Galbraith et al., 1991).

Practice

It was noted on the unit that some children undergoing specific modules of chemotherapy experienced significant problems, such as a mucosal ulceration and fungal infections. In contrast, however, there were significant numbers of children who received specific chemotherapy modules and experienced minimal complications with their oral cavity. Indeed, some children experienced no problems at all. Unfortunately, the current oral care regimens did not reflect this variation in outcomes and in practice many children were receiving inappropriate oral care, i.e. most children received the same oral care, regardless of their chemotherapy protocol or the severity of myelosuppression that they were likely to experience. This regimen consisted of a toothbrush, or foam sponge, toothpaste, oral nystatin and a chlorhexidine (0.2%)-based mouthwash, each being administered four times a day.

Several problems were experienced with this regimen. First, many children complained of chlorhexidine's bitter taste and unpleasant after-taste; this led to problems with adherence. According to Betcher and Burnham (1990) and Rubinstein-Devore (1994), chlorhexidine should be rinsed and remain in contact with the mucosal membrane for at least 30–90 seconds for it to be effective. It was doubtful that many children adhered to this recommendation. In addition, the struggle between parent and child each time oral care was administered was distressing for all. Second, information gained from a conference presentation highlighted a clinical issue when oral nystatin and chlorhexidine were used concurrently; a visible yellow precipitate is produced, rendering the nystatin solution ineffective against candida infections (Barkvoll and Attramadal, 1989; Galbraith et al., 1991; Finlay, 1995). Galbraith et al. (1991) advocated the combination of these two oral care products but recommended that 1 hour be left between their administration. They also recommended a gap of 1 hour between using chlorhexidine and eating or drinking, and a further 20-minute interval after using oral nystatin, so that the effectiveness of these products is not compromised. With this particular regimen, it was very difficult to see when the child would have time to eat! This situation was clearly not acceptable in a population who already had problems maintaining an adequate oral intake and weight (Hanigan and Walter, 1992).

Using action research the working party sought either to validate or to change the current oral care protocol to produce one that would help guide practitioners as to the most appropriate regimen to introduce for the individual child. The steps taken are highlighted in Table 13.2.

Evaluation of the oral care protocol

Diagnosis

There is no doubt that the concurrent use of an OAG (Table 13.3) (Eilers et al., 1988) and an oral care flowchart, or algorithm, proved valuable in providing a more informed and consistent approach to oral care, by both nursing and medical staff working on a paediatric haematology/oncology unit. However, the working party soon became aware, through their observations, reflections on practice and feedback from nurses in the practice setting, that several problems remained unresolved.

Table 13.3 Steps taken to develop and introduce an oral care algorithm

Diagnosis	Action planning	Action taking	Evaluation	Learning specification
All children received the same oral care regimen irrespective of chemotherapy protocol and hence risk factors	Working party reconvened	Sources of knowledge very general, expanded to include information from a panel of experts	Positive response to the oral care protocol and algorithm	Practice no longer ritualized
Children complained of the bitter taste of the chlorhexidine	Review of the literature pertaining to oral complications and their management in the paediatric population	Algorithm and oral care protocol produced with care linked to chemotherapy protocol received	Wide consultation resulted in useful discussion between healthcare professionals and changes were made	Increased confidence and competence in staff
Inappropriate use of chlorhexidine and nystatin when used in combination		Algorithm distributed for consultation supported by a questionnaire		Reduction in conflicting information given to parents

First, there was an issue in relation to the algorithm itself. Many nurses felt that it was not particularly user-friendly and experienced problems using the information to make decisions about the most appropriate oral care regimen to follow. In practice, fluconazole was at times being used indiscriminately. Some children were receiving fluconazole for a longer period than required whereas others were being prescribed the preparation when another antifungal agent may have been more appropriate. Indiscriminate use of fluconazole is of concern, not only because of the cost implications, but also because of the emergence of resistant fungi (Chandrasekar and Gatny, 1994; Hoppe et al., 1994). Second, for babies without teeth, there was confusion about the numerical scoring of this category on the OAG. In practice, nurses were recording the teeth category as not applicable or zero, which altered the overall score system. And lastly, even though nurses were aware of the importance of assessing children's pain, the formal commencement of pain assessment, which would provide continuity of assessment as well as a format for communicating the child's pain status, was lacking. As children frequently do not verbalize pain until it is quite severe (Beck, 1992), good practice would be to monitor pain from a very early stage and intervene promptly with appropriate analgesia. This would allow oral care to continue and therefore possibly limit further deterioration.

Action planning

In view of these concerns, further investigation was warranted to confirm that these problems were widespread and not just isolated reports concerning a few individuals. The working party therefore decided to undertake an evaluation of the use of the oral care protocol so that an accurate picture could be gained. The evaluation consisted of three parts: a structured interview, vignettes and an analysis of documentary evidence from care plans, patient folders and prescription charts. The three approaches were chosen to ensure a comprehensive and inclusive approach to the evaluation.

Action taking

The structured interview was undertaken with a random sample of junior and senior grade nurses on both inpatient and outpatient areas. The sample was selected (by picking entered names from the off-duty rota from a 'hat', sampling 50% from each of the grades). In total 20 junior and 9 senior grade nurses were interviewed. The length of time that staff had been working on the unit varied from 3 months to 10 years.

The interview was conducted by one of the members of the working party. Respondents were approached to request their participation in the evaluation and, if agreed, a mutually convenient time to meet was arranged. No member of staff declined to be involved. All participants were assured of confidentiality. All members of the team were aware that an evaluation of oral care practice was taking place on the unit; however, the detail about the content of the interview had not been discussed with any team members outside the working party. To ensure a consistent approach, a standard statement was read out to each nurse before the interview commenced. The confidential nature of the interview was reaffirmed. Questions were read aloud to the respondents, allowing sufficient time to think, and responses were recorded on to the interview sheet. Questions could be repeated, but no further clarification of a question was provided. However, respondents could be asked to clarify their response if it was not clear to the interviewer.

The vignettes were administered to a purposeful sample of four 'novice' and four 'expert' nurses from the inpatient setting, and two 'expert' nurses from the outpatient setting. The notion of novice and expert was considered in relation to time on the unit as well as time within the specialty.

Documentary analysis was undertaken to include a snapshot from the care plan, patient folder, and prescription chart on random selected days over a period of 1 week within each of the two inpatient areas. Two of the working party members undertook this part of the audit, using a previously prepared guide sheet. Twenty guide sheets in total were completed.

Evaluation of practice

The audit revealed a number of clinical issues, including:

- Although nursing staff were aware of the oral care protocol they did not always refer to the algorithm when planning care.
- Familiarity and knowledge of the steps of the algorithm varied; level of experience and time on the unit made no significant difference to that familiarity.
- The algorithm was not found to be user-friendly, with some nurses finding it difficult to follow the steps.
- Nursing staff found it difficult to apply the algorithm to individual children, particularly if they were unfamiliar with a protocol or where certain children were not identified as a group within the flow diagram.
- There was not enough detail to facilitate decision-making.
- There was indiscriminate use of fluconazole.
- Nursing staff were not always clear on planning care in relation to the score gained from the OAG.
- Some nursing staff were unable to discriminate between prophylactic oral care and those measures required to treat oral complications.
- Nurses did not always have the knowledge to introduce appropriate treatment regimens for oral mucositis.
- There was some confusion over the use of prophylactic oral care agents.

Diagnosis

The evaluation of practice overwhelmingly confirmed that the original areas of concern, notably the indiscriminate use of fluconazole, scoring of the teeth category and pain assessment, were in fact widespread issues within the unit. In addition, other problem areas identified could be attributed to the lack of clarity and omission of detail in the construction of the original algorithm. Its construction began simply as a means of conveying information that was more visually appealing than written material alone. However, no literature was obtained to help guide the algorithm design. Consequently, its construction was rather unsophisticated, which led to a degree of confusion for the user. The algorithm also lacked sufficient detail to guide those for whom it was originally designed, i.e. medical and nursing staff without expert knowledge in this area of care. The algorithm pictorially summarized prophylactic oral care with the written protocol providing much of the detail. However, in practice it seemed as though only the algorithm was being referred to. This resulted in important supplementary details, such as what was meant by normal oral hygiene, and the parameters for using the chlorhexidine mouthwash and fluconazole were not considered. This may explain the finding that 'a number of children did not receive care according to protocol'.

Most of the nurses involved in the evaluation implied that the existing parameters for fluconazole use were misleading. The original algorithm stated that it should be given as an 'inpatient only'. The logic behind this recommendation was that most children were discharged once their neutrophil count had recovered. However, some discharges were delayed for other reasons, such as nutritional problems or further investigations being required, so even though the neutrophil count of these children had recovered they were still, inappropriately, receiving fluconazole.

There were several other issues also indirectly highlighted by the evaluation process. First, it became evident that it was not only the teeth category of the OAG that required reviewing. As the original tool was used in an adult population, dentures were referred to. However, when it was adapted for use in children a normal aspect of childhood development such as teething was inadvertently overlooked. It was also felt that the swallow category, which included 'testing of the gag reflex' – in practice never performed – could not be justified because it may exacerbate feelings of nausea and vomiting as well as being very invasive. In addition, several nurses were not sure how to interpret terminology such as 'angle of the mouth'.

The second area, which promoted discussion, was the fact that the original algorithm did not consider the needs of those children who were febrile and neutropenic. During this time the mouths of these children are vulnerable for two reasons. Foremost, there is a high inverse correlation between the neutrophil count and the degree of mucositis (Kenny, 1990; Burke et al., 1991; Iwamoto, 1991). As the neutrophil count falls the compromised mucosa may provide a site of entry for the migration of normally harmless oral micro-organisms into the bloodstream (Lucas et al., 1997). Second, the mouth itself may be a direct or potential source of infection such as candidiasis, herpes, erythema, ulceration or angular cheilitis (Meurman et al., 1997). Third, there was concern raised that, if a child's diagnosis or treatment schedule did not explicitly appear on the algorithm, there was some confusion as to the most appropriate oral care regimen to implement. The potential outcome was that children would receive inappropriate oral care. Last, even when the OAG score was increasing, there were occasions where this information did not seem to influence or change practice, e.g. an increasing score may indicate deterioration of the mucosa or gingiva, but there was often no evidence that pain assessment or analgesia had been instigated. Moreover, if action was taken, e.g. if a fungal infection became evident, there was confusion as to the most appropriate antifungal agent to use.

Action planning

The aforementioned problems suggested that the first course of action should be directed towards reviewing the literature, so that the main concepts of constructing an algorithm may be identified. Second, information contained within the oral care protocol and algorithm had to be reviewed. Some of the information within the oral care protocol would be more appropriately incorporated into the algorithm itself. It was also obvious that both the protocol and the algorithm required additional information to ensure that children received the most appropriate oral care. Third, the OAG itself had to be reviewed, with additional information being required to make it clearer and more pertinent to the paediatric population. Last, a second, 'therapeutic' algorithm seemed to be required which could help all staff problem-solve by directing them towards the most appropriate interventions.

Action taking

Once the principles of designing an algorithm were clear, the next step was to address the findings and clinical feedback. This culminated in more explicit detail being incorporated into the algorithm, including:

- parameters for the use of fluconazole and Corsodyl
- reminders about using a toothbrush whenever possible
- addressing those children who were febrile and neutropenic
- explicitly categorizing children into treatment groups
- addressing the needs of those children not explicitly listed within any of the three groups, i.e. those with rare malignancies.

It also became evident that changes were required to the OAG that was currently in use. The following changes were made (Figure 13.2):

- If the child has no teeth, score as 1, because that is normal for that particular child.
- Omit 'testing gag reflex'.
- Reword 'angle of mouth' to 'corner of the mouth'.
- Include signs and symptoms of teething.
- Include space on the OAG score sheet to document pain assessment.

Finally, for those children whose mouths show signs of deterioration, the introduction of a second 'therapeutic' algorithm should enhance the care of the child by prompting staff to take the most appropriate action, as indicated by the OAG score.

In addition to refining the original algorithm and producing a therapeutic algorithm, consideration also needs to be given to guidance for children in shared care hospitals. As many children share care between the main centre and their local hospital, dissemination of the new algorithms and the protocol to these 'shared care' hospitals was essential to ensure consistency of care. However, it was recognized that the needs of children at the different centres would vary. There are therefore slight differences between the 'main centre' and 'shared care' algorithms because some children, such as those with infant acute lymphoblastic leukaemia (ALL), are treated only at the main centres. It was, therefore, felt appropriate to omit these details from the shared care algorithms.

Invariably the final algorithm required many drafts as clinical staff, consultants, pharmacy and dental staff were given the opportunity to verify accuracy of detail and clinical appropriateness. After the period of consultation the algorithm was introduced into the practice setting (Figure 13.2 and 13.3).

Learning specification

The algorithms, protocol and OAG were laminated for durability (Banks, 1996) and copies placed in all children's nursing notes. Individual and group teaching sessions are being provided for staff already in post and, as an ongoing initiative; it will also be included in the orientation programme for all staff new to the unit. It is essential that nurses have the knowledge and understanding of the scope and types of oral complications as well as the risks and benefits of the various oral care regimens. Therefore, the main emphasis when teaching will be to concentrate on providing the rationale and the principles for the recommendations made within the oral care protocol and algorithms.

Figure 13.2 Prophylactic oral care for the child with a malignancy: algorithm 1.
AML, acute myeloid leukaemia; ALL, acute lymphoblastic leukaemia; COJEC, cyclophosphamide, cisplatin, etoposide, vincristine, carboplatin; COPADM, cyclophosphamide, methotrexate, daunorubicin, prednisolone; CYM, cytarabine methotrexate: N, neutrophil; NHL, non-Hodgkin's lymphoma; OAG, oral assessment guide; PNET, primitive neuroectadermal tumour.

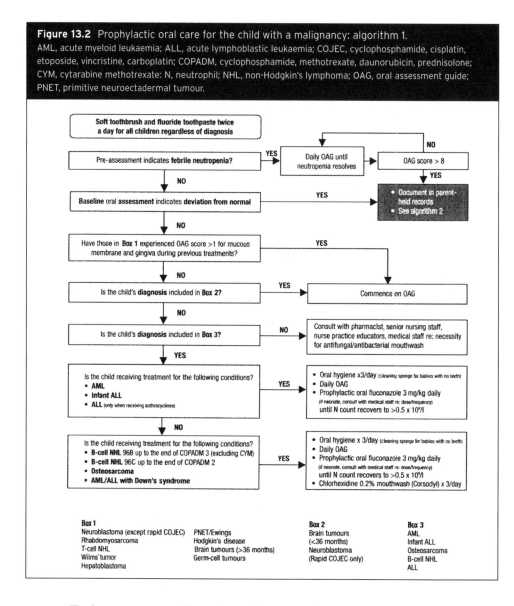

Future areas for development

The process of action research is ongoing. On the unit every opportunity is taken to strive for higher standards and improved outcomes. To achieve this, practice is continually evaluated, and strategies for improvement and future audit and research activity made explicit.

Standardized guidance for oral care in the child with cancer has been produced and introduced on our unit and other units. However, it has

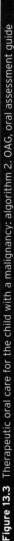

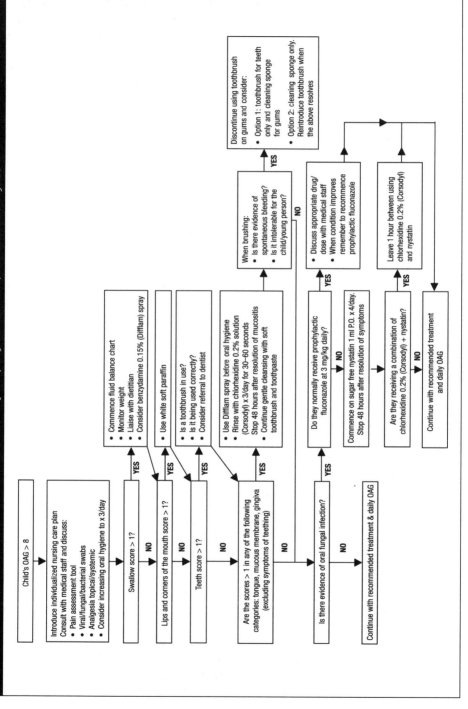

Figure 13.3 Therapeutic oral care for the child with a malignancy: algorithm 2. OAG, oral assessment guide

become clear that the extent of empirical data available in the literature is insufficient and further research into this area is a priority in order to produce evidence-based guidelines. This view has been supported by a recent Cochrane review (Clarkson et al., 2000). Currently, the situation remains that nationally oral care practice remains varied, and that evidence is scarce. Nevertheless, there is evidence to suggest that individual units are questioning their practice and producing unit-specific protocols. However, the following is the consequence of the development of local guidance:

- Much time is wasted re-inventing the wheel.
- Variations in clinical practice may still remain.
- Disagreement between professionals about treatment measures remain unresolved.
- Measurement of clinical outcomes in a multicentre study is impossible.
- Encourages practitioners to disregard the need to develop evidence-based clinical guidelines.

Encouragingly, a multi-professional working party has been established under the auspices of the paediatric oncology nurses forum (PONF) and the UKCCSG to develop evidence-based guidelines.

Conclusion

The use of action research has enabled an enquiry into nurses' understanding and use of a protocol for oral care. By keeping the research open-ended issues from practice could be dealt with through subsequent cycles of diagnosis, action planning, action taking, evaluation and specifying learning. Therefore the practice of oral care has remained a focus of research activity on the unit since the introduction of an oral care protocol over 10 years ago. Action research has thus facilitated the working party to generate a description of the ongoing problems and involve practitioners throughout the process, even though it became clear very early on that the route of the journey could not be predetermined.

Although the current evaluation confirmed the working party's initial areas of concern, it also identified a number of other issues in relation to clarity and omission of detail in the design of the original algorithm and protocol. The working party aimed to resolve the problems in the interest of research-based practice, the end being to improve the practice defined by the group on behalf of its users. Although previous research findings dominated the early stages of the project, action and evaluation became much more prominent towards the end. There was a continual process of evaluation and refinement with the working party members sharing responsibilities on the project, developing skills with the experiences described, allowing for shared learning. What can be highlighted from this work is that collaboration between researchers and practitioners, to solve a practical problem and to change practice, is essential.

As mentioned previously, studies using action research must address two main aims: to create change and improve practice (action) and to develop or refine theory (research) (Susman and Evered, 1978). The study did create change, with an expected outcome that practice will be improved; however, that improvement has yet to be verified. Generation of theory, i.e. a theory of practice (Rolfe, 1996), was possible with the research data collected, contributing to knowledge that influenced the development of the algorithms. The study has face validity using Greenwood's (1994) suggestion that that the findings appear to fit reality. Reliability results from the fact that throughout the study findings were fed back to participants, discussed and reflected upon (Webb et al., 1998), up to the point that members of the healthcare team agreed on the algorithms. Generalizability of the study findings was not an initial aim. Practitioners wishing to relate the findings and use the algorithms bear the onus of making a judgement about the study based on the steps clearly documented about the research process in this chapter.

It was expected that ongoing evaluation and reflection would reveal developments within practice contributing to the ongoing action research cycles. Education now aims to provide the rationale and principles for the recommendations made. Although the oral care protocol developed has been altered and revised for use in other paediatric oncology units, the protocol stands as guidance until evidence-based guidelines are produced. McMahon (1998) stresses that what should be done when no research exists is 'don't do nothing'. In the absence of evidence-based guidelines and in the face of conflicting information about the prevention and management of oral care in children with cancer, this chapter supports the use of expert opinion based on clinical practice as a source of evidence when developing guidance for practice.

Acknowledgements

Thanks to Wendy Nelson, Nicki Morgan and Cathy Crook for their contribution to the activities of the working party.

Thanks to Elsevier Science for permission to reproduce parts of a previously published paper: Nelson et al. (2001).

References

Adams R (1996) Qualified nurses lack of knowledge related to oral health, resulting in inadequate oral care of patients on medical wards. Journal of Advanced Nursing 24: 552-560.

Albright A (1984) Oral care for the cancer chemotherapy patient. Nursing Times 80: 40-42.

Badger TG (2000) Action research, change and methodological rigour. Journal of Nursing Management 8: 201-207.

Banks NJ (1996) Methodology matters – IV. Constructing algorithm flowcharts for clinical performance measurement. International Journal for Quality in Health Care 8: 394-400.

Barkvoll P, Attramadal A (1989) Effects of nystatin and chlorhexidine digluconate on Candida albicans. Oral Surgical Oral Medicine Oral Pathology 67: 279-81.

Beck S (1979) Impact of a systematic oral care protocol on stomatitis after chemotherapy. Cancer Nursing 10: 185-199.

Beck SL (1992) Prevention and management of oral complications in the cancer patient. Issues in Cancer Nursing Practice Updates 1: 1-12.

Betcher DL, Burnham N (1990) Chlorhexidine. Journal of Pediatric Oncology Nursing 7: 82-83.

Burke MB, Wilkes GM, Berg D, Bean CK, Ingwesen K (1991) Cancer Chemotherapy. Boston, MA: Jones & Bartlett Publishers, Inc.

Campbell ST, Evans MA, Mactavish F (1995) The Royal College of Nursing Paediatric Oncology Nursing Forum Guidelines for Mouthcare. London: Royal College of Nursing,

Casey A (1993) Development and use of the partnership model of nursing care. In: Glasper EA, Tucker A (eds), Advances in Child Health Nursing. London: Scutari Press, pp. 183-193.

Chandrasekar PH, Gatny CM (1994) Effect of fluconazole prophylaxis on fever and use of amphotericin in neutropenic cancer patients. Chemotherapy 40: 136-143.

Clarkson JE, Worthington HV, Eden OB (2000) Interventions for preventing oral mucositis or oral candidiasis for patients with cancer receiving chemotherapy (excluding head and neck cancer) (Cochrane Review). In: Cochrane Library, Issue 4. Oxford.

Coleman S (1995a) An overview of the oral complications of adult patients with malignant haematological conditions who have undergone radiotherapy or chemotherapy. Journal of Advanced Nursing 22: 1085-1091.

Coleman S (1995b) An overview of the oral complications of adult patients with malignant haematological conditions who have undergone radiotherapy or chemotherapy. Journal of Advanced Nursing 22: 1085-1091.

Crosby C (1989) Method in mouth care. Nursing Times 85: 38-41.

Daeffler R (1980) Oral hygiene measures for patients with cancer I. Cancer Nursing 3: 347-353.

De Gregorio MW, Lee WM, Ries CA (1982) Candida infections in patients with acute leukemia: Ineffectiveness of nystatin prophylaxis and relationship between oropharyngeal and systemic candidiasis. Cancer 51: 2780-2784.

Dibble SL, Shiba G, MacPhail L, Dodd MJ (1996) MacDibbs mouth assessment. Cancer Practice 4: 135-140.

Dodd MJ, Facione NC, Dibble SL, MacPhail L (1996) Comparison of methods to determine the prevalence and nature of oral mucositis. Cancer Practice 4: 312-318.

Eilers J, Berger AM, Petersen MC (1988) Development, testing and application of the oral assessment guide. Oncology Nursing Forum 15: 325-330.

Finlay I (1995) Oral fungal infections. European Journal of Palliative Care suppl 1: 4-7

Galbraith I, Bailey D, Kelly L et al. (1991) Treatment for alteration in oral mucosa related to chemotherapy. Pediatric Nursing 17: 233-237.

Gibson F, Horsford J, Nelson W (1997) Oral care: practice reconsidered within a framework of action research. Journal of Cancer Nursing 1: 183-190.

Greenwood J (1984) Nursing research; a position paper. Journal of Advanced Nursing 9: 77-82.

Greenwood J (1994) Action research; a few details, a caution and something new. Journal of Advanced Nursing 20: 13-18.

Hanigan MJ, Walter GA (1992) Nutritional support of the child with cancer. Journal of Pediatric Oncology Nursing 9: 110-118.

Holmes S (1991) The oral complications of specific anti cancer therapy. International Journal of Nursing Studies 28: 343-360.

Holmes S (1996) Nursing management of oral care in older patients. Nursing Times 92(9): 37-39.

Hope K (1998-99) Starting out with action research. Nurse Researcher 6: 16-26.

Hoppe JE, Klingebiel T, Niethammer D (1994) Selection of *Candida glabrata* in pediatric bone marrow transplantation recipients receiving fluconazole. Paediatric Haematology and Oncology 11: 207-210.

Iwamoto RR (1991) Alterations in oral status. In: Baird SB, Mccorkle R, Grant M (eds), Cancer Nursing: A comprehensive textbook. Philadelphia: WB Saunders & Co.

Kennedy L, Diamond J (1997) Assessment and management of chemotherapy-induced mucositis in children. Journal of Pediatric Oncology Nursing 14: 164-174.

Kenny SA (1990) Effect of two oral care protocols on the incidence of stomatitis in hematology patients. Cancer Nursing 13: 11-13.

Kitson A (1997) Using the evidence to demonstrate the value of nursing. Nursing Standard 11: 34-39.

Lathlean J (1996) Ethical dimensions of action research. In: de Raeve L (ed.), Nursing Research: An ethical and legal appraisal. London: Baillière Tindall, pp. 32-41.

Lauri S (1982) Development of the nursing process through action research. Journal of Advanced Nursing 7: 301-307.

Lawson K (1989) Oral-dental concerns of the pediatric oncology patient. Issues in Comprehensive Pediatric Nursing 12: 199-206.

Lloyd S (1994) Teaching parents to look after children's teeth. Professional Care of Mother and Child 4: 34-36.

Lucas VS, Beighton D, Roberts GJ, Challacombe SJ (1997) Changes in the oral streptococcal flora of children undergoing allogeneic bone marrow transplantation. British Society for the Study of Infection 35: 135-141.

Macko DJ (1983) Dental complications of cancer and its treatment. In: Altman AJ, Schwartz AD (eds), Malignant Diseases of Infancy, Childhood and Adolescence. Philadelphia: WB Saunders, pp. 177-186.

McMahon A (1998) Developing practice through research. In: Roe B, Webb C (eds), Research and Development in Clinical Nursing Practice. London: Whurr.

Madeya ML (1996) Oral complications from cancer therapy: part 1 - pathophysiology and secondary complications. Oncology Nurses Forum 23: 801-807.

Manley K (1997) A conceptual framework for advanced practice: an action research project operationalising an advanced practitioner/consultant nurse role. Journal of Clinical Nursing 6: 179-190.

Maurer J (1977) Providing optimal oral health. Nursing Clinics of North America 12: 671-684.

Meurman JH, Pyrhonen S, Teerenhovi L, Lindqvist C (1997) Oral sources of septicaemia in patients with malignancies. Oral Oncology 3: 389-397.

Meyer J (1993) New paradigm research in practice: the trials and tribulations of action research. Journal of Advanced Nursing 18: 1006-1072.

Meyer J, Batehup L (1997) Action research in health-care practice: nature, present concerns and future possibilities. NTresearch 2: 175-184.

Miller R, Rubenstein L (1987) Oral health care for hospitalized patients: The nurse's role. Journal of Nursing Education 26: 362-366.

Moore J (1995) Assessment of nurse-administered oral hygiene. Nursing Times 91: 40-41.

Nelson W, Gibson F, Hayden S, Morgan N (2001) Using action research in paediatric oncology to develop an oral care algorithm. European Journal of Oncology Nursing 5: 180-189.

Owen S (1993) Identifying a role for the nurse teacher in the clinical area. Journal of Advanced Nursing 18: 816–825.

Pearson LS (1996) A comparison of the ability of foam swabs and toothbrushes to remove dental plaque. Implications for nursing practice. Journal of Advanced Nursing 23: 62–69.

Peate I (1993) Nurse-administered oral hygiene in the hospitalised patient. British Journal of Nursing 2: 459–462.

Perry AG, Potter PA (1986) Clinical Nursing Skills and Techniques: Basic and intermediate and advanced. Philadelphia: JB Lippincott Co.

Richardson A (1987) A process standard for oral care. Nursing Times 83: 38–40.

Rolfe G (1996) Going to extremes: action research, grounded practice and the theory practice gap in nursing. Journal of Advanced Nursing 24: 1315–1320.

Rolfe G, Philips LM (1995) An action research project to develop and evaluate the role of an advanced nurse practitioner in dementia. Journal of Clinical Nursing 4: 289–293.

Royal College of Nursing (1995) Clinical Guidelines: What you need to know. London: RCN.

Rubinstein-Devore LR (1994) Antimicrobial mouthrinses. Journal of American Dental Association 125(suppl 2): 23–28.

Sonis ST (1983) Epidemiology, frequency, distribution mechanisms and histopathology. In: Peterson D, Sonis ST (eds), Oral Complications of Cancer Chemotherapy. The Hague: Martinus Nighoff Publishers.

Susman G, Evered R (1978) An assessment of the merits of action researches. Administrative Science Quarterly 23: 582–603.

Wallis S (1998) Changing practice through action research. Nurse Researcher 6: 5–15.

Walsh M, Ford P (1989) Nursing Rituals: Research and rational actions. Oxford: Heinemann Nursing.

Webb C, Turton P, Pontin D (1998) Action research: the debate moves on. In: Roe B, Webb C (eds), Research and Development in Clinical Nursing Practice. London: Whurr Publishers.

Chapter 14

Cancer-related fatigue in teenagers: a journey of discovery

Jackie Edwards, Faith Gibson and Beth Sepion

Cancer-related fatigue (CRF) is achieving recognition as a common and disturbing symptom for adults with cancer (Richardson, 1995; Stone et al., 1998). As a result, we are witnessing a growing body of knowledge illustrating the multifactorial nature of this symptom (Ferrell et al., 1996), with increasing evidence revealing the subjective nature of the experience (Richardson and Ream, 1996). However, the current evidence available emanates from results of research with adult patients and limited attention has been paid to the possibility and degree to which children and teenagers with cancer experience fatigue. The question which, at present, remains unanswered asks: Is fatigue the unrecognized symptom in paediatric and adolescent cancer, as the symptoms of pain, nausea and vomiting were some 20 years ago?

So why does the question remain unanswered? Two issues are worth considering. First, there are a number of specific challenges that researchers face when communicating with children and teenagers. The impact of illness on teenagers, in particular, is unique and requires creative approaches from skilled practitioners to facilitate their adherence with treatment regimens and their associated restrictions. Very few nurses specialize in adolescent healthcare and, in general, the training of healthcare professionals may contain little education about the needs of teenagers. It is also interesting to note that, in paediatric oncology, which encompasses a number of defined specialities (e.g. bone marrow transplantation, community nursing), the specific needs of teenagers have received very little attention from researchers. The failure to recognize the uniqueness of adolescence, by healthcare professionals, means that in the past we have made assumptions about the effects of cancer based on studies involving children across a wide age span (Eiser, 1996). Within the clinical environment, communication and non-adherence are acknowledged as difficult areas of care and therefore a major issue facing researchers is the formidable task of identifying methods to encourage participation from teenagers. The use of focus groups (Doswell and Vandestienne, 1996; Galt, 1997; James et al., 1997), draw and write techniques (Wilson and Ratekin, 1990; Pridmore and Bendelow, 1995; Bradding and Horstman, 1999) and sort cards (Hooker, 1997) are innovative ways that have been developed to encourage children and teenagers to tell their own story and to participate in research studies. Yet there remains some uncertainty about how feasible it is to recruit teenagers to participate in research studies.

Second, although the benefits of paediatric clinical research are acknowledged, references to children's legal rights, their ability to give consent and their vulnerability to risks of human experimentation have given rise to concern over the ethics of involving children and teenagers as research participants. The notion that children deserve protection evolved slowly, and this has given rise to the notion of beneficence towards vulnerable individuals (Lee, 1991). It is widely considered that research should be done on children only if comparable research on adults could not answer the same question (British Paediatric Association, 1992). Balanced against this concern is the notion that teenagers should not be excluded from the benefits of research.

This chapter begins by briefly providing some contextual information on paediatric cancer care and assessment, before discussing the current understanding of CRF, drawing on past and current research undertaken in the adult population. The present understanding of this symptom in paediatric oncology nursing practice is highlighted, with personal views from practice being supported with evidence from recent studies undertaken with children and teenagers on and off treatment. The reason for further research is presented. Two research studies that are currently under way are used as a vehicle to describe the approaches taken to develop appropriate research with teenagers and the reasons supporting the approaches that have been taken.

While awaiting the results of research and in the absence of evidence, what should nurses be doing in their practice? Some suggestions about how interprofessional collaborative research can influence practice are made in the final sections of this chapter. Presented as a whole, the journey undertaken by three paediatric oncology nurses is explored to reveal the current status of knowledge about CRF, as well as the challenges, pleasures and rewards of participating in the process of producing evidence that has the potential to support clinical practice.

Background

Cancer therapy for children and teenagers has changed dramatically over the past 20 years. An increase in the intensity of chemotherapy, coupled with the multi-modular approaches to treatment, has increased the cure rates of childhood cancer (Stiller, 1997). At the same time, there has been recognition of the impact, on the quality of life, of treatment and its associated morbidity (Eiser et al., 1995). Thus, an awareness of the impact of symptoms such as pain, nausea and vomiting, and oral stomatitis, to name but a few, has influenced nursing research aimed at providing evidence-based supportive care. Many such symptoms are now viewed in the context of being multifactorial, multidimensional and highly subjective in nature. To date, however, there has been limited recognition of the subtle symptom cancer-related fatigue commonly termed CRF.

Fatigue is a universal human experience – a symptom each and every one of us will encounter after intense physical and/or mental activity. Although psychologists, as a consequence of disease patterns, investigated fatigue as far back as the early nineteenth century, it took until the later part of the twentieth century for CRF to be recognized as a symptom meriting specific attention (Glaus, 2000). This can be attributed in part to the perception that CRF differs in its nature to the 'fatigue' experienced within the general population. There is now a wealth of data within adult cancer care documenting the prevalence and debilitating effects of this symptom (Irvine et al., 1991; Magnusson et al., 1999; Krishnasamy 2000). However, the results of the research involving adult populations have limitations when applied to children because of the latter's unique and diverse needs. Nevertheless learning directly, from nurse researchers, of their experiences, knowledge and proven methodologies when planning and undertaking nursing research in CRF in adult cancer care has provided the basis to start investigations with children and teenagers. In addition, examination of the scientific literature has facilitated a degree of structure and insight, and uncovered innovative research practice that can be incorporated within paediatric oncology nursing practice and research to examine the concept of CRF.

Working within a climate where there is an emphasis on the assessment of quality of life and supportive care, a springboard effect was produced from which to start exploring CRF in teenagers and their families. The potential consequence of a lack of awareness and knowledge by healthcare professionals within clinical practice, which may inadvertently impact on patient management, provided an impetus to begin a journey of discovery. The issues encountered in the journey, to date, have been many and relate to the challenges and the strengths of enabling multiprofessional collaborative research practice between paediatric oncology nurses and adult oncology nurses, as well as the hurdles and rewards of working towards the development of evidence-based clinical practice.

The journey: from idea to research proposal

The journey of enquiry began in 1995 when a paediatric oncology nurse was invited to join an initiative instigated by the European Oncology Nurses Society (EONS) to develop educational material on CRF at a European Nursing Conference on Cancer-Related Fatigue. In turn, discussion and reflection on current clinical practice within paediatric oncology nursing and the lack of empirical evidence of the issues about the relevance of CRF to children with cancer and their families was facilitated. Questions were raised about whether children and teenagers experienced CRF and its lack of recognition.

Interprofessional relationships established at the European conference led to the conception of a research team which included adult oncology nurses and paediatric oncology nurses. The direct result of this relationship was the development of two research studies; this led to the inclusion of a paediatric oncology nurse on a multiprofessional Cancer Fatigue Forum. The first study developed was a multicentred descriptive study to explore the impact of cancer and its treatment on teenagers (with a large focus on CRF). Although this study was still in the development phase, a second study was established that has become a national study to discover the knowledge, perceptions and attitudes of teenagers, carers of teenagers and children, and healthcare professionals about CRF. These studies are ongoing at the time of writing. As mentioned previously, what is reported here is the road from first thought to final research proposals on the journey of exploration of CRF in children and teenagers. The focus of the discussion centres on the first study because many of the methodological issues about researching CRF were addressed in its early stages.

What is known about the symptom CRF?

Relevant information was gathered through a systematic examination of scientific literature. This demonstrated a wealth of information from the adult cancer care setting. A growing body of evidence, which illustrated the enormity of the problem and the gaps in theoretical development, was found to have accrued on CRF. A high prevalence and adverse impact on quality of life have been reported (Vogelzang et al., 1997). This study also reported that a high percentage of patients and their carers viewed the symptom as untreatable and inevitable, with a gap in the perceptions between patients and HCPs of the impact, seriousness and causes of CRF. With the high profile of CRF in the adults' experience of cancer and its treatment, the question of prevalence, perceptions and current treatment strategies within children's cancer care was raised.

A critical review of the literature on the theory and current definitions of CRF illustrates that the major factors reported as hurdles in understanding the nature of the phenomena have been the subjective, multidimensional and multifactorial nature of the symptom (Winningham et al., 1994). An added challenge has also been the lack of a universally accepted definition and theory of the factors influencing the manifestation of CRF (Piper, 1998). Nevertheless, a definition that formed the basis for describing CRF in adults illustrated the unique yet burdensome nature of the symptom, which highlighted the importance of gaining patient-oriented accounts of the experience. One definition proposed that 'fatigue is a subjective, unpleasant symptom which incorporates total body feelings ranging from tiredness to exhaustion creating an unrelenting overall condition which interferes with individuals' ability to function to their normal capacity' (Ream and Richardson, 1997, p. 45). The strength of this definition lies in the manner in which it was formulated, in that the researchers took past defining attributes given by participants that appeared frequently in the literature. As such, the definition is a representation of the body of knowledge that existed at that time, describing the essential qualitative features and providing a depth and richness of understanding of the patients' experiences.

The definition illustrates the broad range in levels of fatigue that a patient may experience from a state of tiredness to that of total exhaustion. This definition was also significant in that it was a reminder to us of the need to put the patient at the centre of 'caring'. Although the family-centred care model (Casey, 1988) is central to paediatric oncology nursing in many settings, a different emphasis was required at this point in time within the discussions. In so much as Ream and Richardson's (1997) definition advocates a truly patient-centred approach, the limitations, when applied to children and teenagers, were recognized in that a proportion of the group would be unable to give verbal accounts of their experiences because of limited cognitive development. Overall, it was felt that attempts to address these limitations within research methodology must be made rather than dismissed. Thus a question arose relating to children's and teenagers' reported experiences of the nature of CRF. The premise is to keep the emphasis on gaining an understanding of the viewpoint of children and teenagers as expressed in their age-appropriate ways, rather than children and young people having to explain their subjective experiences in adult terms.

Stone et al. (1998) go one step further to plot three important distinct dimensions when defining CRF:

- physical sensations (e.g. feeling unable to perform tasks, weariness and unusual tiredness)
- affective sensations (e.g. decreased motivation, low mood and no energy)
- cognitive sensations (e.g. lack of concentration and difficulty thinking clearly).

Subjectively, tiredness from lack of sleep has been further characterized by Stone et al. (1998, p. 1670) as 'feelings of weariness and a perception of decreased capacity for physical or mental work'. This definition could be argued to be a more definitive approach, indicating the impact of fatigue in terms of the effects on functioning, and more relevant to a population who are in remission from cancer, rather than receiving cancer treatment.

The above dimensions illustrate an important point of the subjective and objective views on fatigue, by suggesting that subjective meaning and objective states may not always come together, because a person can feel fatigued without it having an impact on physical functioning. This raises the question of whether people with a chronic illness could perceive themselves as fatigued, but outwardly be viewed to be healthy, because they are able to perform day-to-day tasks. Furthermore, are there individuals or groups of patients in whom CRF is hidden and unspoken? The key message from the debate of the above definitions is that CRF is described by patients as abnormal, prolonged and not relieved by sleep. Take the case example of a 12-year-old girl:

> Laura has been admitted to hospital with a febrile neutropenia as a result of chemotherapy for her cancer, which she received 7 days ago. Her normal pattern of sleep is disrupted because of the need to administer intravenous antibiotics and staff having to monitor her physical status. She reports feeling overwhelmingly tired but is observed carrying out normal activities such as watching television, and socializing with fellow patients, becoming involved in an afternoon party on the ward.

This example illustrates the need for assessment of functional performance alongside gaining descriptive accounts. It was felt important because of the social nature of teenagers in terms of social skills. In some way it was believed that teenagers might be able to adapt and learn to live with fatigue. Thus in order to capture the phenomenon, it was felt that triangulated research methods were needed.

If we turned to the literature on the mechanism of CRF, it became evident that as yet these are unclear. In part this has been attributed to the nature of multiple symptoms experienced during the course of illness and cancer treatments, with symptoms having interrelated and compounded factors (Piper et al., 1996). This suggests that CRF may not be related to one mechanism alone, but various aspects impacting upon one another. This may be the case in teenagers with cancer, where they go through similar biomedical experiences in the disease trajectory to that experienced by adults.

Research on CRF in children and teenagers: what do we already know?

In summarizing the adult literature Curt (2001) states that CRF is the most important untreated symptom in cancer today. He goes on to suggest that this fact is probably the result of the improved management alternatives for other symptoms normally associated with cancer and its treatment, such as pain, oral stomatitis, and nausea and vomiting. The same can probably be stated for CRF in teenagers where symptoms other than CRF have a long history in terms of research and attempts to build an evidence base for practice (Selwood et al., 1999). Current research on CRF is divided between two distinct foci: children and teenagers on treatment and long-term young adult survivors.

A pioneering programme of study from the USA that is ongoing paves the way in beginning to understand the unique experience of children and teenagers on treatment (Hockenberry-Eaton and Hinds, 2000). This study used focus groups to generate descriptive details about the characteristics and nature of CRF from children (7–12 years, $n = 14$), teenagers (13–18 years, $n = 15$), parents (of both age groups, $n = 31$) and staff members (multiprofessional focus, $n = 38$). Focus groups were used to generate detailed descriptive data about the experiences of fatigue. Data were analysed using content analysis described by Krippendorff (1980), and revealed a number of factors that patients, parents and staff believed to cause and alleviate patient fatigue. This seminal work clearly demonstrates that CRF was prevalent in a group of children and teenagers; CRF was illustrated as existing within a context of illness, treatment and cognitive development. The major finding of the study to date has been the different perceptions of the experience of CRF by differing age groups, e.g. 7–12 year olds viewed their experiences within a physical framework, highlighted in one description: 'I see tired in my eyes, and I have a dull face' (Hockenberry-Eaton et al., 1998, p. 176). In comparison the 12–19 year olds viewed CRF with a more global perspective, such as being 'physically tired and mentally challenged' (Hockenberry-Eaton et al., 1998, p. 177). Children answered questions about fatigue in the following way:

- What is it like to feel tired? It is when: I want to lie down; I feel weak; I want to sleep more.
- What makes me feel tired? My treatment for cancer; pain; low blood counts; waking up at night because I am not in my own bed.
- What helps me feel better? Naps and sleeping; being quiet and resting; doing fun things.

Hockenberry-Eaton et al. (1999, p. 9) suggest a tentative definition that attempts to encompass the child's (i.e. those aged 7–12 years) perspective:

> Fatigue is a profound sense of being tired, or having difficulty with movement such as arms and legs, or opening eyes which is influenced by environmental, personal/social and treatment-related factors and can result in difficulties with play, concentration and negative emotions (most typically anger and sadness). The profound tiredness can be acute, episodic or chronic, and is relieved by rest and distraction.

In addition to this work, Langeveld et al. (2000) have studied the concept of fatigue from a survivor's perspective. Semi-structured interviews were undertaken with a purposeful sample of 35 long-term survivors (18–38 years) of childhood cancer who had reported feeling extremely fatigued. In this study fatigue was defined by half of the respondents as having a negative impact on their daily lives. They summarized their key findings as follows:

- Fatigue is described as exerting oneself to the utmost, both physically and mentally.
- Fatigue is present most or all of the time since diagnosis and/or treatment.
- Fatigue is frequently already present on awakening, despite an average of 9 hours sleep per night.
- Fatigue negatively affects daily and social activities.

Both of these programmes of studies have influenced the present work. Primarily they confirmed the belief that it was an important symptom to explore. They also validate concerns associated with the need to develop a knowledge base specifically for this patient group. First, to ascertain whether and how the symptom existed and also to develop specific research tools for this age group. Carrying out research with teenagers presents many challenges such as the number of available participants, the diversity of levels of cognitive development, the impact of the disease and its treatment, gaining consent from parents to recruit the child/teenager and finally their adherence. However, the studies by Hockenberry-Eaton et al. (1998, 1999), Hockenberry-Eaton and Hinds (2000) and Langeveld (2000) overcame these barriers and provided guidelines to assist the development of comparative studies. We felt it was important to carry out studies in the UK to develop a knowledge base relevant to our culture and healthcare approaches, systems and environment.

Conceptual models and theory relating to fatigue

Definitions of fatigue illustrate its complexity, in that there appear to be multidimensional and multifactorial components. There are two conceptual models of fatigue (Piper et al., 1987; Hockenberry-Eaton and Hinds, 2000) that were helpful in further understanding the symptom.

Conceptual models assist research because they are one way of describing and explaining concepts and their relationships, offering a tentative, purposeful and systematic view (McKenna, 1997). Both models assisted in guiding our thinking because they focus on specific characteristics that comprise behavioural, emotional, sensory and cognitive domains. The first model by Piper et al. (1987) illustrates how biological and psychosocial patterns can influence signs and symptoms of fatigue, highlighting the importance for researchers to assess actual changes that may have occurred over the time of illness. The second model by Hockenberry-Eaton and Hinds (2000) illustrates a relationship between contributing factors and mechanisms employed by children to alleviate fatigue. The characteristics in teenagers who are having treatment and those who have completed cancer treatment have yet to be determined.

Mechanisms of fatigue in cancer patients appear unclear at this time. In part this can be attributed to the nature of multiple symptoms experienced during the course of the illness and treatments, with symptoms having interrelated and compounding factors (Piper et al., 1996). However, there are significant differences between the two models, the major difference being that the paediatric model (Hockenberry-Eaton and Hinds, 2000) illustrates the fact that, because fatigue is expressed by children and teenagers as existing within a context of illness, treatment and cognitive development, the emphasis is on developing behavioural coping mechanisms to manage/alleviate the symptom. At one level it may be that the mechanisms used by children as coping strategies are factors that would hinder the expression of the experience to healthcare professionals, raising the question of whether fatigue is disguised by a multitude of variables.

Both models serve to illustrate the multifaceted nature of fatigue in children and adults during cancer treatment. Given the fact that no conceptual model was identified within the scientific literature relating to fatigue in the general population or teenagers who are on treatment or who are survivors of cancer, it is not known whether similar or different facets exist.

As CRF in teenagers and adults on treatment have been described as multifactorial the challenge within a study that includes fatigue experienced after cancer treatment is to isolate it from the more obvious side effects such as respiratory toxicity or neuro-/physiological toxicity after chemotherapy or radiation. It is also important to be able to recognize it within the context of other physical and psychological complications and their impact on function/performance. As such the middle-range theory of unpleasant symptoms (Lenz et al., 1997) was found to be useful in providing a framework that illustrated the cyclical relationship between existing symptoms and the symptom under investigation, and how this can impact further on performance. Three major components of the theory are the symptom that the individual is experiencing, the influencing factors that give rise to or affect the nature of the symptom, and the consequences of the symptom experience. The overarching benefits of this theory lie in illustrating the comprehensive interrelated components in a simplistic manner, providing a platform from which to view fatigue and the impact of additional symptoms. Lenz et al.'s middle-range theory has informed the development of both studies currently in progress.

Research on CRF in teenagers: what do we want to find out and from whom?

The review of the literature on adolescent cancer care and CRF illustrated that there was a need to conduct qualitative research with teenagers who are receiving treatment and those who are childhood cancer survivors. In addressing the background evidence to formulate the studies, no definition was found to exist. This results partly from the infancy of developing a research programme into teenagers' experience of cancer, but also from the fact that current definitions do not have a developmental component pertinent to meeting the needs of teenagers' social and emotional maturity. However, developed models and theories relating to fatigue threw light on the common components of the experience. After gathering scientific evidence the research team took a unanimous decision to explore CRF from the teenagers' perspective. This came as a result of the commonalities between the two specialities of adult cancer care and paediatric cancer care, as well as the fact that little was known of the experience of CRF with this group of patients. The issues facing the teenager defined in this instant, aged 13–19 years, were deemed to be particularly complex. The disease and its treatments, alongside the issues facing a young person who is passing through crucial developmental milestones, can produce significant physical and psychological difficulties (Daum and Collins, 1992; Hanna, 1993; Whyte and Smith, 1997). This, coupled with the impact that a debilitating symptom such as CRF is thought to have on a teenager's ability to cope with issues facing them on a day-to-day basis, was felt to be significant in the way CRF was understood and verbally described. To illustrate further, a typical example of a young person with a non-Hodgkin's lymphoma is reflected in the case study:

> Jake is a 20 year old who is presently receiving chemotherapy. Before his illness he described how active he was, playing football every weekend as well as undertaking a degree at university. Just before he was diagnosed he become more and more tired and listless – one of the reasons he visited his GP. Following the start of chemotherapy, overwhelming tiredness had got progressively worse, to the point that he could not concentrate to watch more than 20 minutes of a football match on television. He described his whole body as 'heavy'. He could not understand why with all the sleep he was getting he was so tired all the time, leaving him feeling frustrated to the point where he stated 'I just can't wait for the chemotherapy to come to an end; only then will I start to feel better'.

It is difficult at this time to conclude confidently that the reasons given for such anecdotal accounts from the clinical area are the direct result of CRF or whether these symptoms are a result of alternative associated factors such as anxiety and depression. Nevertheless, although the literature can be found to allude to such associated indicators (Winningham et al., 1994; Stone et al., 1998), as yet it is unclear whether they are unimportant or significant (Ream and Richardson, 1999). However, it was during our investigations of such literature that the paediatric nurses within the team reflected on the associated myths and misconceptions of children's experience of procedural pain which hampered the delivery of effective pain control for many years. Therefore, it was felt that caution was needed in developing an understanding of CRF based on research findings that may take a period of time to gain.

Recognizing that the pattern of CRF may vary over time (Richardson, 1995), the project team considered the stages at which data would be collected. At this point the knowledge gained from the studies by Hockenberry-Eaton and Hinds (2000) and Langeveld et al. (2000) were particularly useful in reinforcing the need to consider prevalence, duration and pattern of CRF. The fact that long-term survivors reported feeling fatigue indicated a need to consider patients across the trajectory of their cancer experience. The sample therefore includes teenagers on treatment and off treatment for 1–2 years, and those who are more than 5 years off treatment.

Other factors that influenced the sample selected were the wealth of literature reporting the symptom chronic fatigue (Schluederberg et al., 1992). Although much is known about this symptom, how far this reported symptom does or does not resemble CRF remains unknown. By including a non-cancer group in the sample the project team hoped to identify any commonalities for teenagers coping with day-to-day activities such as going to school/college and coping with a hectic social life.

How to research CRF in teenagers?

The complexity of research involving children/teenagers as their own 'story tellers' lies in ensuring that reliable and valid methods are used that will capture the essence of the experience. The use of innovative research initiatives is becoming well documented within the paediatric literature. Methods, such as focus groups, draw and write technique, card sort and semi-structured interviews (Davis and Jones, 1996; McDougall, 1998), have been found to be of benefit. Thus, experience and knowledge of research within paediatric health care highlighted the need for creative methodological approaches of research into CRF.

Although the research questions provided the focus of the studies, selection of appropriate instruments for assessment posed a challenge. A lack of valid and reliable assessment and measurement tools for CRF has hampered investigation within adult cancer care (Richardson, 1998); this problem was further compounded within adolescent care. Although quality-of-life tools have incorporated fatigue measurement (Berglund et al., 1991; Bower et al., 2000) within paediatric cancer care, quality of life has tended to be neglected in measurement instruments (Eiser et al., 1995). Although there are examples of specific fatigue assessment tools such as the paper diary (Faithfull, 1992; Richardson, 1995), hand-grip strength (Sadeh et al., 1991), the Multidimensional Fatigue Inventory (MFI-20) (Smets at al., 1993), the

Functional Assessment of Cancer Therapy – fatigue (Yellen et al., 1997), and the Brief Fatigue Inventory (Mendoza et al., 1999), none had been specifically developed for use with teenagers. Therefore the literature within paediatrics was appraised. As the focus of the initial study was the functional difficulties perceived by teenagers of the problems that they faced living with CRF, it was vital that any instrument, or combination of instruments, was not going to be too lengthy, cumbersome or objectionable to the participants, which could potentially have a negative impact on the experience of fatigue; instead it needed to facilitate willingness for involvement and adherence as well as being sensitive to the trait.

After much searching, two instruments were chosen: the Functional Disability Inventory (Walker and Greene, 1991) and the Perceived Illness Experience (Eiser et al., 1995). The positive attributes of the instruments rested in the fact that they were specifically designed to be appropriate to teenagers across a broad age range, as well as having psychometric properties. The novel idea of building on the diary method by developing a computerized version that incorporated the instrument selected, which overall provided collection of both structured and unstructured data, was seized.

The diary method, also termed 'chronological log' has been used to good effect previously to collect data of perceptions of well-being, ability to maintain 'normal' life and fatigue (Richardson and Ream, 1997). The advantage of using the diary method is that the participant is able to record data close to the occurrence of an event, activity, problem, etc., thus overcoming problems of selective recall (Faithfull, 1992; Richardson and Ream, 1997). This was felt to be important because memories of past experiences may be particularly difficult to recall.

However, the use of diaries for research purposes is not without problems and there have been reports of poor compliance (Fugate Woods, 1981; Faithfull, 1992; Richardson and Ream, 1996, 1997). Clinical observation, however, suggested that many teenagers kept diaries. The addition of a computerized diary was considered by the project team to be one way to facilitate data collection by making the diary completion more interesting and more akin to teenager activities. There was also the belief that the diary approach would also enable the teenager to tell his or her own story in his or her own way. This was supported by the notion of teenagers' egocentricity, with many having the personal belief that 'no one has ever experienced emotions so intensely or lived life so fully' (Eiser, 1996, p. 265).

Planning and decision-making as reported above resulted in the project team selecting to use a paper and electronic diary in which teenagers would be able to report their daily activities alongside perceptions of their general feelings. The structured component of the diary contains items that reflect the intensity of, and the perceived degree of frustration with, fatigue or tiredness as measured by a selection of 10-point numerical scales. In addition to these structured items, space is provided every day for teenagers to jot down other thoughts and feelings that they wish to share with the research team about how they have felt that day. The inclusion of a semi-structured interview aims to enable the researchers to delve deeper into the recordings in the diary, and give the teenagers further opportunities to articulate their perceptions and experiences of the impact of cancer and treatment on them as individuals. Diaries followed by semi-structured interviews are being used with teenagers who have cancer at various stages of the disease trajectory.

In addition to the above, focus groups are used to collect data from teenagers who are survivors of cancer and non-cancer teenagers. As focus groups had been used with success by Hockenberry-Eaton et al. (1998), it was felt to be important to validate further the use of focus groups as an approach to collecting data about CRF from teenagers. Although this method has not yet been used widely in this type of research, it may be a useful means of collecting and triangulating data. The focus groups use questions that have been previously validated in the study by Hockenberry-Eaton et al. (1998). Perceived well-being and ability to maintain 'normal' activities are key variables being explored with teenagers.

As well as the teenager perspective gained in the second study using a survey method, the views of parents and healthcare professionals are also being sought; these views have been found to be helpful in adult studies. In 1996, a study was carried out in the USA (Vogelzang et al., 1997) to examine the extent to which fatigue affects the quality of life of adult cancer patients. The issue was examined from the perspective of the patient, the patient's primary caregiver and oncologists. The research concluded that CRF has a major impact on patients' and caregivers' lives. Most patients (76%) experienced fatigue, as defined by a general feeling of debilitating tiredness or loss of energy, on a regular basis. Fatigue was found to affect many areas of patients' lives, including physical well-being, the ability to work and the ability to experience intimacy with their partner. Of patients 61% said that fatigue affected their life more than the pain associated with cancer. Most patients felt resigned to think of fatigue as a symptom to be endured. In addition to these factors, the study also illustrated gaps between patients and medical colleagues' perceptions of the impact of fatigue, its seriousness and its causes. Patients were more likely to attribute their fatigue to their treatment, but physicians were more likely to attribute a patient's fatigue to the cancer. Furthermore, physicians reported a higher incidence of prescribing treatment for fatigue than patients said they were offered. It is these issues that are specifically being examined in the second study, using an adapted version of a survey questionnaire devised by Stone et al. (2000).

Multicentre collaborative research: advantages and disadvantages

Both the studies under way are multicentre and collaborative. Any study that is multicentred as such necessitates collaboration between multitudes of healthcare professionals and requires clear channels of communication as well as a structure that facilitates staff support. In this regard nursing research is in its infancy. The benefits of such an approach for nursing research within paediatric cancer care in the UK can be seen in the way services are developed. Collaborative practice between tertiary paediatric oncology centres by the United Kingdom Childhood Cancer Study Group (UKCCSG) means that multicentred research can be facilitated, which enables the potential for recruitment of larger numbers of participants within studies. There is also the additional benefit of the ease of raising awareness of research within all the UKCCSG centres because the networks of communication have been formalized. The disadvantage is in ensuring that all the stakeholders and members of staff who agreed to assist in carrying out the research are regularly informed of changes and practicalities of the research. A method employed to ensure that information was given in a timely manner, while at the same time ensuring that the researchers were not overwhelmed by this task, was for members of the team regularly to attend national meetings held with the nurses from the UKCCSG centres (Paediatric Oncology Nurses Forum [PONF]). Using this arena meant that a process could occur whereby information could be communicated through a cascade effect; nurses would disseminate information to the staff in their centres.

The time needed to develop research that is collaborative on such a scale cannot be underestimated. The length of time taken to develop research protocols, for which consensus is required, to raise funds and then to gain ethical approval has taken the team over 4 years. Collaboration, although topical, is viewed as challenging for healthcare professionals (Henneman, 1995). It requires that disciplines share information and expertise in areas in which they may previously have worked independently or competitively, or are currently recognized as expert. In some relationships, e.g. with medical colleagues, collaboration may have to overcome issues of hierarchy. Coluccio and Maguire (1983) describe collaboration as requiring joint decision-making and communication to benefit the patient while respecting colleagues' unique abilities and qualities. It appears that a crucial aspect of collaboration is the balance of power. In collaborative working the power is shared.

As previously mentioned although both studies involved collaboration the collaborative parties involved were different. The study exploring adolescent quality of life combined and used the knowledge and expertise of adult nurses with particular experience in adult cancer fatigue research, and paediatric oncology nurses with knowledge and expertise in adolescent cancers. The logistics of arranging meetings was a challenge because members of the team were based on three different London sites. In the beginning the meetings were arduous, and relationships and roles were negotiated and established as the wealth of expertise and knowledge were bartered. The variety of backgrounds meant that the team had different perceptions and understanding of the ultimate goal of the study and, therefore, even reaching an agreement on this took a number of meetings.

The advantages of the collaboration are evident. The combinations of the different areas of knowledge relating to the key issues underpinning the study are clearly visible. The variety of different ways and appropriate tools that have been used to develop the current knowledge base on adult cancer fatigue were explored and relevant ones were adapted, using adolescent development theory and cancer knowledge, to design the current study.

Having established a cohesive collaborative relationship to design the study, a different form of collaboration was required to carry it out. As the number of adolescents with cancer is small, especially compared with the adult cancer population, it was necessary to recruit patients from three centres in the London area. The logistical nightmare this time was for the researcher:

- To have access to the patients, ethical agreement had to be obtained from each centre. The information required from each centre was slightly different and each took different lengths of time to be completed successfully. It was easier at the two sites where members of the research team were based.
- Once ethical agreement had been gained the researcher had to establish relationships with the staff in the centres in order to have access to information about potential participants.
- The researcher then had the difficulty of trying to be in three different centres on the most appropriate days, thus combining multicentre and multidisciplinary collaboration.

The second study involved similar collaborative working as the above in that it is multicentre but also required collaboration between the different healthcare professionals within each centre. For a comparable investigation to that of the adult study (Stone et al., 2000), all 22 regional paediatric oncology centres were asked to participate in the collection of data from healthcare professionals. At the same time four of the centres collected data from patients and their carers. The organization and implementation of this required a person, known as the local researcher, on site to coordinate the collection. As previously mentioned this was organized through the PONF, with each centre identifying a member to accept the responsibility. This meant that it was a nurse-led project and, therefore, had the potential to fall into difficulties of hierarchical conflict. As a result of existing collaboration between the PONF and the UKCC-SG this has not been evident. The most important aspect of collaboration for the researcher in this study has been the establishment of effective communication with the local researchers in order to support them.

One of the difficulties encountered since the start of these studies, and one that is highlighted in the literature, is the potential effect on practice when a research question is identified or when an absence of evidence to underpin current practice becomes apparent. This raising of awareness can affect the health carer's approach and/or attitude to the management of the symptom. Evidence-based practice is topical; it is the ultimate aim of healthcare professionals to demonstrate that their practice is based on the best available current evidence (Muir Gray, 1999). However, when searching for the evidence to underpin current approaches to the care of adolescent cancer patients, there is little available. Most of the current approaches to care are based on the desire to return the patient to being able to live life within the realms of being 'normal'. Emphasis is made to facilitate the maintenance of normal activities of daily living.

To prevent the patient from falling too far behind with school/college work, the patient is encouraged to return to school as soon as possible and while in hospital teachers continue to offer academic tutoring. The tension lies between caring for and coping with the present treatment and its side effects/implications, and preparing for and living with the end of treatment and the known potential long-term side effects. Although there is evidence that the amount of schooling that a child/adolescent misses out on as a result of treatment, etc. for cancer will impact on issues such as peer maintenance, attainment of school grades and subsequently career choices (Charlton et al., 1991), we do not have an understanding of the short or long-term implications of the management of fatigue in teenagers. There is the temptation to transfer the knowledge about the management of this symptom in adults to teenagers. A large proportion of adults, including healthcare professionals, view teenagers as small, immature adults and may be tempted, therefore, to feel it appropriate simply to apply findings from studies undertaken with adults. However, teenagers are still growing, physically and cognitively, whereas adults are in a state of repair so that physiologically their needs are different. Also adolescent goals, motivation and support mechanisms are still in the development stage, which again may influence their ability to comply with management strategies. Older teenagers may be further through their adolescent trajectory and may, therefore, have resources other than their parents to help them. However, 12–16 year olds may be at the start or in the middle of this emancipation and have no or limited resources to assist them in decision-making about important treatment issues or day-to-day activities.

Current practice must consider these issues and the way in which healthcare professionals facilitate informed choice for teenagers must be examined (Campbell, 2001). The attitude of sticking to known practices can result in 'if you always do it the same way you will always get what you got'. Although this may be acceptable for some patients it may not be for all. We are only just beginning to gain an understanding of the long-term implications of surviving child/adolescent cancer. The physical side effects are well documented as are some of the psychological effects (Eiser and Jenney, 1996); however, we need to question how much of our current practice is based on evidence gained specifically from the age group with which we are working.

It is vital, therefore, that teenager-specific research is carried out. The difficulty is always the number of available 'subjects', the development of research tools that attract adolescent adherence, and the ability to recruit and retain a valid sample. These are challenges that can be overcome through collaborative studies. They are only the start of the journey. Critics of qualitative research argue, correctly, that the findings of these studies are often not generalizable; however, Payne (2000) suggests that size is not always important and that small studies can be useful in developing theory. They are a way to make a start and they have the potential to produce data that challenge current thinking and approaches to care; they may also act as pilot or preliminary studies (Payne, 2000). There is also the issue that, if new evidence supports the notion to change the approach/management of adolescent cancer, the teenager will not necessarily comply if it goes against their normative behaviour or makes them appear different. And finally, if the evidence suggests a complete turnabout in the current approach to the care of this patient group, do we have the resources and the power to influence change? Once a sound theory has been developed, its various components can be tested using quantitative approaches.

Conclusion

Overcoming daily difficulties since starting the development of the two studies has been a considerable challenge. Much has been learned specifically about undertaking research with teenagers and collaborating on research studies. Fatigue, as a consequence of cancer treatment in teenagers, is currently poorly understood. The aim of both the studies described in this chapter is to add to the body of knowledge about symptoms experienced during and after treatment. Our ability to deliver effective care and contribute to teenagers' overall quality of life rests on our understanding of the totality of their cancer experience. How far fatigue influences their experience will, it is hoped, be illuminated by the two studies.

Acknowledgements

Thanks to Alison Richardson and Emma Ream, our research colleagues, who have contributed vast knowledge and skills and have facilitated our thinking on this complex subject.

References

Berglund G, Bolund C, Fornander T, Rutqvist LE, Sjoden P (1991) Late effects of adjuvant chemotherapy and post operative radiotherapy on quality of life among breast cancer patients. European Journal of Cancer 27: 1075-1081.

Bower JE, Ganz PA, Desmond KA, Rowland JH, Meyerowitz BE, Belin TR (2000) Fatigue in breast cancer survivors: occurrence, correlates, and impact on quality of life. Journal of Clinical Oncology 18: 743-753.

Bradding A, Horstman M (1999) Using the write and draw technique with children. European Journal of Oncology Nursing 3: 170-175.

British Paediatric Association (1992) Guidelines for the Ethical Conduct of Medical Research Involving Children. London: British Paediatric Association.

Casey A (1988) A partnership with child and family. Senior Nurse 8: 8-9.

Campbell A (2001) Informed choice for adolescents. Paediatric Nursing 13: 41-42.

Charlton A, Larcombe IJ, Meller ST et al. (1991) Absence from school related to cancer and other chronic conditions. Archives of Disease in Childhood 66: 1217-1222.

Coluccio M, Maguire P (1983) Collaborative practice: becoming a reality through primary nursing. Nursing Administration Quarterly 7: 59-63.

Curt GA (2001) Fatigue in cancer. British Medical Journal 322: 1560.

Daum AL, Collins C (1992) Failure to master early developmental tasks as a predictor of adaptation to cancer in the young adult. Oncology Nursing Forum 19: 1513-1518.

Davis A, Jones L (1996) Environmental constraints on health: listening to children's views. Health Education Journal 55: 363-374.

Doswell WM, Vandestienne G (1996) The use of focus groups to examine pubertal concerns in preteen girls: initial findings and implications for practice and research. Issues in Comprehensive Pediatric Nursing 19: 103-120.

Eiser C (1996) The impact of treatment: adolescents' views. In: Selby P, Bailey C (eds), Cancer and the Adolescent. London: BMJ Publishing Group, pp. 264-275.

Eiser C, Jenney EM (1996) Measuring symptomatic benefit and quality of life in paediatric oncology. British Journal of Cancer 7: 1313-1316.

Eiser C, Havermans T, Craft A, Kernham J (1995) Development of a measure to assess the perceived illness experience after treatment for cancer. Archives of Disease in Childhood 72: 302-307.

Faithfull S (1992) The diary method for nursing research: a study of somnolence syndrome. European Journal of Cancer Care 1: 13-18.

Ferrell BR, Grant M, Dean GE, Funk B, Ly J (1996) Bone tired: the experience of fatigue and its impact on quality of life. Oncology Nurses Forum. 23: 1539-1547.

Fugate Woods N (1981) The health diary as an instrument for nursing research: problems and promise. Western Journal of Nursing Research 3: 76-93.

Galt M (1997) Illicit drug availability in rural areas and attitudes toward their use - young people talking. Health Education Journal 56: 17-34.

Glaus A (2000) Fatigue in patients with cancer - from an orphan topic to a global concern. Supportive Cancer Care 9: 1-3.

Hanna KM (1993) Health behaviors of adolescents who have been diagnosed with cancer. Issues in Comprehensive Pediatric Nursing 16: 219-228.

Henneman E (1995) Nurse physician collaboration: a post structuralist view. Journal of Advanced Nursing 22: 359-363.

Hockenberry-Eaton M, Hinds PS (2000) Fatigue in children and adolescents with cancer: Evolution of a program of study. Seminars in Oncology Nursing 16: 261-272.

Hockenberry-Eaton M, Hinds PS, Alcoser P et al. (1998) Fatigue in children and adolescents with cancer. Journal of Pediatric Oncology Nursing 15: 172-182.

Hockenberry-Eaton M, Hinds P, Brace O'Neill J et al. (1999) Developing a conceptual model for fatigue in children. European Journal of Oncology Nursing 3: 5-11.

Hooker L (1997) Information needs of teenagers with cancer: developing a tool to explore the perceptions of patients and professionals. Journal of Cancer Care 1: 160-168.

Irvine DM, Vincent L, Bubela N, Thompson L, Graydon J (1991) A critical appraisal of the research literature investigating fatigue in the individual with cancer. Cancer Nursing 14: 188-199.

James DCS, Rienzo BA, Frazee C (1997) Using focus groups to develop a nutritional educational video for high school students. Journal of School Health 67: 376-379.

Krippendorff K (1980) Content Analysis: An introduction to its methodology. Newbury Park: Sage Publications.

Krishnasamy M (2000) Fatigue in advanced cancer - meaning before measurement? International Journal of Nursing Studies 37: 401-414.

Langeveld N, Ubbink M, Smets E (2000) 'I don't have any energy': the experience of fatigue in young adult survivors of childhood cancer. European Journal of Oncology Nursing 4: 20-28.

Lee L (1991) Ethical issues related to research involving children. Journal of Paediatric Oncology Nursing 8: 24-29

Lenz ER, Pugh LC, Milligan RA, Gift A, Suppe F (1997) The middle-range theory of unpleasant symptoms: an update. Advances in Nursing Science 19: 14-27.

McDougall P (1998) Teenagers and nutrition: assessing levels of knowledge. Health Visitor 21: 63-64.

McKenna H (1997) Nursing Theories and Models. London: Routledge.

Magnusson K, Moller A, Ekman T, Wallgren A (1999) A qualitative study to explore the experience of fatigue in cancer patients. European Journal of Cancer Care 8: 224-232.

Mendoza TR, Shelley Wang X, Cleeland CF et al. (1999) The rapid assessment of fatigue severity in cancer patients: use of the brief fatigue inventory. Cancer 85(5): 1186-1196.

Muir Gray JA (1999) Evidence-based Health Care: How to make health policy and management decisions. Edinburgh: Churchill Livingstone.

Payne S (2000) Research involves small steps not giant leaps [Editorial]. International Journal of Palliative Nursing 6: 56.

Piper BF (1998) The groopman article reviewed. Oncology 12: 345-346.

Piper BF, Lindsey AL, Dodd MJ (1987) Fatigue mechanisms in cancer patients: developing nursing theory. Oncology Nurses Forum 14: 17-21.

Piper B, Dibble S, Dodd M (1996) The revised Piper Fatigue Scale: confirmation of its multidimensionality and reduction in number of items in women with breast cancer. Oncology Nursing Forum 23: 352 (abstract 172).

Pridmore P, Bendelow G (1995) Images of health: exploring beliefs of children using the 'draw-and-write' technique. Health Education Journal 54: 473-488.

Ream E, Richardson A (1997) Fatigue in patients with cancer and chronic obstructive airways disease: a phenomenological enquiry. International Journal of Nursing Studies 34: 44-53.

Ream E, Richardson A (1999) from theory to practice: designing interventions to reduce fatigue in patients with cancer. Oncology Nurses Forum. 26: 1295-1303.

Richardson A (1995) Fatigue in cancer patients: a review of the literature. European Journal of Cancer Nursing 4: 20-37.

Richardson A (1998) Measuring fatigue in patients with cancer. Support Cancer Care 6: 94-100.

Richardson A, Ream E (1996) Fatigue in patients receiving chemotherapy for advanced cancer. International Journal of Palliative Care 2: 199-204.

Sadeh A, Lavie P, Scher A, Tirosh E, Epstein R (1991) Actigraph home monitoring sleep disturbed and control infants and young children: A new method for pediatric assessment of sleep-wake patterns. Pediatrics 87: 494-499.

Schluederberg A, Straus SE, Peterson P et al. (1992) Chronic fatigue syndrome research: definition and medical outcome assessment. Annals of Internal Medicine 117: 325-331.

Selwood K, Gibson F, Evans M (1999) Side effects of chemotherapy. In: Gibson F, Evans M (eds), Paediatric Oncology: Acute nursing care. London: Whurr, pp. 59-128.

Smets EMA, Garssen B, Schuster-Uitterhoeve ALJ, Haes JCJM (1993) Fatigue in cancer patients. British Journal of Cancer 68: 220-224.

Stiller CA (1997) Aetiology and epidemiology. In: Plowman PN, Pinkerton CR (eds), Paediatric Oncology: Clinical practice and controversies. London, Chapman & Hall Medical, pp. 3-26.

Stone P, Richards M, Hardy J (1998) Fatigue in patients with cancer. European Journal of Cancer 34: 1670-1678.

Stone P, Richardson A, Ream E, Smith AG, Kerr DJ, Kearney N (2000) Cancer-related fatigue: inevitable, unimportant and untreatable? Results of a multi-centre patient survey. Annals of Oncology 11: 971-975.

Vogelzang NJ, Breitbart W, Cella D et al. (1997) Patient, caregiver, and oncologist perceptions of cancer-related fatigue: results of a tripart assessment survey. Seminars in Hematology 34: 4-12.

Walker LS, Greene JW (1991) The functional disability inventory: measuring a neglected dimension of child health status. Journal of Pediatric Psychology 16(1): 39-58.

Whyte F, Smith L (1997) A literature review of adolescence and cancer. European Journal of Cancer Care 6: 137-146.

Wilson D, Ratekin C (1990) An introduction to using children's drawings as an assessment tool. Nurse Practitioner 15: 23-35.

Winningham M, Nail LM, Barton Burke M et al. (1994) Fatigue and the cancer experience: The state of the knowledge. Oncology Nurses Forum 21: 23-36.

Yellen S, Cella D, Webster K, Blendowski C, Kaplan E (1997) Measuring fatigue and other anaemia-related symptoms with the functional assessment of cancer therapy (FACT) measurement system. Journal of Pain and Symptom Management 13: 63-74.

Chapter 15

The experience of children with a central venous catheter

Linda Sanderson

Cancer is a rare childhood illness, which in many cases, can now be cured (Pinkerton et al., 1994). The improved survival of children with cancer has been partially attributed to intensive chemotherapy regimens and better supportive care (Hollis, 1997). To deliver intensive chemotherapy regimens safely, monitor the effects on the child's blood and effectively give supportive products, e.g. blood products, antibiotics and parenteral nutrition, most children have a central venous catheter (CVC) inserted (Sepion, 1990).

In the clinical situation, children with cancer respond to their CVC in a variety of ways from calm acceptance to rage at having their catheters handled. This anecdotal evidence suggests that, to the child, a CVC is much more than a management tool; it is something that is endorsed by meaning.

Much has been written about CVCs from the perspective of the technical handling of the lines (Hollis, 1992; Bravery and Hannan, 1997), dealing with complications (Marcoux et al., 1990; Baranowski, 1993) and managing the child with the least distress (Leese, 1989); only Dale (1992) focused on the child's experience of a CVC, the Hickman line in particular. A child's response to a CVC could be affected by his or her understanding of the illness, fear of medical procedures, limited coping strategies or the impact of the CVC on body image. All of these explanations would be influenced by the child's developmental stage. By referring to relevant literature, research and theory, it is possible to build up an explanation of why a child may respond to a CVC in a certain way, but a vital piece of the picture would be missing – the child's own story of his or her experience. Benner and Wrubel (1989) suggest that the illness experience can be understood only by listening to the patient's story, which then allows the nurse to offer a more sensitive approach to care.

The aim of this research was to gain a deeper, more sophisticated understanding of the child's lived experience of having a CVC, so that care can be given more sensitively and tactfully to children in the future, e.g. in preparing the child for a CVC and handling the CVC. It is imperative to listen to the child's story of their lived experience of having a CVC and this should be of interest to any healthcare professional working in the field of paediatric oncology because so many such children have a CVC. Children with other long-term illnesses may also have a CVC and, therefore, the results of this study may be generalizable to children other than those with cancer (Bravery and Hannan, 1997).

Research methodology

A phenomenological approach was used to address the research question:

> What is the lived experience of having a central venous catheter for children with cancer?

A phenomenological approach to research 'explores the meaning of individuals' lived experience through their description' (Holloway and Wheeler, 1996, p. 209). Holloway and Wheeler's (1996) definition of phenomenology is seductively simplistic! On first reading, phenomenology seemed to be a straightforward and appropriate research approach because I was keen to hear the child's description of his or her lived experience of having a CVC. Other nurses have also grasped at phenomenology as a research approach because it is congruent with their primary concern – the patient's subjective experience of illness (Jasper, 1994; Tatano Beck, 1994; Hallett, 1995). However, it soon became apparent to me that phenomenology is not an easy research option; entries from my diary capture my frustration:

> This has been a traumatic week, I have had a real panic about not being able to understand phenomenology. I have lost sight of my project and I am thinking about throwing the whole thing in.
>
> I still find the whole language of phenomenology alien.

I took some comfort from the fact that others had also found this a difficult approach (Taylor, 1995). I used a diary throughout the period of the research; not only did it allow me to organize the work to be undertaken, it also allowed me to reflect on the impact that the research was having on me and my nursing practice.

Initially my interest in phenomenology was based on the value that I placed on subjective experience. I have never had a CVC so I thought that it was essential to hear from the children what this experience was like. The value that I placed on individual, subjective experience as a valuable source of knowledge is consistent with human sciences, often explored by qualitative research methods, rather than natural sciences, which are underpinned by quantitative research methods (Holloway and Wheeler, 1996). Crotty (1996) suggests that phenomenological research, which emphasizes subjective experience, is of value to nurses, but he suggests that this is a 'new' phenomenology rather than 'traditional' phenomenology. Crotty urges nurse researchers to explore phenomenology in more depth, to go beyond the subjective experiences and see the world from a different point of view (pp. 24–25); he suggests that this can be achieved by articulation and application of the philosophical underpinnings of phenomenology to research projects.

'Traditional' phenomenology embraces two significantly different views of human beings: transcendental phenomenology and existential phenomenology. Edward Husserl (1859–1938) is considered to be the founder of transcendental phenomenology and his philosophical life work attempts to explain the origin of absolute truth, which is found within the human, prereflective, prejudice-free consciousness (Ray, 1994), whereas Martin Heidegger (1889–1976), a pupil of Husserl, diverted from Husserl's search for absolute truth, and became more concerned with the ontological question of what it is to be a person in the world (Leonard, 1994).

Max Van Manen is a contemporary phenomenological researcher who appears to be less interested in phenomenological philosophy and more interested in practical phenomenological research. He emphasizes the importance of phenomenological research, which increases perceptiveness, and understanding of everyday experiences (Van Manen, 1997, p. 350).

Van Manen (1990) combines aspects of both descriptive and interpretative phenomenology (Cohen and Omery, 1994). His work was particularly relevant to this study because of his interest in phenomenological research with children. Van Manen's interest in children was as a teacher and a parent rather than as a nurse, but as there was only one example of phenomenological research with children in the nursing literature (Hockenberry-Eaton and Minick, 1994) I felt that it was appropriate to apply his ideas.

Van Manen's work is pragmatic and he provides a useful framework for approaching phenomenological research. His pragmatism was a little disconcerting at times, e.g. when he proclaimed that 'human science is often used interchangeably with phenomenology and hermeneutics' (Van Manen, 1990, p. 2); however, he goes on to explain clearly what he means by hermeneutic phenomenological human science and I based my methodology on this structure.

According to Van Manen (1990), phenomenological research is the:

1. *The study of lived experiences*: Van Manen suggested that subjective experience is experience that has been reflected on or conceptualized, i.e. lived experience. However, this reflection or conceptualization stems from the life world, i.e. pre-reflective meaning; if this pre-reflective meaning can be articulated it can lead to a deeper understanding of the experience.

2. *The explication of phenomena as they present themselves to consciousness*: Van Manen proposed that a person is connected to the world via their consciousness. To be conscious of some 'thing' (real, imaginary or subjectively felt) is to be aware of some aspect of the world that has significance to the person. The only way a person can know the world is through their consciousness but this knowledge is always retrospective. A person cannot reflect on his or her experience while experiencing it so the researcher attempts to describe a phenomenon as it comes into consciousness.

3. *The study of essences*: for Van Manen essence means 'a description of phenomena' (1990, p. 39) which must be linguistic in nature. The essence of a lived experience is concerned less with the factual status of a particular instance, e.g. how many times does a child cry when having their CVC handled, than with the child's description of the experience of having the CVC handled. If the essence of an experience is adequately described, it will show the significance of that experience in a deeper manner and so enhance understanding.

4. *The description of the experiential meanings we live as we live them*: Van Manen used this aspect of phenomenological research to differentiate from other types of social research. Phenomenological research is the only approach that aims to discover the meaning of an experience as it is lived. Van Manen (1990, p. 11) was arguably inconsistent or inaccurate in his use of language; presumably he was referring to retrospective meaning, because a person cannot reflect on experience as they are experiencing it.

5. *The attentive practice of thoughtfulness*: thoughtfulness epitomizes phenomenological research. I encountered this thoughtfulness as I grappled with phenomenology. The children in this study appeared to be thoughtful as they talked about their lived experience of having a CVC; I was thoughtful as I described and interpreted their data and I hope that this research will provoke thoughtfulness in others.

6. *The search for what it means to be human.* Here there are echoes of Heideggerian existential phenomenology because Van Manen suggested that his approach to research can help the researcher to understand more fully what it means to be a human being in the world. This meaning, he suggested, takes account of the cultural and historical background of the person.

7. *A poetizing activity:* initially I felt uncomfortable with the word poetizing because it suggested to me that research could be plucked from creative thought rather than based in lived experience. However, Van Manen explained that phenomenological research is unlike other research because the results cannot be summarized or concluded; like a poem they must be taken as they are. The language of phenomenological research is original language; it is language that describes and interprets pre-reflective meaning so, argued Van Manen, it has a poetizing quality that makes the reader think and feel about a phenomenon in ways that they have never thought or felt before.

Van Manen (1990) summarized phenomenological research as systematic, explicit, self-critical and intersubjective: systematic because of the modes of questioning used, explicit because of the attempt made to describe the structure of meaning embedded in lived experience, self-critical because the whole research is constantly under review and intersubjective because the researcher needs the 'other', i.e. research participant and reader, in order to validate the phenomena described. The aim of the study was:

> To describe and interpret the meanings that children with cancer ascribe to their lived experience of having a central venous catheter in order to offer a more tactful and sensitive approach to care.

Method

The method for this research was planned and undertaken with the following considerations in mind:

1. The research question and the underpinning phenomenological methodology influenced all aspects of data collection and analysis.

2. Children in general, and children with an illness in particular, represent a vulnerable group of research participants (Koocher and Keith-Spiegel, 1994; Wender, 1994). All decisions about the research method respected the child and were aimed at minimizing any potential harm.

3. Qualitative research, including phenomenological research, should be judged against the criteria of credibility, dependability, transferability and confirmability (Sandelowski, 1986; Guba and Lincoln, 1989; Koch, 1994).

Ethical considerations

Historically, children have been considered as the 'possessions' of adults with little ability to participate effectively in the decisions affecting them (Taylor and Adelman, 1986; Alderson, 1993). These presumptions have led either to reluctance on the part of researchers to include children in their work or to the inclusion of children in research without their participation in any of the decision processes (Moore and Ruccione, 1989; Lederer and Grodin, 1994). Over the last 10 years this view of the child has been challenged by the United Nations' Convention on the Rights of the Child (Franklin, 1995), the Children Act 1989 (Lyon and Parton, 1995), the British Paediatric Association (1992) and the work of Priscilla Alderson (1993).

This study respected and sought to understand the child's view of the world, so it was inevitable that the research process was undertaken with the child's interests always in mind. The British Paediatric Association (1992) considers research that involves questioning children as being of 'minimal risk' to the child. However, the four ethical principles of respect for autonomy, non-maleficence, beneficence and justice were used to promote the involvement of the children in a thoughtful manner (Beauchamp and Childress, 1994).

The principle of the respect for autonomy was mainly concerned with ensuring that the children were given the opportunity willingly to assent to, or dissent from, participation in the study. Weithorn and Scherer (1994) refer to assent as 'a child's affirmative agreement to participate in research' (p. 143) which is based on adequate, understandable information, the child's competence to understand the information and express a preference, and that the agreement is given voluntarily.

Non-maleficence is the ethical principle that is concerned with doing the child no harm. It was difficult to predict fully the harm that this research could impose on the child. It was anticipated that talking about having a CVC might arouse emotions in the child that may not have previously been addressed, although Faux et al. (1988) suggest that this may be a benefit for the child if handled appropriately. Other opportunities for beneficence, or 'doing good', include giving the child an opportunity to practise decision-making skills, increase his or her sense of control and make him or her feel important.

The final ethical principle to be considered was that of justice. Purposive sampling unfortunately meant that not every child with a CVC was given the opportunity to tell his or her story, which can be perceived as being unjust. The steps taken to address the principle of justice and the other ethical principles, as they related to this research, are given in Table 15.1.

Table 15.1 Addressing the ethical principles

Respect for autonomy	The children were given a written and verbal explanation of the research which encouraged their questions
	Children aged 6–11 were considered able to assent to research (Alderson, 1993) but their understanding was assessed by asking them to explain why they had been asked to participate in the study
	An age-appropriate consent form was used
	The initial contact with the child was via parents which, in two cases, allowed the child to use parents to dissent to participate in the research
	Written and verbal emphasis that the child did not have to participate in the study
	The child decided on who could know what they had said in the interview, so their anonymity was respected
	Four children did not wish to participate in the study; this decision was respected
Non-maleficence	Respect for autonomy, as above
	Interviewer alert to signs of distress which led to stopping the interview in one case
	Research scrutinized by three gatekeepers
	Support mechanisms available in the children's cancer unit if required
Beneficence	Respect for autonomy, as above
	Children were genuinely thanked for their participation
	Children seemed to enjoy participating in the study
Justice	A report of the study went into the children's cancer unit newsletter. Children, not involved in the study, were given the opportunity to write to me about their experience of having a CVC

Selection of research participants

Phenomenological research aims at describing and interpreting the essential structure of a lived experience; consequently the research participants are selected because they have experienced particular phenomena, i.e. they are a purposeful sample (Holloway and Wheeler, 1996). With the research question in mind, the following criteria were used for selecting research participants:

- They must have a CVC.
- They must be aged between 6 and 11 years.
- They must be undergoing treatment for a malignant disease.

After careful consideration of the advantages and disadvantages of the decision, children receiving treatment at the paediatric oncology unit where I work were invited to participate in the research. Schutz (1994) warned of the potential difficulties of researching in an environment where the participants know the researcher. This is particularly pertinent in qualitative research where the researcher is considered to be the research tool (Tatano Beck, 1994; Morse and Field, 1996). The main concern is that the 'power' position of the researcher may affect voluntary consent; the data generated, and in the case of children, cause confusion (Moston, 1987; Faux et al., 1988).

As a nurse on the inpatient paediatric oncology unit, it was a concern that I would be in a powerful position compared with the research participants. This issue was addressed by a variety of strategies:

- The initial contact with the families was by letter followed by telephone because I felt that it would be easier for them to say 'no' to participation if I were not sitting in front of them.
- Assent to participate in the research was obtained from each child (see Ethical considerations above).
- The interviews took place in the outpatient setting, or in the child's home in one case, and I was out of uniform.
- The children chose whether to invite their parents into the 'interview room'.

These strategies appeared to be effective because five children (of 25) decided not to participate in the study (four girls and one boy). Having addressed the disadvantages of researching in the 'home' clinical environment, it is important to point out that there was also an important advantage. The relationship that I had previously built up with the children in the inpatient environment helped to establish trust and rapport, which were essential elements for the success of interviews as a data collection method (Faux et al., 1988; Seidman, 1991).

After establishing the selection criteria for inviting children to participate in the study, a list of 'eligible' children was produced by the data manager of the children's cancer unit. A total of 25 children fulfilled the criteria for participation in the study: 16 girls and 9 boys. Before contacting them access was negotiated with the relevant gatekeepers.

Access to research participants

As a researcher in the clinical environment in which I worked, I had contact, from time to time, with the children invited to participate. Care was taken not to abuse this privileged position; permission was sought from three gatekeepers before the children were approached to invite them to participate in the research. Holloway and Wheeler (1996) define gatekeepers as 'Those individuals that have the power to permit access to an organization, a setting or people in the setting' (p. 208); the three gatekeepers identified for this research were:

- local ethics committee
- healthcare professionals
- parents.

The local ethics committee was responsible for the protection of research participants; they were formally approached via the ethics committee proposal. The process took 3 months to complete and the proposal was accepted without any amendments.

Letters were sent to several healthcare professionals whom I perceived to be gatekeepers; these included consultants responsible for the children's medical treatment, the senior nurses in the unit and the operations manager for children's services. Not only was it polite to seek permission to approach the research participants (Holloway and Wheeler 1996), I also respected the gatekeeper's knowledge of the child's current health status and perceived ability to participate in the study.

The final 'gatekeepers' to liaise with were the parents of the children whom I had decided to invite to participate. Faux et al. (1988) point out that it is polite to seek parental permission and it was impossible to imagine how this study could have been undertaken without it. However, Weithorn and Scherer (1994) warn that children may feel pressurized to participate in research because their parents have agreed. To guard against this it was important to emphasize to the parents that their permission was being sought to ask their child if they wished to participate, not to ask their permission to interview their child. When I spoke to the parents on the telephone, we made an appointment to meet and again I reiterated that I would explain the study to the child and let him or her decide if he or she wanted to participate.

When permission had been received from all three gatekeepers, the children were invited to participate. Table 15.2 includes a list of the children who were interviewed; all of their names have been changed and their diagnosis has been excluded to protect their identity.

Table 15.2 The children interviewed in the study

Name	Age (years)	Type of central venous catheter
Susan	10	Implanted port
Gemma	9	Double-lumen tunnelled catheter
Helen	8	Implanted port
Alice	6	Double-lumen tunnelled catheter
Lucy	6	Double-lumen tunnelled catheter
Steven	10	Single-lumen tunnelled catheter
Julie	8	Implanted port
Wendy	6	Implanted port
Samantha	7	Implanted port
Katie	7	Implanted port

The final potential gatekeepers to the study were the children; their cooperation was central to the success of the project, and strategies used to facilitate their cooperation are discussed under 'Ethical considerations' above.

Data collection

The interview is a data collection technique that is often used in phenomenological research where 'the researcher is hoping to "borrow" the lived experience of a particular phenomena [sic] in order to more fully understand that experience' (Van Manen, 1990, p. 28). Van Manen (1990) does not give a structured formula for undertaking interviews in phenomenological research because he believes that the research question must drive the method. However, he advises that the researcher must facilitate interviewees to tell their personal stories of their lived experience in as much detail as possible.

Other authors, such as Faux et al. (1988), Alderson (1993) and Bernheimer (1986), give suggestions and guidance about interviewing children, which proved useful. I also took advice from the clinical psychologist linked to the paediatric oncology unit about interviewing children.

To help the children relax, which I felt was vital if they were to tell me their personal stories about living with a CVC, I spent some time with them in the waiting area of the outpatient clinic just chatting about school or holidays. When I felt that the child was comfortable with me around, I invited him or her into a quiet room so we could 'chat' about the CVC. All the children were given the option of their parents coming to the quiet room as well; only Lucy, Wendy and Samantha wanted their parents present.

Once in the quiet room I asked the child to explain to me why he or she thought that I wanted to talk to him or her; this was an opportunity to check the child's understanding of the study. The interviews were audio-taped, so I showed the recorder to the children and let them decide where we should place it.

The interviews were semi-structured; there were areas that I thought would be useful to explore, e.g. Why does the child think he or she has a CVC? Who does he or she tell about it? How does it feel having the CVC handled? However, I was keen to allow the child to explain the lived experience of having a CVC in his or her own way. Some of the children were confident in telling their story, e.g. Susan and Gemma; other children required more encouragement, e.g. Lucy and Samantha.

To assist children to tell their stories in as much detail as possible, I used a variety of approaches. I suggested that they think of a particular situation, e.g. 'What is it like when the nurses take blood from your line?', or I asked them to explain the CVC to an imaginary third person, e.g. a 'Spice girl' or another boy or girl; in one case I asked a child to draw a picture of herself, which enabled her to talk about her CVC.

All of the interviews were tape-recorded; this allowed me to concentrate on what the children were saying, and I felt that making notes while the children were talking might distract them. Rose (1994) warned that a tape-recorder can intimidate the interviewee but, on the whole, the children seemed unperturbed by it; many of them had used tape-recorders at school. Samantha was a notable exception; she talked happily with me before the tape-recorder was switched on but then became very shy when the recorder was on. After about 7 minutes, I felt that Samantha was no longer happy to participate in the study so I thanked her and switched off the recorder. Once the recorder was off Samantha relaxed again and started to tell me about her CVC; with her permission I made notes of what she had said and I added this on to the end of the interview script for analysis. An advantage of using a tape-recorder was that the child could listen to what he or she had said; this was an opportunity for the child to add anything further or delete parts of the interview if he or she wanted to. None of the children altered what was on the tape but they all listened carefully to the replay.

Technical problems can be a disadvantage when tape-recording interviews (Rose 1994); fortunately there was only one such problem in this study. One interview did not record but, immediately after the interview, I made notes about the significant aspects of the interview; this method of data collection is an approach taken by some researchers (Holloway and Wheeler, 1996).

I transcribed each of the interviews, which was a time-consuming activity. However, transcription of the interviews helped me to immerse myself in the data, which, as Seidman (1991) suggested, is helpful in the data analysis.

Analysis of the data

The aim of the research was to describe and interpret the meanings that children with cancer ascribe to their lived experience of having a CVC. To achieve this aim the interviews were analysed in such a way as to explicate the meanings that the children put on their lived experience of having a CVC.

Van Manen (1990) talks of phenomenological reflection as a way of grasping the essential meaning of something. This reflection demands that the researcher becomes immersed in the data and then attempts to 'explicate the structure of meaning of the lived experience' (Van Manen 1990, p. 77). Van Manen believes that the structure of meaning of a lived experience can best be approached by thinking of the phenomena as being composed of units or themes. However, these 'themes' are more than a collection of words, they arise from a desire to make sense of something, they reflect the sense that has been made of phenomena and they can arise only from an openness in the description of the phenomena. A theme, according to Van Manen (1990, p. 88), is the process of 'insightful invention, discovery and disclosure'. Other authors have referred to this creative insight as intuiting (Moustakas, 1994; Crotty, 1996).

Hycner (1985) suggested that there has been reluctance on the part of phenomenological researchers to articulate clearly how 'themes' are derived from the data because of a fear that a stepwise approach would be too restrictive; certainly Van Manen (1990) gives only a brief outline of approaches that may be taken by the researcher. As a novice researcher I sought more guidance about analysing the data that I had obtained from the children, so I used Colaizzi's (1978) analytical approach, which other nurse researchers had also used (Tatano Beck, 1994).

All the interviews were analysed using the following approach, based on Colaizzi (1978), until an exhaustive description of the lived experience of having a CVC was achieved:

- The recording of each interview was listened to several times, and the transcripts read to get an overall feel for the child's experience.
- Significant statements from each interview were identified and transcribed, in full, on separate sheets of paper. I identified significant statements as anything in the interviews that pertained to the lived experience of having a CVC.
- From each significant statement meanings were formulated. This was the creative aspect of phenomenological research, and it was essential to ensure that the formulated meanings actually reflected the interview data.
- The formulated meanings were organized into clusters of themes. Meanings common to several interviews were drawn together but the differences in the interviews were left apparent.

To validate the exhaustive description that I achieved, it was discussed with children who had a CVC to see whether they could recognize my description. The parents of five children were approached to ask permission to discuss the 'exhaustive description' with their children. All the parents agreed and the children were asked if they were interested in hearing about my 'project'. The five children with whom I discussed the exhaustive description included two girls who had previously been interviewed, one girl aged 7 (Girl 1) and two boys aged 9 and 6 years (Boy 1 and Boy 2).

The themes and exhaustive description are discussed in greater detail below.

Findings and discussion

Van Manen (1990) suggested that the essential structure of phenomena, e.g. the lived experience of having a CVC, can be reported in units of meaning or themes to promote thoughtfulness about every aspect of the phenomena (p. 78). The lived experience of having a CVC for children with cancer included the following themes:

- vulnerability
- differentness
- restrictions
- information
- decisions
- taken-for-grantedness.

Thematic formulations give structure and shape to the lived experience of having a CVC. Each of these themes represents a 'part' of the 'whole' of the lived experience of having a CVC and, therefore, they should be considered together and not in isolation (Van Manen, 1990, p. 88).

Vulnerability

> I was scared me (Gemma)

It became apparent, from listening to the children's stories, that there were times in the lived experience of having a CVC when the children felt particularly vulnerable. The children used words such as 'scared' (Gemma, Helen, Steven), 'frightened' (Wendy) and 'nervous' (Samantha) to express their vulnerability.

The situations that appeared to highlight the feelings of vulnerability for the children were when they had something 'pushed' into their central venous catheter, e.g. the Port-A-Cath needle, antibiotics, saline or heparin solution, or something 'pulled' out of the CVC e.g. the Port-A-Cath needle or blood. For the children with an implanted port, a feature of their stories concerned the needle, which has to be pushed into the implanted port in order to have blood taken or medicine given. With the use of local anaesthetic cream over the implanted port, the children appeared to be in agreement that this did not hurt, but they still felt vulnerable because of the pushing associated with the insertion of the needle:

> I felt it being pushed in, and it felt, it felt like it was being pushed in quite hard and it felt, I could feel it but now it doesn't feel as though it is being pushed in quite so hard. (Susan)
>
> When you've got the Emla cream on it hurts a little bit . . . . The pressing feels funny. (Samantha)

Having a needle pushed into an implanted port was only one aspect of the lived experience of having a CVC that seemed to make the children feel vulnerable. Lucy explained how her CVC was used to 'put things through'; other children described the sensations and 'tastes' that they experience when 'things' were pushed into their CVC:

> ... but if you put saline in or, or the other one in it's sometimes cold ... in the line, up here [points to clavicle]. And the Heplock sometimes tastes a bit ... like salty water .... If I have a drink I don't mind it but ... other times I go 'yuk'. (Alice)

> You can't feel anything but when they put that like salty water in you can taste it. (Steven)

The children with a tunnelled catheter appeared to feel particularly vulnerable when having the dressing replaced over their CVC (Alice) or when they were connected to an intravenous infusion machine, because they were worried that their CVC may fall out (Steven). Gemma was very clear about what she thought would happen if her CVC fell out:

> All blood would rush out [pause], but me sister said in bed, she said if I pull it out what would happen and I said all blood would come out, she didn't talk about it then. (Gemma)

Susan, who had an implanted port, explained what it felt like to have the needle removed from the 'port':

> It's a strange feeling like when you're about to go home and they take the needle out you can feel it being pulled out and then they just put a plaster on and it's all gone. (Susan)

Susan was also concerned that she would bleed when the needle was removed. The younger children in the study did not seem to feel as vulnerable when their needle was removed as Susan; this may reflect a developmental difference in body knowledge. Susan obviously had a complex understanding of where the CVC was placed inside her body, whereas the younger children tended to explain the position of the CVC in terms of the external features. This developmental aspect of children's understanding of their internal body parts was demonstrated by McEwing (1996) in her research involving 'healthy' children.

For Helen, Julie and Samantha, their lived experience of having a CVC included feelings of vulnerability associated with the operation to insert the CVC:

> I was just really scared and I was shivering ... when I was going to have the Port-A-Cath put in and being put to sleep, I got really scared. (Julie)

The vulnerability that appeared to be a 'part' of the lived experience of having a CVC is not referred to in any of the literature reviewed concerning the use of CVC in children, but it may be linked to the child's perceived level of control over the situation. A number of people have 'access' via the CVC to the child's body, which could be perceived by the child as having limited control over their body. Susman et al. (1987) suggested that a child's reasoning about illness may be decreased if they do not feel in control; therefore, at a time when a nurse/parent requires the child's cooperation, e.g. when giving the child a drug via their CVC, the child may feel particularly vulnerable and unable to understand that the drug may help him or her get better, leading to distress and less cooperation.

The child's vulnerability may also reflect a lack of knowledge about the function of the internal body, e.g. if blood is being 'pulled' from the CVC, the child may believe that they will not have any blood left; even very young children understand the importance of blood (McEwing, 1996). The children in this study with an implanted port were concerned about the 'pushing' that accompanied the insertion of a needle; this may reflect their lack of knowledge about the structure and function of the rib cage. The implanted port is normally inserted on the anterior aspect of the rib cage so, when the needle is inserted, the flexibility of the rib cage may lead the child to feel as though he or she is going to be squashed which, understandably, could make him or her feel very vulnerable.

Bibace and Walsh (1980) proposed an explanation of a child's understanding of illness based on their cognitive development. In the age group 6–11 years, Bibace and Walsh suggested, children tend to view illness as being caused by either contamination from an external source, person or object, or from an external cause that has entered their body, i.e. internalization. Children in this age group with a CVC may feel particularly vulnerable if they fear that germs can be introduced into their body via their CVC. This point may be particularly pertinent in children with cancer, who are regularly told that they may have to come back into hospital with an infection because of their vulnerable immune system (Pinkerton et al., 1994).

Vulnerability is one aspect of the lived experience of having a CVC that has not been articulated in the literature previously, as far as I am aware, and it emphasizes the importance of listening to children in order to give more sensitive care. There are steps that can be taken in practice, which may minimize a child's feelings of vulnerability; these are summarized in the conclusion.

Vulnerability is an aspect of the lived experience of having a CVC which seemed to be most apparent in relation to the healthcare setting, although children with cancer also have lives away from the hospital which is when their 'differentness' became most apparent.

Differentness

> She let me go and get changed in the corner. (Helen)

According to Price's body image model (1990), it could be assumed that a CVC would alter children's body reality and, possibly, their body ideal, which has the potential to lower self-esteem (Harter, 1998). In the CVC literature, there is an assumption that the tunnelled catheter is more of a problem to the child's body image than the implanted port because of the external catheter (Marcoux et al., 1990; Baranowski, 1993). In this study it was apparent that both types of CVC could make the child feel 'different', although the implanted port does not have an external catheter; to the children with the implanted port it was a 'big lump under the skin' (Wendy).

The differentness that the children felt was most apparent when they discussed the reactions of their friends and family to their CVC. Helen was initially 'scared' to show her friends her implanted port and so she asked her teacher if she could 'get changed in the corner'. The response of friends to the children's CVC emphasized their difference, e.g. Steven's friends were 'shocked', Gemma's friend thought the CVC was like a 'worm sticking out' and Samantha's friends were very curious about her CVC:

> My friends keep saying can I have a look at your Port-A-Cath all the time.

Most of the children were aware that other children did not want to have a CVC, which again emphasized their difference; however, Katie appeared unconcerned by her CVC and she thought that the 'Power Rangers' might also have a CVC occasionally. When the exhaustive description was discussed with Girl 1 (age 7) she said that she did not feel different to her friends.

Differentness has the potential to isolate children (Price, 1993; Cluroe, 1997) and the CVC certainly appeared to alter the children's relationship with their friends. Alice and Samantha described how they had to ask their friends not to push or pull them because of their CVC. Helen had had some difficulty at school with her friends; the CVC was a contributing factor:

> It were about allsorts they just kept looking at me and laughing. (Helen)

Of course a CVC is just one aspect of cancer that could make children feel different; alopecia may be another, but the children focused their stories on the lived experience of having a CVC; only Gemma related this to being ill and Samantha to having leukaemia.

Writers such as Susan Sontag (1991) emphasize the enormous impact that cancer can have on a person's life, not only because the illness can physically make a person different, but also because society's negative attitudes to cancer magnify the differences. It would appear from the analysis of the data in this study that the children did not relate their differentness to their illness as such; rather they in part related it to having a CVC.

School-aged children have an increasing ability to evaluate themselves because of their developing cognitive ability and the opportunities they have to compare themselves with others (Harter, 1998, p. 586). Disparity between perceived and ideal self is an accepted part of 'growing up' (Glick and Zigler, 1985), but a CVC may increase the disparity, leading to lowered self-esteem. A related, but distinct, aspect of the lived experience of having a CVC, which the children discussed, concerned the restrictions imposed on their activities by their CVC.

Restrictions

> But I can't, so I feel left out a lot. (Julie)

In the literature it is clearly recognized that a child should not go swimming with a tunnelled catheter *in situ* (Marcoux et al., 1990), although this is acceptable with the implanted port (Hollis, 1992). It is recommended that the child should not participate in contact sports with the implanted port (Bagnall and Ruccione, 1987). Most of the children interviewed in this study commented on the things that they were not able to do because of their CVC, with the exception of Wendy who said that she had been able to do anything that she wanted to do with her implanted port *in situ* and Katie who did not mention this aspect of the lived experience of having a CVC at all.

All of the children with a tunnelled catheter, except for Alice, mentioned that they could not go swimming. Steven discussed how he had chosen a tunnelled catheter over an implanted port because he had wanted to play football, i.e. a contact sport. It became apparent from talking to the children that there were other restrictions on activities, which were not mentioned in the literature but which were important aspects of the lived experience of having a CVC, e.g. Julie 'felt quite upset' because she could not play football or gymnastics with her CVC *in situ*, and Helen and Gemma were worried about doing physical education at school in case they damaged their CVC in some way. Boy 1, after listening to the exhaustive description, said that he was glad he could go swimming with his CVC but he missed being able to play football 'properly'.

Living with a CVC also restricted less obvious activities for some of the children, which again were not mentioned in the literature reviewed. Susan mentioned that her CVC sometimes interrupted her sleeping, Gemma, Alice and Steven all mentioned that their CVC altered the way that they bathed, and Lucy mentioned that she could not have a shower.

These restrictions again emphasize the children's differentness from their friends, which may lead to lowered self-esteem as previously discussed. However, James's theory on the formation of self (as discussed by Harter, 1998) suggested that restrictions will affect a child's self-esteem only if it prevents them from achieving their pretensions. On the whole the children in this study had dealt with the restrictions imposed by taking up hobbies that they could pursue, e.g. Julie had taken up the violin, or they had altered their behaviour to incorporate the restrictions, e.g. Lucy had a bath instead of a shower.

The lived experience of having a CVC appeared to include potentially negative themes, i.e. vulnerability, differentness and restrictions, and it also involved the children in making some important decisions.

Decisions

In the paediatric oncology unit where this study was undertaken, it was normal practice to offer the children a choice of CVC except for those children who required very intensive treatment; it is recommended that they have a double-lumen tunnelled catheter. In this study Gemma, Alice and Lucy would not have been able to choose which CVC to have; Gemma commented on this:

> I would have liked a Port-A-Cath better than a Hickman line . . . I don't know why, but I just would.

Of those children who had a choice, only Steven chose a tunnelled catheter over an implanted port. All of the children, except for Katie, had clear reasons for choosing one type of CVC over the other. Susan, Julie and Samantha chose the implanted port because they did not want a line 'dangling' from their body. Helen, Wendy and Samantha included being able to go swimming in their reasons for choosing the implanted port. Steven chose the tunnelled catheter because he was a keen football player and also because 'I don't need to have needles put into my skin'. Alice did not have a choice about which CVC to have – she had to have a tunnelled catheter – but she appreciated not having needles put into her skin.

Children with cancer have a CVC inserted near to the time of the diagnosis of their illness so this theme, which forms part of the lived experience of having a CVC, highlights the decision-making abilities that children have if they are given information. The ability of children to make important decisions has been discussed at length in the literature about the ability of children to assent to research, e.g. Lederer and Grodin (1994) and Weithorn and Scherer (1994). Alderson (1993) focused the debate in the healthcare setting when she interviewed children about their involvement in the decision to have major limb-lengthening surgery. Alderson (1993, p. 196) concluded, 'that there should never be a case for excluding children from decision making because excluding children can increase fear'. Young children can be courageous and wise and those children with a long-standing illness have unique knowledge that is essential to the decision-making process. The children in this study demonstrated their wisdom when they discussed their reasons for choosing a particular CVC.

Another important decision that the children in this study had made was concerned with whom they told about their CVC. Each of the children, except for Katie, had chosen a particular group of people to tell about their CVC. Susan had told only her close family; Helen, Lucy, Steven, Samantha and Wendy had told a small group of friends. Alice had told her close family and those friends who had visited the house, Gemma had told her teacher and her best friend. Julie appeared to be a little upset because she had been unable to decide whom to tell:

> I didn't tell anybody but mummy told [friend] and then it just started getting spreaded. (Julie)

It may be that the children used their discretion in choosing 'who to tell' about their CVC as a means of gaining control over their situation and minimizing the impact of their differentness. This is an important aspect of the lived experience of having a CVC and it has implications for parents, healthcare professionals in the hospital setting and those who liaise with the community: children need to be involved in the decision about who to tell about their CVC. Helen highlighted the importance of being able to choose whom she told about her CVC:

> People who don't know you and you've got a jumper or a tee-shirt on they don't know it's there. (Helen)

For children to be able to make the decision about which CVC to have, and who to tell about their CVC, it was important that they had adequate information at an appropriate level for them to understand.

Information

'Information' is a distinct theme, rather than a subtheme of 'decisions', because it became apparent that the information the children had used to make sense of their CVC was not just concerned with making decisions. Several of the children had had to explain their CVC to their friends and family, i.e. Susan, Steven, Julie and Samantha.

The older children, e.g. Susan and Steven, explained the positioning and functioning of their CVC in complex detail, whereas the younger children, e.g. Katie and Lucy, explained their CVC in terms of what could be seen and what was done to the CVC. These differences possibly reflect the children's cognitive development (Newcombe, 1996) but they emphasize that children of all ages require information to make sense of their situation. Perrin and Gerrity (1981) suggested that children are unable to make sense of many medical terms, but this study supports the work of Alderson (1993) where children could comprehend if the information was made understandable to them.

Taken-for-grantedness

> It doesn't feel like anything (Lucy)

Phenomenological enquiry aims to explicate the essential structure of a lived experience, to describe and interpret everyday, taken-for-granted experiences in order to have a greater understanding of the phenomena (Van Manen, 1990). A phenomenological approach was taken in this study to address the question 'What is the lived experience of having a CVC for children with cancer?', so it is interesting that one of the themes of that lived experience is 'taken-for-grantedness'.

Although there appeared to be occasions when the children were aware of their CVC, i.e. when they were vulnerable, different or restricted, this was not the whole lived experience of having a CVC. There was a sense of taken-for-grantedness of the CVC as the children told their stories, which appeared to have developed over time:

> I could feel it but now it doesn't feel as though it is being pushed in quite so hard, it just feels normal. (Susan)

> Just tell 'em about when it goes into you it does hurt at first but then you get used to it and then it's OK. (Gemma)

> If you have it tucked in you might forget it's tucked in. (Alice).

The interview with Katie epitomized the theme of 'taken-for-grantedness'; for 40 minutes we played and chatted but she said very little about having a CVC. I did not feel that Katie found it difficult to talk about her CVC; she just gave the impression that there were far more important things to think about even though she had agreed to talk about her CVC. Katie had had her CVC in for almost 2 years so perhaps the 'taken-for-grantedness' was a result of the coping strategies that she had developed over that time to minimize the effects of 'vulnerability', 'differentness' or 'restrictions'.

Other children appeared to have adopted coping strategies to deal with their CVC; perhaps their increased perceived ability to 'cope' meant that their CVC was less of a threat and, therefore, demanded less attention (Lazarus, 1976). The coping strategies that the children had adopted included pretending that the CVC was a washing line (Gemma), using distraction when the CVC was being handled (Helen), becoming very familiar with the details of the CVC (Lucy) and becoming involved in the practicalities of living with a CVC (Alice and Lucy).

Researchers such as Susman et al. (1987) and Neff and Beardslee (1990) have been surprised by the ability of children to adapt to living with cancer, but Bearison and Mulhern (1994) and Eiser (1990) emphasized that research into children's coping with illness should be moving away from a 'pathology oriented' model, i.e. how many psychological problems the child has (Bearison and Mulhern, 1994, p. 36), to an approach that recognizes that children with illness are 'normal' children who are coping with many stresses. The lived experience of having a CVC was just one aspect of the lived experience of having cancer for the children interviewed, but the theme of 'taken-for-grantedness' highlights the strength and adaptability of children to deal with apparently difficult situations.

Exhaustive description of the lived experience

Most children with cancer have a CVC inserted shortly after their diagnosis and it remains *in situ* for the duration of their treatment. As an experienced nurse in the paediatric oncology unit, I was very aware of the medical benefits of the CVC in terms of managing the disease and treatment, but I was intrigued by the different ways in which children responded to their CVC being handled. I felt that it was essential to listen to the children's stories about their lived experience of having a CVC to gain a deeper understanding of this important aspect of having cancer.

The phenomenological approach to the study allowed the children to tell their own stories, in their own way, but it became apparent that there were commonalities in the lived experience of having a CVC for the ten children interviewed and the five children who commented on the findings of the study. The exhaustive description of having a CVC included themes that had not previously appeared in the literature, so it is hoped that this study will lead to thoughtfulness in the readers and further discussions with children about their lived experience of having a CVC.

The lived experience of having a CVC incorporated several 'parts', but it is essential that these are not considered in isolation. One 'part' of the lived experience of having a CVC was 'vulnerability'. Vulnerability, if considered in isolation, may lead to the impression that children with cancer need constant protection and supervision. This was not the case for the children interviewed; perhaps they needed support when they were feeling particularly vulnerable but another 'part' of the lived experience of having a CVC was 'taken-for-grantedness'. 'Taken-for-grantedness' highlighted the ability of children with cancer to carry on with their lives, but if this 'part' was taken in isolation it may lead to an assumption that children with a CVC do not need information or support because they just get on with their life. If the 'whole' of the lived experience of having a CVC is considered, then appropriate and sensitive care can be offered to the children.

The exhaustive description of the lived experience of having a CVC for children with cancer included vulnerability at times, an awareness of being different, restrictions on activities and the need for information in order to make important decisions at times when the CVC is taken-for-granted.

Limitations of the study

This study addressed a subject that was previously unexplored in the literature, and it has culminated in the exhaustive description of the lived experience of having a CVC for children with cancer, although there were limitations to the study:

- The study was undertaken in my own place of work, so the children were familiar with me before the study. This not only may have made the children feel obliged to participate in the study but also may have prevented them from fully discussing their lived experience of having a CVC. On the other hand, I felt that there was an advantage to knowing the children – it helped to build trust and rapport, which was essential for them to participate fully in the interviews. However, only two of the children linked having a CVC to having an illness; this may truly reflect the lived experience of having a CVC or it may reflect the fact that they knew I knew what was wrong with them. Strategies were used to address this problem, e.g. the children were asked to explain their CVC to an 'imaginary person'.

- Three of the children were interviewed with their parents present, which may have altered their responses. I felt that it was essential that the children were able to decide whether they wanted their parents present at the interview, if that made them feel more comfortable.

- Nine of the ten interviews took place in the outpatient setting; the children may have given a different response if they had been in their own home environment. The parents mainly took the decision about where the interview should take place. If I had insisted on the interview taking place away from the hospital, i.e. at their home, I am sure that some of the parents would have felt obliged to say 'yes', but an important aspect of this study was ensuring that participation was voluntary for the children and the parents.

- There were four children who did not want to participate in the study; I perceived that these children had had some difficulty in living with their CVC; perhaps if they had told their story it may have altered the exhaustive description presented.

- Only one boy participated in the interviews; this reflected the available 'possible' participants at the time of the study. To address this apparent bias the validation of the study included a further two boys.

Conclusion

There are many examples of existing literature that could help to explain why a child may respond in a particular way to having their CVC handled in some way. However, the extant knowledge is inanimate; it does not capture what it is like to live with a CVC. Only a child who has a CVC is, I believe, able to describe the lived experience of having a CVC.

The research question addressed in this study 'What is the lived experience of having a CVC for children with cancer?' is a 'meaning' question and as such it cannot be solved and 'done away with' (Van Manen, 1990, p. 23). The exhaustive description, which emanated from the children's stories, should help the reader to understand more fully the lived experience of having a CVC, but it is hoped that this description will continue to provoke thoughtful reflection in the reader.

Analysis of the children's stories led to an exhaustive description of having a CVC, which included vulnerability at times, an awareness of being different, restrictions on activities, a need for information in order to make important decisions and times when the CVC is taken-for-granted.

Implications for practice, education and research

Reflection on this description of the lived experience of having a CVC has led to a deeper understanding, which has implications for practice, education and further research.

Practice

- Explanation to the child of what is going to happen with their CVC and discussion with the child about how they can be involved may give them an opportunity to take control and, therefore, feel less vulnerable.
- Exploration with the child of ways in which they could minimize their fear of their CVC being pulled out, e.g. taping the CVC securely or wearing a close-fitting vest.
- Children who feel vulnerable when having a needle 'pushed' into their CVC may be able to sit more upright and learn to expand their rib cage to resist the feeling of being squashed. Helen (age 8) had learned this technique:

    Cos when it goes in I think it's going to hurt but it doesn't but they push it and I'm scared and I pull my tummy in meself. (Helen)

- Not all paediatric oncology units offer the children a choice of CVC – they all receive a tunnelled catheter (Tweddle et al., 1997). It may be prudent to revisit that particular policy in light of this research.
- In the unit where this research was undertaken, it has recently become practice to offer the older children a choice of a double-lumen tunnelled catheter or a double-implanted port; it may be relevant to offer such a choice to the younger children as well, if that is surgically possible.
- Children should be given the opportunity to be involved in the decision about who to tell and when to tell them about their CVC.
- Children are capable of being involved in the decision about which CVC to have; the information they are given needs to be understandable and relevant. It may be useful to explore the possibility of developing an 'information video' for children, featuring children who have a CVC.
- 'Taken-for-grantedness' is an optimistic aspect of the lived experience of having a CVC, especially for newly diagnosed children. The findings of this study have already been disseminated to children and their families via the children's cancer unit newsletter.

Education

- The current approach to the education of 'children's nurses' emphasizes the importance, and skill, of enabling children to participate in their own care (Campbell and Glasper, 1995, p. 27). The findings of this study will endorse that particular aspect of nurse education and provide valuable reflective material.

- When discussing the response of children to medical procedures with healthcare professionals, this study may provide reflective material to consider the limitations of extant knowledge and emphasize the importance of listening to children.

Research

- This study adds to a small but growing body of literature that demonstrates that, with appropriate sensitivity and respect, children can successfully participate in qualitative research.
- This study explored a small aspect of the child's lived experience of having cancer. Van Manen (1990, p. 167) recommends that the researcher be focused on a well-defined subject for their study, so that they do not become overwhelmed by the responses to their questions. There are other aspects of the lived experience of cancer that could be usefully explored in a study of this size, e.g. the lived experience of alopecia, of having a nasogastric tube, of nausea. If a more substantial research project was to be undertaken, e.g. for a PhD, it would be possible to explore the lived experience of having cancer for the child.
- Although the phenomenological approach was appropriate to explore the research question in this study, the limitations of such an approach must be acknowledged. A phenomenological approach is not appropriate to test hypotheses or to study the responses of large numbers of children; alternative research approaches should be adopted for those scenarios.

References

Alderson P (1993) Children's Consent to Surgery. Buckingham: Open University Press.

Bagnall H, Ruccione K (1987) Experience with totally implanted venous access devices in children with malignant disease. Oncology Nurses Forum 14: 51–55.

Baranowski S (1993) Central venous access devices. Current technologies, uses and management strategies. Journal of Intravenous Nursing 16: 167–194.

Bearison DJ, Mulhern RK (1994) Pediatric Psychooncology. Oxford: Oxford University Press.

Beauchamp TL, Childress JF (1994) Principles of Biomedical Ethics, 4th edn. New York: Oxford University Press.

Benner P, Wrubel J (1989) The Primacy of Caring. Stress and coping in health and illness. California: Addison-Wesley.

Bernheimer LP (1986) Use of qualitative methodology in child health research. Child Health Care 14: 224–232.

Bibace R, Walsh ME (1980) Development of children's concepts of illness. Pediatrics 66: 912–917.

Bravery K, Hannan J (1997) The use of long term central venous access devices in children. Paediatric Nursing 9: 29–35.

British Paediatric Association (1992) Guidelines for the Ethical Conduct of Medical Research Involving Children. London: British Paediatric Association.

Campbell S, Glasper A (eds) (1995) Whaley and Wong's Children's Nursing. New York: Mosby.

Cluroe S (1997) Altered body image in children. In: Salter M (ed.), Altered Body Image. The nurse's role, 2nd edn. London: Ballière Tindall, Chapter 5.

Cohen MZ, Omery A (1994) Schools of phenomenology: implications for research. In: Morse JM (ed.), Critical Issues in Qualitative Research Methods. London: Sage, Chapter 8.

Colaizzi PF (1978) Psychological research as the phenomenologist views it. In: Valle R, King M (eds), Existential-Phenomenological Alternatives for Psychology. New York: Oxford University Press, Chapter 3.

Crotty M (1996) Phenomenology and Nursing Research. Melbourne, Australia: Churchill Livingstone.

Dale E (1992) Learning to live with 'wiggly'. Nursing Times 88: 42–44.

Eiser C (1990) Psychological effects of chronic disease. Journal of Child Psychology and Psychiatry 31: 85–98.

Faux SA, Walsh M, Deatrick JA (1988) Intensive interviewing with children and adolescents. Western Journal of Nursing Research 10: 180–194.

Franklin B (1995) Preface. In: Franklin B (ed.), The Handbook of Children's Rights. Comparative policy and practice. London: Routledge, pp. ix–xiii.

Glick M, Zigler E (1985) Self image: a cognitive-developmental approach. In: Leahy R (ed.), The Development of Self. London: Academic Press, Chapter 1.

Guba EG, Lincoln YS (1989) Fourth Generation Evaluation. London: Sage Publications.

Hallett C (1995) Understanding the phenomenological approach to nursing research. Nurse Researcher 3: 55–65.

Harter S (1998) The development of self representations. In: Damon W, Eisenberg N (eds), Handbook of Child Psychology, Vol 3, 5th edn. New York: John Wiley & Sons, Chapter 9.

Hockenberry-Eaton M, Minick P (1994) Living with cancer: children of extraordinary courage. Oncology Nurses' Forum 21: 1025–1031.

Hollis R (1992) Central venous access in children. Paediatric Nursing 4: 18–21.

Hollis R (1997) Childhood cancer into the 21st century. Paediatric Nursing 9: 12–15.

Holloway I, Wheeler S (1996) Qualitative Research for Nurses. London: Blackwell Science.

Hycner RH (1985) Some guidelines for the phenomenological analysis of interview data. Human Studies 8: 279–303.

Jasper MA (1994) Issues in phenomenology for researchers of nursing. Journal of Advanced Nursing 19: 309–314.

Koch T (1994) Establishing rigour in qualitative research: the decision trail. Journal of Advanced Nursing 19: 976–986.

Koocher GP, Keith-Spiegel P (1994) Scientific issues in psychosocial and educational research with children. In: Grodi MA, Glant LH (eds), Children as Research Subjects. Oxford: Oxford University Press, Chapter 2.

Lazarus R (1976) Patterns of Adjustment, 3rd edn. London: McGraw Hill.

Lederer SE, Grodin MA (1994) Historical overview: pediatric experimentation. In: Grodin MA, Glantz LH (eds), Children as Research Subjects. Oxford: Oxford University Press, Chapter 1.

Leese D (1989) My friend Wiggly. Paediatric Nursing May: 12–13.

Leonard VW (1994) A Heideggerian phenomenological perspective on the concept of person. In: Benner P (ed.), Interpretive Phenomenology. London: Sage Publications, Chapter 3.

Lyon C, Parton N (1995) Children's rights and the Children Act 1989. In: Franklin B (ed.), The Handbook of Children's Rights. Comparative policy and practice. London: Routledge Chapter 3.

McEwing G (1996) Children's understanding of their internal body parts. British Journal of Nursing 5: 423–429.

Marcoux C, Fisher S, Wong D (1990) Central venous access in children. Pediatric Nursing 16: 123–133.

Moore IM, Ruccione K (1989) Challenges to conducting research with children with cancer. Oncology Nurses' Forum 16: 587–589.

Morse JM, Field PA (1996) Nursing Research. The application of qualitative approaches, 2nd edn. London: Chapman & Hall.

Moston S (1987) The suggestibility of children in interview studies. First Language 7: 67–78.

Moustakas C (1994) Phenomenological Research Methods. Thousand Oaks, CA: Sage.

Neff EJ, Beardslee CI (1990) Body knowledge and concerns of children with cancer as compared with the knowledge and concerns of other children. Journal of Pediatric Nursing 5: 179–189.

Newcombe N (1996) Child Development. Change over time, 8th edn. New York: Harper Collins College Publishers.

Perrin EC, Gerrity PS (1981) 'There's a demon in your belly': Children's understanding of illness. Pediatrics 67: 841–849.

Pinkerton CR, Cushing P, Sepion B (1994) Childhood Cancer Management. London: Chapman & Hall Medical.

Price B (1990) Body Image. Nursing concepts and care. London: Prentice Hall.

Price B (1993) Diseases and altered body image in children. Paediatric Nursing 5: 18–21.

Ray MA (1994) The richness of phenomenology: philosophic, theoretic and methodological concerns. In: Morse JM (ed.), Critical Issues in Qualitative Research Methods. London: Sage, pp. 117–135.

Rose K (1994) Unstructured and semi-structured interviewing. Nurse Researcher 1: 23–32.

Sandelowski M (1986) The problem of rigor in qualitative research. Advances in Nursing Science 8: 27–37.

Schutz SE (1994) Exploring the benefits of a subjective approach in qualitative nursing research. Journal of Advanced Nursing 20: 412–417.

Seidman IE (1991) Interviewing as Qualitative Research: A guide for researchers in educational and social sciences. New York: Teacher's College Press.

Sepion B (1990) Intravenous care for children. Paediatric Nursing 2: 14–16.

Sontag S (1991) Illness as a Metaphor. London: Penguin.

Susman EJ, Dorn LD, Fletcher JC (1987) Reasoning about illness in ill and healthy children and adolescents: cognitive and emotional developmental aspects. Developmental and Behavioural Pediatrics 8: 266–273.

Tatano Beck C (1994) Phenomenology: its use in nursing research. International Journal of Nursing Studies 31: 499–510.

Taylor BJ (1995) Interpreting phenomenology for nursing research. Nurse Researcher 3: 66–79.

Taylor L, Adelman SH (1986) Facilitating children's participation in decisions that affect them: from concept to practice. Journal of Clinical Child Psychology 15: 346–351.

Tweddle DA, Windebank KP, Barrett MA, Leese DC, Gowing R (1997) Central venous catheter use in UKCCSG oncology centres. Archives of Disease in Childhood 77: 58–59.

Van Manen M (1990) Researching Lived Experience. Human science for an action sensitive pedagogy. New York: SUNY Press.

Van Manen M (1997) From meaning to method. Qualitative Health Research 7: 345–359.

Weithorn LA, Scherer DG (1994) Children's involvement in research participation decisions: psychological considerations. In: Grodin MA, Glantz LH (eds), Children as Research Subjects. Oxford: Oxford University Press, Chapter 5.

Wender EH (1994) Assessment of risk in children. In: Grodin MA, Glantz LH (eds), Children as Research Subjects. Oxford: Oxford University Press, Chapter 6.

Chapter 16

Disease and treatment-related distress among children aged 4-7 years: parent and nurse perceptions

Mariann Hedström and Louise von Essen

To give children with cancer optimal care it is important to explore their psychosocial concerns. The aim of the present study was to investigate which events children aged 4–7 years, regardless of whether on or off treatment for cancer, perceive as distressing or positive in relation to disease and treatment.

There are various descriptions of child distress in relation to cancer experiences. In a study by McGrath et al. (1990), 77 children with cancer (ages 2–19) and/or their parents rated the children's pain in relation to the disease, diagnostic and monitoring procedures and treatment. Three-quarters of the children experienced severe pain from procedures, half experienced pain from treatment and a quarter reported pain from disease. These results agree with those found by Ljungman et al. (1999), who interviewed 55 children with cancer (aged 1–19) and/or their parents. The results demonstrated that pain caused by treatment and procedures was a greater problem than pain resulting from disease itself and that younger children (<5 years) were more concerned about procedural pain than older children. This finding supports the results of a study by Dahlquist et al. (1994), which illustrate that children under age 8 experience significantly higher levels of distress during invasive procedures than older children. It seems safe to conclude that medical procedures are more troublesome for pre-school-age children than for older children. The reason might be related to the fact that children aged 8 or older, more often than younger children, are able to use autonomous cognitive strategies to cope with pain and fear (Reissland, 1983). Thus, children aged 7 or younger may be more distressed by medical interventions than older children.

Hockenberry-Eaton and Minick (1994) interviewed 21 children (aged 7–13) about having cancer. Knowledge of the illness and treatment made it easier to adjust to the diagnosis and treatment, and provided a sense of control. In addition, feeling cared for and special, but normal, helped the children through treatment. In a study by Collins et al. (2000), 159 children with cancer, aged 10–18 years, rated their symptoms according to a modified version of the Memorial Symptom Assessment Scale (MSAS 10-18). The most common symptoms were: lack of energy, pain, drowsiness, nausea, cough and lack of appetite, as well as psychological symptoms such as sadness, nervousness, anxiety and irritability. Symptoms associated with high distress for more than 40% of the children who experienced them were: difficulty swallowing, insomnia, mouth sores, 'I do not look like myself', hair loss, skin changes and vomiting.

Thus, it appears that several well-performed studies have been conducted that attempt to investigate the perceived distress of children with cancer. Variations in the findings might be related to methodological differences, as well as the complexity of the issues studied. Some of these studies focus on one or a few issues whereas others attempt to describe the situation on a more general level. Most of them, however, focus on children older than 7 years. To the author's knowledge, few studies have investigated the symptom experience of pre-school-age children with cancer. One obvious problem is that these children have limited verbal and cognitive capacities to express themselves. By interviewing parents as well as nurses, it might be possible to achieve an adequate picture of young children's experiences in relation to disease and treatment. As Varni et al. (1995) have pointed out, no informant should be considered more accurate than another, because disparate reports may reflect child situation and behaviour under different conditions.

The following research questions were posed: according to parents and staff:

- What is perceived as distressing when being told the diagnosis?
- What is perceived as distressing or positive when receiving chemotherapy and when coming for follow-up?
- What is perceived as particularly distressing in relation to disease and treatment?

Method

Setting and participants

This study is part of a project titled 'Care of children and adolescents with cancer', involving children, their parents and nurses from two of the six paediatric cancer centres in Sweden, Uppsala and Linköping. Swedish-speaking parents with a child 4–7 years, diagnosed with a malignancy at least one month before potential inclusion, and not participating in a parallel study investigating the psychosocial situation of bone marrow-transplanted children, were eligible.

Thirty-three families were eligible in Uppsala; two of these declined to participate. In Linköping, eight families were eligible; parents from one of these did not accept participation. Parents who declined participation were not asked to state a reason for this. Thirty-eight parents were interviewed; three of these interviews were lost as a result of technical failure. Of the interviewed parents 22 were mothers (aged 26–41) and 13 were fathers (aged 29–45). One nurse/nurse assistant was to be interviewed about each child whose parents accepted participation. All registered nurses and nurse assistants (non-registered staff with at least 2 years of education) who worked regular hours at the units were asked to participate; none declined; 38 nurses were interviewed (aged 23–60), 37 of whom were female, 29 registered and nine nurse assistants. In the following discussion, nurses and nurse assistants are referred to as nurses. The demographic characteristics of the children (n = 38) are described in Table 16.1.

Interview

The interviews were semi-structured, audio-taped and transcribed verbatim. An interview guide was used and questions were asked about the time of diagnosis, an especially distressing event, receiving therapy, coming for follow-up, important aspects of care and assistance at home. The interviewers (the last author and a second person) were supportive and follow-up prompt questions were sometimes asked in order to make the participants elucidate or develop their answers. The following questions have been chosen for discussion in this chapter:

- Was there anything distressing for the child when told the diagnosis?
- Has anything been distressing or positive for the child when receiving chemotherapy?
- Has there been anything that is distressing or positive for the child when coming for a follow-up (concerns children who have completed therapy)?
- Has anything been particularly distressing for the child?

Background data were collected by questionnaires, whereas a coordinating nurse at each site collected demographic data for the children such as diagnosis, treatment and time since diagnosis, from the medical records.

Table 16.1 The children interviewed in the study

	Mean	SD	Range	n	Percentage
Sex					
Boys				22	58
Girls				16	42
Age at investigation (years)[a]	5.5	1.2	4-7		
4-5 years				18	49
6-7 years				19	51
Age at diagnosis (years)	3.7	1.4	1-7		
Months from diagnosis to investigation	22.2	16.6	1-60		
1-12				16	42
13-36				14	39
37-				8	19
Diagnosis					
Leukaemia				20	53
Lymphoma				7	18
Rhabdomyosarcoma				5	13
Wilms' tumour				3	8
Other				3	8
Treatment					
Chemotherapy				38	100
Surgery				10	26
Radiotherapy				2	5
Bone marrow transplantation				1	3
Therapy status					
Treatment				15	39
Follow-up				23	61
Times of admission[b]					
1-5				7	19
6-10				9	24
11-20				13	35
21-40				8	22
Siblings					
Yes				34	89
No				4	11
Study site					
Uppsala				31	82
Linköping				7	18

a Age = one drop-out.
b Times of admission = one drop-out

Procedure

Ethical approval was obtained from the local research ethics committees at the faculties of medicine in Uppsala and Linköping. Parents of children aged 4–7 years with a cancer diagnosis, and scheduled for admittance to the hospital in Uppsala for treatment or a clinical control, received an invitation letter one week before the visit. The aim and the procedure of the study were presented in the letter, which was signed by the oncologist in charge and the coordinating nurse at each site. The parents were informed that participation was voluntary and that non-participation would not influence the care of their child. On admission in Uppsala, the parents received further information about the study from the coordinating nurse, who asked whether one of the parents was willing to participate. In Linköping, parents were contacted by telephone and asked to participate by the coordinating nurse. On the day of the parent interview, a nurse who had cared for the child on at least three occasions was interviewed on the same day or as close as possible to the parent interview day.

Data analysis

Data were analysed by the first author using content analysis, a method that uses a set of procedures to draw valid inferences from a text by objective and systematic identification of specified communication characteristics. Answers to open-ended questions are suitable for this technique (Weber, 1990). Words and sentences in the interviews were classified into content categories, which are supposed to reflect central messages in the text. Sentences classified in the same category are presumed to have similar meanings, either based on the precise meaning of the words or on words sharing similar connotations.

The analysis was performed using the following steps:

- The transcribed text was read and the statements by each individual in response to each of the interview questions were identified.
- Sentences or parts of a sentence that contained information relevant to the study questions were identified and defined as recording units. Recording units were transcribed separately and contrasted with each other.
- Recording units were grouped into categories reflecting central text messages. Criteria for distinguishing the categories were that they were positively different from one another. At this stage, some of the categories were judged to be misleading (by the authors and a third person) and were re-formulated.

- Boundaries of each category were defined and descriptions of the central characteristics of each category were developed.

No matter how many times a certain recording unit was mentioned by a person, it was calculated as mentioned only once by that specific person in the presentation of the results.

Interrater agreement for categories

With access to the statements, the recording units and the category descriptions, a second assessor (the third person referred to above) assigned the recording units to the categories. The authors and the second assessor discussed boundaries between categories and their content, and a few changes were made in order to clarify the coding system and to make the categories clearer. Finally, a comparison of the assessors' categorizations was done using the Kappa method (Howell, 1997). The Kappa values for the six questions varied between 0.94 and 1.0, which indicate almost perfect agreement (Brennan and Hays, 1992).

Results

The discussion below follows a presentation of categories and number of included recording units, by parents and nurses, with response to each of the interview questions (see Table 16.2 for a detailed presentation). Quotations representing the typical content of a category are usually presented. Numbers within parentheses after quotations denote case numbers and /. . ./ indicates an excluded insignificant statement.

Being told the diagnosis

Just over half of parents (n = 20 of 35) and nurses (n =24 of 38) did not think, or did not know, if the child they were interviewed about had found it distressing to be told the diagnosis. It was mentioned that, at the time of the diagnosis, the child was too young to understand the seriousness of the disease or too ill to care. Three children were not aware of their diagnosis at the time of the interview.

Seeing their parents sad and worried when the family was told the diagnosis a few children reacted, according to four parents and nine

Table 16.2 Categories, total number of persons mentioning recording units in categories and number of parents (*n* = 35) and nurses (*n* = 38) mentioning recording units in categories

Question	Category	No. of people	No. of parents	No. of nurses
1. Was there anything distressing for the child when told the diagnosis?[a] (three children did not know their diagnosis)	Nothing distressing/Do not know	44	20	24
	Concerned parents	13	4	9
	Understanding the seriousness	6	6	0
	The same disease as . . .	2	0	2
2. Has anything been distressing for the child when receiving chemotherapy?[b]	Physical concerns	43	24	19
	Confinement	18	7	11
	Nothing distressing/Do not know	16	4	12
	Altered self-image	11	9	2
	Worry before medical procedures	4	3	1
3. Has anything been positive for the child when receiving chemotherapy?[c]	Nothing positive/Do not know	38	16	22
	To get well	27	14	13
4. Has anything been distressing for the child when coming for a follow-up (parents: n = 21, nurses: n = 23)?[d]	Nothing distressing/Do not know	21	7	14
	Physical concerns	20	11	9
	Memories and concerns	10	3	7
5. Has anything been positive for the child when coming for a follow-up (parents: n = 21, nurses: n = 23)?[e]	Connection	19	8	11
	Nothing positive/Do not know	15	7	8
	Check-up	9	6	3
	A special day	5	1	4
6. Has anything been particularly distressing for the child?[f]	Physical concerns	41	25	16
	Feelings of alienation	11	9	2
	Confinement	10	2	8
	Worry before medical procedures	9	2	7
	Nothing distressing/Do not know	10	1	9
	Altered self-image	8	7	1
	Understanding the seriousness	4	1	3
	Lack of parental support	4	0	4
	Fear in relation to complications	3	2	1

Drop-outs: a Three parents, three nurses. b Two parents. c Five parents, three nurses. d One parent, two nurses. e Two parents. f One parent.

nurses, with confusion or shame or became withdrawn. Statements about such reactions were categorized as 'Concerned parents', e.g.

> /. . ./ when his mom and dad cried over the information they got, he understood that something was terribly wrong. You understand that even if you are very young. /. . ./. (Nurse 4)

According to parents six children became distressed when told the diagnosis because they understood the seriousness, 'Understanding the seriousness', e.g.

> Immediately she started asking questions about what I would do if she died. /. . ./ That was what was on her mind, I think. (Mother 35)

According to nurses, two children became distressed when told the diagnosis as they had previous experiences of friends and/or family members being treated for cancer. These statements were referred into the category 'The same disease as . . .'.

Distressing aspects of receiving chemotherapy

Four parents and approximately a third of the nurses did not think, or did not remember, that anything had bothered the child when receiving chemotherapy.

According to the parents, two-thirds of the children, and according to the nurses half of the children, had experienced various aspects of 'Physical concerns' when receiving chemotherapy. Side effects (such as nausea and vomiting, painful mouth sores, constipation, headache, allergic reactions and infections caused by decreased immunodefence system) and painful medical procedures (such as nasogastric tubes, Port-A-Cath punctures, intramuscular injections and chemotherapy administrated intrathecally) were mentioned.

Seven children, according to their parents, and eleven, according to their nurses, had suffered from being kept in restricted space, mostly as a result of the drip-feed, having to take tablets or to urinate very often for 3–4 days, or being dependent on the nurses. These sources of distress were categorized as 'Confinement', e.g.

> That he gets stuck in his room. He wants to go to the play therapy. It is awfully hard for him to become shut up there. (Nurse 32)

Physical and mental fatigue, hair loss, appetite loss, changes in mood, not being able to be still and bed-wetting were categorized as 'Altered self-image', e.g.

> She became weak, down-hearted and quiet during one or two days. /.../ Not during the treatments but a week later. (Father 27)

According to the parents nine children had suffered from altered self-image caused by chemotherapy; however, only two nurses mentioned this kind of distress.

'Worry before medical procedures' was mentioned as distressing for three children according to parents and one child according to nurses.

Positive aspects of receiving chemotherapy

Approximately half of the parents and two-thirds of the nurses did not think that, or did not know if, the child they were interviewed about had found anything positive with regard to receiving the chemotherapy. Most of the remaining children had, according to parents and nurses, understood that treatment was necessary and that it could reduce pain and help the child 'to get well':

> He has told me this. 'One gets well when one gets medicine.' (Mother 20)

Distressing aspects of coming for follow-up

The results are based on the answers from those parents ($n = 21$) and nurses ($n = 23$) who were interviewed about children who had completed treatment and attended for follow-up.

Seven children, according to parents, and fourteen, according to nurses, had not experienced anything distressing with regard to coming for follow-up. 'Physical concerns' caused by various punctures, examinations and palpations had distressed approximately half of the children according to their parents and nurses.

> The only thing he finds hard is when they insert the needle in his Port-A-Cath. (Father 14)

A few children, according to three parents and seven nurses, were reluctant or concerned about coming for a follow-up because it reminded them of the disease or because they did not really understand why a check-up was necessary. These statements were referred to the category 'Memories and concerns':

> I think she finds it hard because it is all coming back to her. All her memories of how it was to be here. (Nurse 5)

Positive aspects of coming for follow-up

Approximately a third of the children had, according to parents and nurses, found nothing positive with regard to coming for follow-up.

Meeting friends and staff, talking about what had happened, getting attention and spending time in play therapy were positive aspects in relation to coming for a follow-up for eight children, according to parents, and for eleven, according to the nurses. These aspects were categorized as 'Connection', e.g.

> That she could go to the play therapy and connect to the people she got to know before, those who work here. (Nurse 33)

For some children, six according to parents and three according to nurses, the 'check-up' provided the child with a sense of security. Some parents emphasized that their own positive attitude towards the check-up was transmitted to the child, e.g.

> I tell him that we have to come here so they can take a lot of tests and see that he is not ill again /.../ I think it's good and I think I convey that feeling to him. (Mother 10)

For one child according to parents and for four according to nurses, the day of the follow-up was perceived as 'a special day', an occasion to have a day off from school, travel by train and/or have one's parents all to oneself for a day.

Particularly distressing events

One parent and nine nurses did not think that, or did not remember if, there had been any particularly distressing event for the child about whom they were interviewed. However, 'Physical concerns' had been particularly distressing for as many as 25 children according to parents and 16 according to nurses. Chemotherapy side effects (e.g. nausea, vomiting, fever, mouth sores, altered taste sensations, pain, infections), painful medical procedures (e.g. various punctures, bone marrow examinations, nasogastric tubes, repeated surgery, removal of sticking plasters) and suffering caused by the disease itself (e.g. breathing difficulties and abdominal or skeletal pain) are included in the category.

'Feelings of alienation', i.e. missing siblings, peers, home and things, everyday life such as day-care centre as well as feelings of being different and being among strangers were reported as particularly distressing for nine children according to parents and for two according to nurses, e.g.

> It was hard to explain to him that 'your friends are not to visit you today because you are very sensitive to infections and they all have runny noses. Because if you catch a cold we must go to the hospital'. That was harder for him to understand than that he had to eat medicine to get well. (Mother 25)

Problems caused by the child's loss of autonomy or independence were categorized as 'Confinement', e.g. not being able to refuse treatments, having to take tablets, being held during interventions or having to keep still while the drip-feed was running, had particularly distressed two children according to their parents and eight according to the nurses.

> And he has kicked and turned and cried and said that he doesn't want this. /. . ./ I know he finds it troublesome to be stuck and he knows that when he gets a needle in his Port-A-Cath he gets drip-feed and tubes and devices. (Nurse 11)

Two children according to their parents and seven according to the nurses had been particularly distressed by 'Worry before medical procedures', e.g.

> When she got needles in her Port-A-Cath, she was very anxious in advance and during the procedure she was panicking. /. . ./ I know she sometimes got sedatives. (Staff 15)

Changed appearance and behaviour caused by disease and treatment, e.g. hair loss, excessive weight gain and clumsiness, fatigue and weariness, non-controllable temper, immense appetite or loss of appetite were reported as particularly distressing and were categorized as 'Altered self-image', e.g.

> When she got the treatment and lost her hair and became swollen and ate very much. /. . ./ I think she found that distressing, and in the beginning when she lost her hair, she was apathetic and sat still, did not want to do anything. One couldn't touch her. (Mother 35)

According to parents seven children had perceived the altered self-image as particularly distressing, whereas only one nurse mentioned that a child had suffered particularly from altered self-image.

A few children had, as reported by one parent and three nurses, felt agony of death or sadness as a result of 'Understanding the seriousness of the disease', often in connection with a relapse:

> It was especially hard when he came back with a relapse. I think he understood that there was something serious happening. /. . ./ He was sad, he was over-excited, he was aggressive. (Nurse 37)

According to the nurses four children had found 'Lack of parental support' particularly distressing. This category includes descriptions of situations in which the child was left with a feeling of insecurity because the parents' insecurity or distrust made them unable to support the child:

> He refused to take tablets so he had a nasogastric tube. Then it was decided that it was to be removed but his mother did not want that. /. . ./ She was so convinced that he wouldn't make it and it's hard for a child to believe he can do it if not even his mother believes he will manage. It was hard for him that she did not support him. (Nurse 34)

Two children according to parents and one according to a nurse had been particularly distressed by fear and grief as a result of complications of the disease and treatment, 'Fear in relation to complications', e.g.

> He had an enormously high blood pressure so he had to take medicine. /. . ./ A cardiologist came to see him. I know that was distressing for him because the heart is so important. (Nurse 2).

Discussion

Being told the diagnosis

Most parents and nurses did not think that, or did not know if, the child had found it distressing to be told the cancer diagnosis. Some of the children were reported to be too young to understand or too ill to care. As for the nurses, most of them had not been present at this occasion. However, one might assume that there are a remarkably high number of parents who have a limited insight into their child's reactions. It has been proposed that the entire family should be deeply affected at the time of the diagnosis (Bracken, 1986) and it is possible that the parents were preoccupied with their own reactions and thus did not observe the child closely. Most of the reported distressing aspects with regard to being told the diagnosis dealt with the parent's anxiety and the child's understanding of the seriousness of the disease.

Receiving chemotherapy

Physical concerns appear, according to parents and nurses, to be the aspect of receiving chemotherapy that distresses most children aged 4–7 years whether or not they are on treatment for cancer. However, aspects of confinement and altered self-image were also frequently mentioned.

According to parents half of the children and according to the nurses about two-thirds had found nothing positive in relation to receiving chemotherapy. However, for the remaining children it had some positive value, because they understood that it could help them get well. A further analysis (post hoc) of the data revealed that almost all parents of children with leukaemia reported that the child found it positive to receive the chemotherapy, whereas none of the parents of children with solid tumours reported that the child thought so (χ^2 = 16.25, degree of freedom or d.f. = 1, p < 0.001). This result suggests that children with leukaemia in general understand the need for chemotherapy treatment (Ross, 1989), whereas many children with solid tumours do not. The reason for this is not known, but it could be assumed that, when informing a child with a solid tumour about the disease, the information about the 'lump that must be removed' is emphasized so much that the child does not understand why any treatment other than surgery is needed. This interpretation is tentative; however, the authors found the result interesting and worth further study.

Coming for a follow-up

Coming for follow-up caused physical concerns for about half the children and reminded some about the disease and related experiences. However, for some children the occasion is related to positive aspects such as meeting friends and staff at the ward, getting to know that everything is well and having the possibility of a special day.

Particularly distressing events

Pain, often in relation to procedures, and problems about changes in self-perception and personal life, as well as fears of interventions, complications and restrictions, were mentioned as particularly distressing for the children. Most of the particularly distressing aspects were described as physical, e.g. side effects and painful medical procedures. This finding supports earlier findings by Ljungman et al. (1999) and McGrath et al. (1990), who have concluded that pain resulting from treatment and procedures is a greater problem than pain caused by the disease itself. Statements included in the 'Physical concerns' vary from being concerned with severe skeletal and muscular pain, to pain caused by the removal of sticking plasters. The results indicate that something possibly regarded as a trivial matter such as removal of sticking plasters might be perceived as an especially distressing event in relation to childhood cancer.

The categories 'Feelings of alienation' and 'Altered self-image' include many parental statements. These results imply that even very young children miss their everyday life, feel left aside and worry about their appearance. This issue is not substantially described in the literature. Parents and nurses presented relatively equivalent experiences on most aspects. Parents, more often than nurses, mentioned physical concerns, altered self-image and alienation as particularly distressing for the children whereas nurses, more often than parents, mentioned aspects of fear and psychosocial concerns. The reason for this might be that an event is perceived as particularly distressing by the caregiver if he or she feels helpless in relation to it, e.g. the parents may feel helpless while the child is in pain (Ferrell et al., 1994) because they have few or even no means of alleviating the pain. On the other hand, parents often have a greater possibility than nurses of calming and comforting a frightened child. Reissland (1983) found that young children (aged 4–7) are dependent on parents to cope with fear and pain. Nurses mentioned situations when the children's distress was accentuated or caused by the parents' insecurity, distrust or inability to support the child as particularly distressing. It is not difficult to imagine that, when parents fail to support a young child on or off treatment for cancer, the child will be put in an extremely difficult situation.

Methodological reflections

On consideration of how the interrater agreement for the categories was established, one might argue that there is a risk of inflated Kappa values. The risk could be the result of the fact that the categorization of some recording units was changed in order to clarify the coding system after an additional assessor had assigned the recording units to categories, but before the Kappa calculation was done. However, the authors consider the risk minimal because not more than 10 changes were made as a result of this procedure.

Another methodological issue to consider is that, as a result of the study design, some data concerned distress experienced several years ago whereas other data concerned recent or present experiences. This circumstance might be regarded as a methodological shortcoming if recent experiences are considered more 'true', i.e. more valid, than data about experiences from a long time ago. However, this circumstance may also be considered as a methodological advantage because it gave the authors the possibility to illuminate the investigated phenomena from various time perspectives.

The degree of fit of the results is, in the author's opinion, supported because the interviewed nurses, when taking part in the results, have recognized the presence of the inductively derived aspects of distress.

Conclusion

The results indicate that, for pre-school-age children, the worst aspects of receiving chemotherapy, coming for a follow-up and the entire cancer experience were various aspects of physical concerns. In addition, feelings of alienation, confinement, worry before medical procedures as well as altered self-image were perceived as particularly distressing.

Implications for nursing care

Nurses should be aware that feelings of alienation and altered self-image can be serious problems for children as young as 4-7 years. To help the children cope with these problems and promote a hope for the future, nurses should communicate that most of these changes are a result of treatment and therefore temporary. When possible, nursing staff should encourage the family to let the sick child meet friends and do normal things. It is assumed that, when parents fail to support the sick child, the child will be extremely vulnerable. Nurses are a most valuable resource of support for the family and need to put extra effort into helping parents rise to the demand of being the mainstay in caring for their child with cancer.

Acknowledgements

We would like to express our sincere gratitude to the parents who agreed to share their experiences with us, and to acknowledge the support of Dr Anders Kreuger, and the staff at the paediatric oncology ward at the Uppsala University Children's Hospital and the Linköping University Hospital. We wish to thank Karin Enskär for interviewing the participants from Linköping and Inger Skolin for assisting in assessing the categories. This study was supported by grants from the Swedish Children's Cancer Foundation.

References

Bracken JM (1986) Children with Cancer. New York: Oxford University Press.

Brennan PF, Hays BJ (1992) The Kappa statistic for establishing interrater reliability in the secondary analysis of qualitative clinical data. Research in Nursing and Health 15: 153-158.

Collins JJ, Byrnes ME, Dunkel IJ et al. (2000) The measurement of symptoms in children with cancer. Journal of Pain and Symptom Management 19: 363-377.

Dahlquist LM, Power TG, Cox C, Fernbach DJ (1994) Parenting and child distress during cancer procedures: a multidimensional assessment. Children's Health Care 23: 149-166.

Ferrell BR, Rhiner M, Shapiro B, Dierkes M (1994) The experience of pediatric cancer pain, part 1: impact of pain on the family. Journal of Pediatric Nursing 9: 368-379.

Hockenberry-Eaton M, Minick P (1994) Living with cancer: children with extraordinary courage. Oncology Nursing Forum 21: 1025-1031.

Howell D (1997) Statistical Methods for Psychology. Belmont, CA: Duxbury Press.

Ljungman G, Gordh T, Sorensen S, Kreuger A (1999) Pain in paediatric oncology: interviews with children, adolescents and their parents. Acta Paediatrica 88: 623-630.

McGrath PJ, Hsu E, Capelli M, Luke B, Goodman JT, Dunn-Geier J (1990) Pain from pediatric cancer: a survey of an out-patient oncology clinic. Journal of Psychosocial Oncology 8: 109-124.

Reissland N (1983) Cognitive maturity and the experience of fear and pain in hospital. Social Science and Medicine 17: 1389-1395.

Ross S (1989) Childhood leukemia: the child's view. Journal of Psychosocial Oncology 7(4): 75-90.

Varni JW, Katz ER, Colegrove R, Dolgin M (1995) Adjustment of children with newly diagnosed cancer: cross-informant variance. Journal of Psychosocial Oncology 13(4): 23-37.

Weber R (1990) Basic Content Analysis. London: Sage Publications.

Chapter 17

Parental home administration of cytosine chemotherapy

Pippa Chesterfield

With the development of multimodal treatment and intensive chemother-apy regimens, childhood leukaemia is now considered a life-threatening chronic illness with phases of remission and relapse. Potentially curative treatment for childhood acute lymphoblastic leukaemia (ALL) involves periods of daily bolus intravenous injections of cytosine arabinoside (cytosine) chemotherapy. This has implications for the National Health Service (NHS), families and outpatient workload. Hospital staff poten-tially have to administer the cytosine injections, with the subsequent cost implications. Family life and the child's schooling are further disrupted, with frequent hospital appointments and travel expenses adding to the demands of caring for a chronically sick child. As a result, parents may be offered the opportunity to administer bolus doses of cytosine chemother-apy via a central venous catheter at home. Therefore, an understanding of the lived experience of these parents is of relevance to both nursing and the wider NHS in delivering effective, efficient and safe health care.

A literature search revealed none related to the lived experience of par-ents giving intravenous chemotherapy to their child at home. Indeed, there was no lived experience research related to parental involvement in giving home intravenous therapy of any kind. However, there were three papers describing home intravenous chemotherapy (Jayabose et al., 1992; Close et al., 1995; Hooker and Kohler, 1999). Only two studies involved parental administration of chemotherapy at home (Jayabose et al., 1992; Hooker and Kohler, 1999), neither of which explored the lived experience of parents.

The lived experience of parents administering chemotherapy to their child at home cannot be taken out of the social and political context of healthcare. Currently, in the UK, paediatric nursing practice is based on a philosophy of partnership in care, with many parents taking on aspects of their child's care previously considered to be the domain of nursing. It is clear, however, that there are many factors influencing partnership (Palmer, 1993; Casey, 1995; Coyne, 1995). There is a dearth of literature both on how parental participation can be facilitated and on exploration of the meaning of situations for parents (Coyne, 1995). Coyne (1995), reviewing the literature, highlights the need for lived experience research of parental perspectives as a way forward in facilitating partnership in care. At present, cost containment is high on the agenda in the NHS. Parental administration of home chemotherapy may be seen as a cost-containment strategy. Thus, there is the potential for healthcare to be driven by economic factors rather than the needs of these families, so it was both timely and appropriate to gain a deeper understanding of the experiences of parents administering chemotherapy to their child at home, at the same time developing evidence-based practice for nursing consistent with current Department of Health directives (DoH, 1997, 1998, 1999).

The study design

Approval for the study was gained from the local hospital ethics committee of the United Kingdom Children's Cancer Study Group (UKCCSG) centre from where parents would be recruited. A naturalistic/interpretive research approach to the study was taken. Naturalistic/interpretive research, as well as nursing, values uniqueness, and views with subjectivity the individual as being intentional, goal oriented and context relevant (Heron, 1981; Dahlberg and Drew, 1997). This approach was congruent with the research question and consistent with my own personal philosophy. The study was based on lived experience research underpinned by a Heideggerian/Gadamerian phenomenological philosophy. The emphasis within phenomenology is on the meaning and understanding of phenomena and the lived experience of being for the individual (Knaack, 1984; Thorne, 1991; Beck, 1994; Morse and Field, 1996; Van Manen, 1997). Heidegger, a student of Husserl, expanded and adapted Husserl's ideas (Koch, 1995), developing hermeneutic or interpretive phenomenology. Hermeneutics is the theory and practice of interpretation; this approach becomes necessary when there is the possibility of misunderstanding, which is pertinent to this study. Gadamer developed Heidegger's ideas further, with the development of the fusion/expansion of horizons (Thompson, 1990; Walsh, 1996; Walters, 1996; Annells, 1999). The horizon of an individual is the understanding of being in the world.

Fusion of horizons occurs when two individual horizons meet and intersect, creating understanding between individuals. Consequently, fusion or expansion of horizons acknowledges the horizons of both the researcher and the participants, which can fuse to give understanding. The concept of fusion/expansion of horizons and shared understanding is particularly pertinent to nursing and this study, if care is to be negotiated (Beck, 1994; Pascoe, 1996; Walsh, 1996; Dahlberg and Drew, 1997; Annells, 1999).

Congruent with a phenomenological approach to research, the main literature review was delayed until data collection and analysis had commenced (Morse and Field, 1996). This is to try to prevent bias and pre-suppositions. However, a limited review of the literature was carried out at the proposal stage, in order to develop the research question and to identify other studies within the area of interest.

A CINAHL and Medline review of the literature from 1982 to 2000 was undertaken. The search was broad in order to retrieve all potentially relevant papers, which could then be reviewed for pertinence to this specific study. The review included all related topics such as:

- home intravenous therapy
- care by parent
- partnership in care
- parental perspectives
- phenomenology
- lived experience research
- childhood cancer
- childhood chronic illness.

The literature provided a theoretical understanding of the likely feelings, tasks and challenges facing families of children with chronic conditions and the adaptive strategies used by families. However, this did not provide an understanding of the lived experience of parents carrying out complex care for their chronically ill child at home. Nor did the literature provide evidence on which to base healthcare practice.

Phenomenology does not offer research methods to be used. These are developed in relation to the question asked. Six mothers and three fathers who had all administered bolus cytosine chemotherapy via a central venous catheter to their child at home were recruited to the study. A semi-structured audio-taped interview with prompts and probes was used to collect data (see Appendix at the end of the chapter). This allowed parents to tell their story as they wished. Data analysis incorporated thematic analysis of the interviews and a further phase of deeper interpretation. Benner (1994) and Van Manen (1997) identify thematic analysis with exemplars as an approach to data analysis, which involves moving between the whole to the parts of the data. The interviews were transcribed verbatim and themes identified. Once themes and exemplars from each interview had been identified, these were compared with the other interviews to gain an overview of the lived experience of the parents before identifying commonalities and differences between interviews and experiences of individual parents. Fourteen themes were identified:

1. The need to help their child
2. Being guided by their child
3. Letting their child get on with life
4. Managing the many other aspects of life
5. Getting it right
6. Caring with confidence
7. Giving their child a toxic drug
8. Sheer practical dexterity and hygiene
9. Is the line going to work?
10. It becomes second nature, part of everyday routine
11. Administering chemotherapy: a way of regaining care of their child
12. Awareness of the workload of the ward and costing
13. Choice
14. A sense of mastery.

To confirm the themes found and to allow parents the opportunity to elaborate further, a second interview was completed. All the parents were able to identify the themes that evolved from the first interviews. For the purpose of this chapter, only the themes identified by the parents and implications for nursing and healthcare are discussed.

The experience of parents

Although there were common themes for all parents these were expressed in different ways by the parents, coupled with many individual experiences. A parent's role is to care for his or her child; however, this aspect of care was an unusual aspect of parenting. From parents' comments, administration of cytosine chemotherapy at home cannot be isolated from the whole experience of parenting a child with cancer:

> It's just part of coping. I mean giving chemotherapy, it's just part of how you're coping with the whole situation really . . . it's just isolating one aspect of your child's illness. (Mother 2)

The need to help their child

With the threat to their child's life posed by cancer they wanted to do anything they could to help their child, e.g. parents stated:

> It just felt as though I was doing something, no matter how small it was, to help my daughter's recovery. (Mother 1)

The will to do anything they could to help their child outweighed the anxiety of giving chemotherapy, as one father said:

> The will to want to do it [give cytosine], to help him was more than I don't want to do it . . . all I want to do is be there for him. . . I'd have a go at anything, as long as everything goes OK, but if something should happen that I lost him, I could turn round and say 'well I did my bit, you know I tried'. (Father 3)

Being guided by their child

The child's relaxation when the parent gives the chemotherapy enabled parents to have the confidence to administer the chemotherapy at home; parents commented:

> He seems to be a lot more relaxed having it done here within the home and with me doing it than he normally is in the hospital. (Father 1)

> His confidence in me does me the world of good. (Father 3)

Letting their child get on with life

Giving chemotherapy enabled parents to allow their child to get on with life and reduced the disruption caused by treatment. Administering chemotherapy at home allowed the child to go to school and reduced the time spent travelling to hospital and waiting in clinic:

> It makes it a much easier existence for [child's name] and certainly when he's out of the ward environment, he wanted to be as normal as possible. (Mother 4)

> I wanted to do it for him, because it meant that he didn't miss as much school. (Mother 6)

A serendipitous finding in getting on with life for the two teenage boys having chemotherapy at home was the facilitation of integration and understanding of friends. Friends were able to observe and see what treatment meant for the teenager:

> This has helped the sort of bonding at school and the camaraderie. (Father 2)
>
> With giving chemo at home he relays that to his friends . . . they now can actually relate to the problem that he's got. (Father 3)

To enable their child to continue with his or her life, parents tailored times of administering chemotherapy to the needs of the child; one mother gave her son chemotherapy in the morning before school, whereas another gave the chemotherapy in the evening so that the child could sleep off the flu-like symptoms that resulted from cytosine chemotherapy:

> We discovered that he gets flu-like symptoms a couple of hours after the cytosine, so at the period of time when he was having it in hospital, and then going off to school he was getting quite unwell, quite sick at school, and then he had to come home. So in fact what we do with cytosine is we give it at night before he goes to bed so he can sort of sleep those symptoms off. (Mother 4)

Managing the many other aspects of life

Parents had to manage the many other aspects and demands of life that continued on a day-to-day basis, becoming skilled jugglers of time and meeting everyone's needs. By giving chemotherapy at home this enabled family routines to continue, e.g. the child's siblings could go to school and other commitments could continue such as work, thus reducing the disruption to the whole family:

> It makes life easier for the child certainly and therefore it's easier for the whole family. (Mother 6)

The instinct of the parents to help their child was balanced by a sense of responsibility to get it right.

Getting it right

All parents felt immense responsibility for this aspect of care. They were responsible for giving potentially dangerous drugs with life-threatening implications to their child whom they love. One father expressed this feeling of responsibility to get it right as:

> Your son's life is in your hands . . . you are sort of playing god . . . should I be doing this, am I qualified enough . . . what happens if I do this wrong? (Father 2)

A mother commented:

> I was very conscious that the responsibility was there for me and I was the one that was giving her drugs and I wanted to get it right. (Mother 1)

This was expressed in many different ways by parents. It was often on their minds all day both before and after they had given the chemotherapy:

> The whole day I was thinking 'did I do this right, did I do that right?', and I kept looking back in the notes that they'd given me. (Mother 6)

> I was very much tuned in to what time this job needed to be given and the next time. (Mother 1)

They checked and double-checked drugs and read the guidelines doing everything strictly by the book:

> Double-checking, referring back to the notes that you have from the hospital, making sure that you're doing things you know strictly by the book. (Father 3)

For some parents the issue of administering chemotherapy through a central venous catheter created an added sense of responsibility:

> It just frightened me that I was putting this medicine straight into his body. (Mother 6)

To take on this responsibility confidence was essential for these parents.

Caring with confidence

Gaining confidence was integral to the empowerment of parents administering chemotherapy at home. This ranged for the parents from being given written information and practical teaching to the confidence of the hospital staff in the parent's abilities to administer the chemotherapy:

> We were given training to do all of that at the time, and we felt confident that the training we were given was good. (Mother 4)

> I felt that the hospital if they didn't feel that I was capable of doing it and being sensible with the drugs wouldn't have given me the opportunity. (Mother 1)

Having someone to come and be with them at home when they first gave chemotherapy was helpful for parents in gaining confidence:

> I was glad the Macmillan Paediatric Nurse came out and watched me to know that you felt I was competent to do it, which made me feel more confident to know I'd got it right. (Mother 6)

One mother who had not had anybody visit her at home when she first gave chemotherapy felt that this would have been helpful:

> There isn't a lot of backup at home if anything happens. I mean could they have district nurses coming around, or could they have someone to come around and check with you? (Mother 2)

However, the experience of being taught and having someone observe them both at home and in the hospital could be stressful for parents:

> Although it made me more nervous, it was probably in the long run better to have someone watching you and making sure you did it absolutely perfectly. (Mother 5)

> It's like going for a driving test. (Father 3)

The will to help their child and the confidence that they could get it right enabled parents to give such a toxic drug as cytosine chemotherapy.

Giving my child a toxic drug

All parents were aware of the toxicity of the drug that they were giving their child. This added to the sense of responsibility for all parents:

> Initially you think, oh chemo, I'm never going to be able to go near this or do this, and that's sort of a magical, mythical thing that everybody has about chemo. (Father 2)

> I mean basically you're dumping toxic waste into your child's body, and you don't know for definite, how it's going to affect them, you don't know if at one time they're not going to have a side effect to it. So the one thing that's running through your mind is what would happen if they, this time, had a side effect to it. (Mother 3)

> With chemo we were trebly sure, you know making absolutely certain it was the right stuff and the right amount. (Father 1)

The stricter protocol with the wearing of gloves and disposal of equipment, combined with the visual cues of a black bag, all served as reminders of the significance of chemotherapy:

> You're aware of the black bag with the chemo in, and it having its little place in the fridge where you know exactly where it is. And everyone in the family was aware of what it was and what it was doing there and why it was there. (Mother 1)

> I felt very nervous of putting a toxic drug in my child's body that required me putting gloves on. I think I found that very upsetting . . . I couldn't believe that these children are getting drugs that are so toxic you need to wear gloves. (Mother 2)

Even with all the feelings of responsibility and the knowledge of the significance of the drug that they were giving, parents willingly took on the challenge of this aspect of care to help their child.

Sheer practical dexterity and hygiene

For parents, learning the practical skills and becoming familiar with handling equipment were all aspects of the experience:

> Initially it was the technicalities and trying to remember all the bits and pieces, the hygiene and what you drew up and which needles went on first. (Mother 6)

> Sheer dexterity of doing it all, or preparing it was enough of a problem. (Father 2)

However, this varied for parents depending on their past experience with using the central line. For some parents they were already used to flushing the line, giving antibiotics and taking blood. Chemotherapy comes prepared in syringes, whereas antibiotics required preparation, making the experience of giving chemotherapy context dependent:

> It wasn't that bad for me, because I'd done the other things, because I'd already been involved with working with his line, and got used to

drawing up Hepsal and actually injecting into his line. The chemo wasn't that different to me. (Father 2)

Not only were dexterity and hygiene an issue, but also parents were conscious of the potential for problems with the central line.

Is the line going to work?

For some parents knowledge of their child's central venous catheter was integral to the experience. This involved tacit knowledge, such as whether the line was stiff, and concerns related to the line being blocked:

I will then know exactly what goes on, so when he has problems with the line being stiff or blocked, I'll realize that because I did it last week and the week before . . . so it's a continuity. (Father 2)

I felt nervous more for the sake that I was hoping that the line wouldn't block. (Father 3)

For the parents giving chemotherapy on a 9-week cycle, it was important to have the line checked by the nurses. This gave the parents reassurance before giving chemotherapy, as there had been a 7-week gap:

Somehow it's sort of like it's been, the car's been in for a service, so you do the chemo after they've checked it. (Father 2)

Although giving chemotherapy at home to their child was a significant experience for parents, after initial apprehension it became incorporated into a new everyday routine.

It becomes second nature, part of everyday routine

From initial nerves and 'butterflies in the tummy' when giving chemotherapy at home, parents incorporated this unusual aspect of being a parent into a new everyday routine:

As your confidence grows and your child grows with you, that book gets shut up and put away because you know it, and it comes second nature to you. (Father 3)

It's another routine that you put into a routine that you never had. You know it's a case of 'well I've got to find a space to do it'. (Mother 3)

It's as though you'd been doing it all your life . . . chemo just really becomes a part of life. (Mother 5)

For some parents, with each gap in giving chemotherapy it was like starting again to regain their confidence:

> I've had quite a large break in between giving him the injections . . . it's been about 2 or 3 months . . . so when I go to hospital obviously I'm going to be watching them and double-checking with them, so that when I get home I'm feeling confident in myself again. (Mother 3)

Incorporating chemotherapy into the everyday routine of caring for a child with cancer helped parents regain the care of their child.

Administering chemotherapy: a way of regaining care of their child

Parents felt that they handed over their child to people whom they did not know when their child was diagnosed with cancer:

> I think from sort of day one when you know we were given the news we lost a certain amount of responsibility. (Mother 4)

> Suddenly you've got somebody that you've never met before, saying give me your child for the next 2 years and they can't guarantee that they can give you back your child. (Father 2)

Administering chemotherapy was a way of participating in their child's treatment and regaining care of their child:

> It's literally kids being taken away and being dealt with by other people. So it's nice to get back into participating. (Father 3)

> You begin to feel part of it. A lot of the time you feel quite distant and obviously you want to do as much as you can for your child, and giving chemo does help you in that respect. (Father 1)

> It's something I wanted to do because it's my part of control of his disease. (Mother 3)

For parents who had taken on the responsibility for giving chemotherapy at home, if their child was admitted to hospital, it was like losing their child again, because the nurses then took on this task:

> It's like losing him again, you've done so much for him and then it just stops. (Father 3)

> It's easy to sort of sit back and watch the medical staff doing their job. (Mother 2)

> Whereas if the hospital does it, then you feel a bit left out, as though you're not doing anything to help. (Mother 5)

For one father who wanted to continue to give his son's chemotherapy in hospital, he did not feel that he could ask to give it. This was exacerbated by the fact that no one negotiated this aspect of care with him. However, he also qualified this by saying that it enabled him to relax if the nurse gave the chemotherapy:

> I wouldn't like to be known on the ward as the father that you know wants to do everything, although most fathers would . . . but there again the nurses and the doctors, they've got their jobs to do, and it makes me relax . . . I can sit there with him and relax. (Father 3)

Awareness of the workload of the ward and costing

Some parents were also aware of the workload of the ward and pressures on the staff. By taking on this aspect of care they felt that they were reducing the workload of the staff:

> It's a little bit easier for the ward because it's something else that they don't have to do. (Father 1)

> I do feel that there is pressure up at the hospital for people to do things like that, because I think economically you know it saves money, and for the nurses it saves time. (Mother 2)

Choice

Although these parents had chosen to take on this role, they were also aware that this was not right for everybody:

> It's something where you've got to think about, something that's got to be right for you. (Mother 3)

Parents needed to have this aspect of care negotiated *and* be given choice:

> It was suggested to me at the hospital, if I wanted to do chemotherapy it was an option, but if I didn't want to then I didn't have to. (Mother 3)

> I feel there's so much support I don't feel that I have to do anything I don't want to do. (Mother 6)

One mother who felt that she had not been given the choice stated:

> With giving the chemo there wasn't any preliminary. It was just 'right this is what you have got to do, and I'll show you, and I'll get the syringes and this what you have to do' . . . I think it would have been helpful if you had like a discussion. (Mother 3)

For parents who took the decision to give their child chemotherapy at home there were potential personal benefits. There was the potential for this lived experience to provide an opportunity for personal development and satisfaction for parents.

A sense of mastery

Parents had a great sense of satisfaction that they have helped their child and mastered this aspect of care:

> It gives you a great sense of satisfaction, or it did me. (Father 3)

> It is like, it's like sort of like a butterflies stomach feeling and there's tremendous tension, but there's sort of elation in some ways that you're helping. (Father 2)

> At the beginning I thought well I wouldn't be able to manage it, but at the end I felt pleased that I did do it, whereas if I'd left it to the hospital I felt you know I didn't try to help her and I felt good that I did and pleased with myself. (Mother 5)

The aim of phenomenology is to gain a deeper understanding rather than to develop theory or to offer recommendations for practice. The themes identified enable readers to gain deeper understanding of the experience of parents administering cytosine chemotherapy to their child at home. However, implications for nursing and healthcare did evolve from the parents' stories.

Implications for nursing and healthcare

It is clear that, although partnership in care is the espoused philosophy, in practice this was not always the case. Nurses have a distinct role to play in facilitating home chemotherapy by parents. It is important for parents to be given the choice and to have discussions before taking on this aspect of care. This should be an ongoing process, which starts with an initial discussion of parental home administration of chemotherapy, because individual parents differ and their experience changes over time. Re-negotiation is specifically needed if their child is readmitted to hospital or when there has been a long gap between courses of chemotherapy. A relationship of trust and understanding is required between the parent and nurse, if effective negotiation is to take place. Comprehensive teaching programmes, including written information and practical teaching, are needed. A positive approach from the nurse is required if parents are to be empowered to take on this aspect of their child's care. A home visit by a professional familiar with the administration of chemotherapy when parents first give chemotherapy at home is needed to boost the parent's confidence. To achieve this, the nurses' role and focus will need to change – they need to become more facilitative and educational rather than taking over and doing for children and their families (Palmer, 1993; Neill, 1996).

Parental home administration of chemotherapy is one strategy in implementing nursing's key values into practice. Two key concepts and values in paediatric nursing are family-centred care and partnership in care (Casey, 1988; Coyne, 1995). Through parental home chemotherapy administration, partnership in care is promoted with maintenance of family functioning and support networks. Parental administration of chemotherapy to their child at home has potential benefits for all family members. Parents may feel more positive about the experience of having cared for a child with cancer in the future. If their child dies they may feel that they have done everything to help their child, helping to facilitate a healthy grieving and bereavement process. The sick child's normal development will have been maintained, with care being given by familiar carers and thus maintaining their sense of security. In addition, siblings will potentially not feel so isolated from family members. As a result, the adverse psychological consequences for the whole family of childhood cancer sufferers may be reduced. Home administration of chemotherapy may result in fewer referrals to mental health services such as child and family guidance. However, having identified the positive benefits, nurses need to be aware of potentially negative outcomes of home chemotherapy by parents. Parents may feel responsible if their child becomes ill, relapses or dies, if they have given them chemotherapy. Nurses need to ensure appropriate and quick referral to other agencies such as counselling services at any time during the child's illness or during long-term follow-up of the child and family.

In the current healthcare climate of cost containment, parental home administration of chemotherapy is an effective cost-containment strategy that is acceptable to some parents. In the short term nursing time will be used teaching parents, but in the long term nursing time will be saved as parents take on this aspect of care. Having identified that there are positive benefits for families and cost containment for the NHS, this concept could be expanded. Parents could administer other chemotherapy drugs at home after appropriate teaching, support and discussion with families, e.g. parents could give intravenous bolus vincristine, thus reducing hospital visits and time away from home. In the future teenagers could take on this aspect of their own treatment. This could be beneficial in helping teenagers to regain some control of their lives and would develop their self-efficacy and locus of control related to healthcare behaviour. It could also help teenagers to understand treatment and help future adjustment, because many will be long-term survivors of cancer.

Although the findings were not unexpected, they add to the empathetic and aesthetic knowledge of nursing identified by Carper (1978). The study also adds depth and richness to the theoretical body of nursing knowledge specifically and healthcare professionals in general. The findings develop evidence on which nurses can base their practice in line with current Department of Health directives mentioned previously, which reinforce the centrality of the patient and his or her carer in treatment and care.

Strengths and limitations of the study

The story told by the parents in this study enhances the understanding of the lived experience of parents administering chemotherapy to their child at home. However, the findings need to be treated with caution. My ability as an interviewer may have limited the data available for discussion. I may have missed cues, thus not encouraging parents to expand on relevant issues. Nevertheless, on reading the transcripts I did not seem to have missed many cues. Parents may have found it difficult to articulate their experiences, or they may have disassociated part of the experience as a result of the existential issues involved with childhood cancer. They may have been unwilling to tell me things that they found embarrassing. However, as I had known the parents for at least 12 weeks and because of my role as a nurse involved with chemotherapy and caring for their child, this helped in creating a relationship of trust. A complete stranger who had no understanding of caring for a child with cancer could have found it difficult to develop a relationship with these parents and connect with their experiences. Overall my insider–outsider situation with parental administration of chemotherapy was an asset.

For some parents the non-directive nature of the interviews was difficult, because they wanted to answer direct questions. Conversely, the non-directive nature of the research approach and methods used allowed the parents to tell their stories as they wished. The parents were also given other opportunities to elaborate their stories both in writing and at a second interview. The research approach taken was appropriate for the question asked, adding credibility to the findings. The findings seem to be intuitively right and support the current body of theoretical knowledge.

The study only begins to explore the topic of parental administration of chemotherapy to their child at home. The sample was small, consisting of a socially and culturally biased group of white British parents, limiting the transferability of the study findings. There are many areas that require further research, e.g. parents from different cultures may have different experiences. Also the sample here was a group of parents who had chosen to take on this aspect of care. What is the lived experience of those parents who choose not to administer chemotherapy to their child? The experiences of fathers were limited in this study. However, the experiences of both mothers and fathers seemed similar; this would require confirmation in further studies. The age of the child and position in the family may also be a factor influencing the lived experience of parents, which requires further research.

The experience cannot be taken in isolation from other members of the family. What is the experience of other family members? What is the experience of the parent in the family not giving the chemotherapy? Does parental administration of chemotherapy facilitate long-term adaptation of family members following the lived experience of childhood cancer in the family? What is the long-term lived experiences of each member of the family? All these issues need exploration to gain a deeper understanding of the lived experience of parents administering intravenous chemotherapy within the context of the family experience of childhood cancer.

Gaining an understanding of nurses' lived experience of giving chemotherapy and experience with parental administration of chemotherapy would help us understand the situational differences for nurses and parents, e.g. nurses may see parental administration of chemotherapy as parents taking away their nursing role and trivializing what nurses do. From an understanding of the different perspectives, parental and nursing horizons could be fused or expanded.

The research: a personal perspective of the experience

Consistent with a phenomenological perspective, the researcher cannot be disassociated from the research process and end product. It is therefore appropriate to offer a personal perspective of the experience. At the outset I had a theoretical knowledge of the research approach taken. I was aware, through discussion and reading, that to understand phenomenological research was to do phenomenological research. Through completing this piece of research I gained a deeper understanding of the philosophical underpinnings and concepts of this approach. From a broader perspective I was aware that the research process was not linear and as smooth as research articles suggested. As a very clinically oriented nurse, research was something that was abstract and rather esoteric. At the start I was unsure whether I would enjoy the experience of completing a piece of research. On reading my research journal, I can see changes in my understanding and eventual enjoyment of the experience.

I had an idealistic impression of the research process and soon realized that I had to take a more realistic and pragmatic approach. Although I had a clear idea of what I was going to do at the beginning, this changed and I needed to adapt with the research evolving over time, e.g. although I thought I would use an opening statement with the first interviews, in practice this did not happen. My ideas did not always prove useful, with the theory not working in practice. The idea of sending the written transcripts to parents in order to give them the opportunity to write down their ideas, which might have added to the data for interpretation, did not work in practice. The research process was not smooth; I experienced problems related to recruitment and arranging interview times. Although I understood conceptually that data collection and analysis were integrated phases, through completion of the research I understood this experientially. Although I was aware that writing up my interpretation was part of the process of interpreting, I gained invaluable experiential understanding of this through the process of writing up the study. Ownership and connection with the study came with time. I realized I owned and was connected to the study when I started to enjoy the experience and talked about the study at work. As a consequence I realized research cannot be disconnected from the researcher; it is a very personal experience.

The experience of actually completing this piece of research has had many benefits. It was both a privilege and a pleasure to spend time with these parents listening to their stories. The understanding of these parents' lived experiences of administering chemotherapy to their child at home has benefited my practice. From this understanding, I am able to connect and be present for these parents. I am also less likely to take parental administration of chemotherapy for granted and therefore negotiate more with families. I have gained a deeper and richer understanding of the research process and more specifically phenomenology as a philosophy and research approach. Ultimately this experience has added richness to my evolving experience of being.

Conclusion

The study was small and does not offer generalizations or prescriptions for practice. There are many areas related to parental administration of chemotherapy to their child that require further research, e.g. the experience of other family members and families who choose not to administer chemotherapy at home. Longitudinal studies identifying the changing experience for family members need to be undertaken. However, there are clear emerging implications for families and healthcare professionals from the current study. There are potential benefits for families who choose to administer chemotherapy at home. Nurses have a distinct role to play in facilitating this aspect of care. There is now evidence on which nurses can base their practice in this aspect of care. Within a climate of stringent cost containment, parental home administration of chemotherapy can be one strategy used to contain healthcare costs. The understanding gained of parents' experiences helps to develop healthcare that is sensitive to the needs of children with cancer and their families.

References

Annells M (1999) Hermeneutic phenomenology: philosophical perspectives and current use in nursing research. Journal of Advanced Nursing 23: 705-713.

Beck CT (1994) Phenomenology its use in nursing research. International Journal of Nursing Studies 31: 499-510.

Benner P (1994) The tradition and skill of interpretive phenomenology in studying health, illness and caring practices. In: Benner P (ed.), Interpretive Phenomenology: Embodiment, caring and ethics in health care and illness. London: Sage Publications. pp 99-127.

Carper BA (1978) Fundamental patterns of knowing in nursing. Advances in Nursing Science 1: 13-23.

Casey A (1988) A partnership with child and family. Senior Nurse 8: 8-9.

Casey A (1995) Partnership nursing: influences on involvement of informal carers. Journal of Advanced Nursing 22: 1058-1062.

Close P, Burkey E, Kazak A, Danz P, Lange B (1995) A prospective, controlled evaluation of home chemotherapy for children with cancer. Pediatrics 95: 896-900.

Coyne IT (1995) Parental participation in care: a critical review of the literature. Journal of Advanced Nursing 21: 716-722.

Dahlberg K, Drew N (1997) A lifeworld paradigm for nursing research. Journal of Holistic Nursing 15: 303-317.

Department of Health (1997) The New NHS Modern Dependable. London: HMSO.

Department of Health (1998) A First Class Service: Quality in the new NHS. London: HMSO.

Department of Health (1999) Clinical Governance: Quality in the new NHS. London: HMSO.

Heron J (1981) Philosophical basis for a new paradigm. In: Reason P, Rowan J (eds), Human Inquiry: A sourcebook of new paradigm research. Chichester: John Wiley & Sons Ltd, pp. 19-35.

Hooker L, Kohler J (1999) Safety, and acceptability of home intravenous therapy administered by parents of pediatric oncology patients. Medical and Pediatric Oncology 32: 421-426.

Jayabose S, Escobedo V, Tugal O et al. (1992) Home chemotherapy for children with cancer. Cancer 69: 574–579.

Knaack P (1984) Phenomenological research. Western Journal of Nursing Research 6: 107–114.

Koch T (1995) Interpretive approaches in nursing research the influences of Husserl and Heidegger. Journal of Advanced Nursing 21: 827–836.

Morse JM, Field PA (1996) Nursing Research: The application of qualitative approaches, 2nd edn. London: Chapman & Hall.

Neill SJ (1996) Parent participation 2: findings and their implications for practice. British Journal of Nursing 5: 110–117.

Palmer SJ (1993) Care of sick children by parents: a meaningful role. Journal of Advanced Nursing 18: 185–191.

Pascoe E (1996) The value of nursing research of Gadamer's hermeneutic philosophy. Journal of Advanced Nursing 18: 1309–1314.

Thompson JL (1990) Hermeneutic inquiry. In: Moody LE (ed.), Advancing Nursing Science through Research, Vol 2. London: Sage Publications Ltd, pp 223–280.

Thorne SE (1991) Methodological orthodoxy in qualitative research: analysis of the issues. Qualitative Health Research 1: 178–199.

Van Manen M (1997) Researching Lived Experience: Human science for an action sensitive pedagogy, 2nd edn. New York: State University of New York Press.

Walsh K (1996) Philosophical hermeneutics and the project of Hans Georg Gadamer: implications for nursing research. Nursing Inquiry 3: 231–237.

Walters AJ (1996) Nursing research methodology: transcending Cartesianism. Nursing Inquiry 3: 91–100.

Appendix: Interview guide

Opening statement:
I am interested in understanding what it was like for you having to give your child chemotherapy at home.

Questions:
Can you tell me about when you heard you might be able to give cytosine at home?
What made you opt to give [child's name] cytosine at home?
What were the important issues for you?
By the end of the course of cytosine did you feel differently?

Probes/Prompts:
Can you explain that to me?
Can you give me an example?
What do you mean by that?
Is there anything else you want to add/say?

Clarification:
I am not sure I understand, do you mean _ _ _ _ _ _?
Have I understood correctly?

Index